# Psychiatric Neuroethics

# International Perspectives in Philosophy and Psychiatry

Series editors: Bill (K.W.M.) Fulford, Lisa Bortolotti, Matthew Broome, Katherine Morris, John Z. Sadler, and Giovanni Stanghellini

**VOLUMES IN THE SERIES:**

**Philosophy, Psychoanalysis, and the A-Rational Mind**
Brakel

**Unconscious Knowing and Other Essays in Psycho-Philosophical Analysis**
Brakel

**Psychiatry as Cognitive Neuroscience**
Broome and Bortolotti (eds.)

**Free Will and Responsibility**
*A Guide for Practitioners*
Callender

**Reconceiving Schizophrenia**
Chung, Fulford, and Graham (eds.)

**Darwin and Psychiatry**
De Block and Adriaens (eds.)

**The Oxford Handbook of Philosophy and Psychiatry**
Fulford, Davies, Gipps, Graham, Sadler, Stanghellini, and Thornton

**Nature and Narrative**
*An Introduction to the New Philosophy of Psychiatry*
Fulford, Morris, Sadler, and Stanghellini (eds.)

**The Oxford Textbook of Philosophy and Psychiatry**
Fulford, Thornton, and Graham

**The Mind and Its Discontents**
Gillett

**Psychiatric Neuroethics**
*Studies in Research and Practice*
Glannon

**The Abraham Dilemma**
Graham

**Is Evidence-Based Psychiatry Ethical?**
Gupta

*Thinking Through Dementia*
Hughes

**Dementia**
*Mind, Meaning, and the Person*
Hughes, Louw, and Sabat (eds.)

**Talking Cures and Placebo Effects**
Jopling

**Vagueness in Psychiatry**
Keil, Keuck, and Hauswald

**Philosophical Issues in Psychiatry II**
*Nosology*
Kendler and Parnas (eds.)

**Philosophical Issues in Psychiatry III**
*The Nature and Sources of Historical Change*
Kendler and Parnas (eds.)

**Philosophical Issues in Psychiatry IV**
*Classification of Psychiatric Illness*
Kendler and Parnas (eds.)

**Discursive Perspectives in Therapeutic Practice**
Lock and Strong (ed.)

**Schizophrenia and the Fate of the Self**
Lysaker and Lysaker

**Embodied Selves and Divided Minds**
Maiese

**Responsibility and Psychopathy**
Malatesti and McMillan

**Body-Subjects and Disordered Minds**
Matthews

**Rationality and Compulsion**
*Applying Action Theory to Psychiatry*
Nordenfelt

**Diagnostic Dilemmas in Child and Adolescent Psychiatry**
Perring and Wells (eds.)

**Philosophical Perspectives on Technology and Psychiatry**
Phillips (ed.)

**The Metaphor of Mental Illness**
Pickering

**Mapping the Edges and the In-between**
Potter

**Trauma, Truth, and Reconciliation**
*Healing Damaged Relationships*
Potter (ed.)

**The Philosophy of Psychiatry**
*A Companion*
Radden

**The Virtuous Psychiatrist**
Radden and Sadler

**Addiction and Weakness of Will**
Radoilska

**Autonomy and Mental Disorder**
Radoilska (ed.)

**Feelings of Being**
Ratcliffe

**Experiences of Depression**
*A Study in Phenomenology*
Ratcliffe

**Recovery of People with Mental Illness**
*Philosophical and Related Perspectives*
Rudnick (ed.)

**Values and Psychiatric Diagnosis**
Sadler

**The Oxford Handbook of Psychiatric Ethics**
Sadler, Van Staden, and Fulford

**Madness and Modernism**
Sass

**Disembodied Spirits and Deanimated Bodies**
*The Psychopathology of Common Sense*
Stanghellini

**Lost in Dialogue**
*Anthropology, Psychopathology, and Care*
Stanghellini

**One Century of Karl Jaspers Psychopathology**
Stanghellini and Fuchs

**Emotions and Personhood**
Stanghellini and Rosfort

**Essential Philosophy of Psychiatry**
Thornton

**Naturalism, Hermeneutics, and Mental Disorder**
Varga

**The Healing Virtues**
*Character Ethics in Psychotherapy*
Waring

*Empirical Ethics in Psychiatry*
Widdershoven, McMillan, Hope, and Van der Scheer (eds.)

*The Sublime Object of Psychiatry: Schizophrenia in Clinical and Cultural Theory*
Woods

*Alternate Perspectives on Psychiatric Validation: DSM, ICD, RDoC, and Beyond*
Zachar, St. Stoyanov, Aragona, and Jablensky (eds.)

# Psychiatric Neuroethics
## Studies in Research and Practice

Walter Glannon

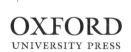

OXFORD
UNIVERSITY PRESS

# OXFORD
UNIVERSITY PRESS

Great Clarendon Street, Oxford, OX2 6DP,
United Kingdom

Oxford University Press is a department of the University of Oxford.
It furthers the University's objective of excellence in research, scholarship,
and education by publishing worldwide. Oxford is a registered trade mark of
Oxford University Press in the UK and in certain other countries

© Oxford University Press 2019

The moral rights of the author have been asserted

First Edition Published in 2019

Impression: 1

Published in the United States of America by Oxford University Press
198 Madison Avenue, New York, NY 10016, United States of America

British Library Cataloguing in Publication Data
Data available

Library of Congress Control Number: 2018941859

ISBN 978-0-19-875885-3

Printed in Great Britain by
Ashford Colour Press Ltd, Gosport, Hampshire

*For Yee-Wah*

# Advance praise

'This book is extraordinary as it addresses central and sometimes controversial issues in psychiatry, including its model of the mind–brain relation and ethical issues such as euthanasia. Walter Glannon, one of the leading experts in the philosophy of psychiatry, delivers an outstanding book which will, I am sure, become standard reading in the field and beyond.'

*Georg Northoff*
*Mind, Brain Imaging and Neuroethics Research Unit*
*University of Ottawa Institute of Mental Health Research, Canada*

'As the big pharma have withdrawn from investing in the development of psychopharmaceuticals, the therapeutic void needs to be filled, and one of the ways to do so is by noninvasive and invasive neuromodulation. Walter Glannon bravely takes the lead in addressing and providing ethical guidance in how to embrace the new technology in real-world settings. A must-read and highly needed work for everybody who is interested or involved in the treatment of psychiatric brain disorders.'

*Dirk De Ridder*
*Neurological Foundation Professor of Neurosurgery*
*University of Otago, New Zealand*

'In *Psychiatric Neuroethics: Studies in Research and Practice*, Walter Glannon combines a philosophical sensibility with an appreciation of psychiatry as a psycho-biological science of the brain as well as the mind. With precision, Glannon adroitly teases out ethical conflicts, treating a range of psychiatric interventions such as psychosurgery, neuromodulation, control of psychopathic behavior, and rationales for assisted suicide for psychiatric and neurodegenerative conditions. His critical analysis is an original contribution to psychiatry and neuroethics.'

*Laurence R. Tancredi*
*Clinical Professor of Psychiatry*
*New York University School of Medicine, USA*

'Walter Glannon's *Psychiatric Neuroethics* provides keen insights into the intersecting domains of brain science, mental health practice, philosophy, ethics, and law. In addressing longstanding philosophical questions about the nature of the mind, self, and psychiatry as a discipline, Glannon presents a detailed examination of the ways in which ongoing neuroscientific research has been used, or in some cases misused, in the understanding, classification, diagnosis, and care of mental illness. This book affords a prudent perspective on neuroethical issues, questions, and possible solutions that are important in guiding applications of brain science in the clinical practices of the field-in-evolution that is psychiatry.'

*James Giordano*
*Professor, Departments of Neurology and Biochemistry Chief,*
*Neuroethics Studies Program Pellegrino*
*Center for Clinical Bioethics Georgetown*
*University Medical Center, USA*

# Acknowledgments

I thank my editors at Oxford University Press, Martin Baum, Charlotte Holloway, and Janine Fisher, for supporting and guiding this project. Three anonymous reviewers and the editors of the International Perspectives in Philosophy and Psychiatry (IPPP) series gave me helpful comments on the book proposal. For their comments on earlier versions of Chapter 5, I thank Nicole Vincent, Allan MacCay, Karen Rommelfanger, and Syd Johnson. Special thanks go to John Sadler for extensive and very helpful comments on earlier versions of Chapters 3 and 4 and to Dirk De Ridder for equally extensive and helpful comments on earlier versions of Chapters 4 and 5. Some sections of the book have appeared previously in journal articles and book chapters. I have benefited from the thoughtful and constructive reviews of the referees.

I presented some of the ideas in the book to audiences at the Neuroethics Unit of the Institut de recherches cliniques de Montreal, a conference on neuromodulation at the Brocher Foundation in Hermance, Switzerland, the Department of Neurosurgery of the University of Zurich Hospital, a philosophy colloquium at the University of Turku, and a conference on Neurointerventions and the Law at Georgia State University.

For discussion and correspondence, I am grateful to Jean-Pierre Changeux, Dirk De Ridder, Thomas Fuchs, Christian Ineichen, Nir Lipsman, Georg Northoff, Roger Pitman, Ulrike Rimmele, John Sadler, Daniel Schacter, Sigrid Sterckx, Teresa Yu, and Adam Zeman. I am especially grateful to John Sadler for encouraging me to submit my project proposal for consideration in the IPPP series and his continued support.

# Contents

Introduction  *1*

**1** A paradigm for psychiatry  *15*

**2** Disorders of consciousness, memory, and will  *51*

**3** Treating psychiatric disorders: Less invasive and noninvasive interventions  *87*

**4** Psychiatric neurosurgery  *135*

**5** Neuromodulation: Control, identity, and justice  *185*

**6** Intervening in the psychopath's brain  *219*

**7** Euthanasia and assisted suicide for psychiatric disorders  *251*

**8** Prediction and prevention  *291*

Epilogue: Psychiatry, neuroscience, philosophy  *327*

References  *333*
Index  *369*

# Introduction

In 2013, data from the World Health Organization (WHO) World Mental Health Surveys indicated that mental illness constituted 7.4% of the global burden of disease and that its incidence and burden would increase exponentially in the future (Alonso, Chatterji, and He, 2013; Becker and Kleinman, 2013). This followed a 2012 estimate by the WHO that depression would be the leading cause of the global burden of all diseases by 2030 (World Health Organization, 2012). Schizophrenia, which is the most functionally disabling psychiatric disorder, affects approximately 24 million people worldwide. Mental illness is untreated or undertreated in many countries. These facts and estimates underscore the need for continued research that will lead to a better understanding of psychiatric disorders. This research may in turn lead to the development of safer and more effective therapies that will relieve or prevent the burden of disease experienced by millions of people.

*Psychiatric Neuroethics* is an analysis and discussion of questions at the intersection of psychiatry, neuroscience, philosophy, and law that have arisen from advances in psychiatric research and clinical psychiatric practice in the last 30 years. Are psychiatric disorders diseases of the brain, caused by dysfunctional neural circuits and neurotransmitters? What role do genes, neuroendocrine and neuroimmune interactions, and a person's response to the environment play in the development of these disorders? How do different explanations of the etiology and pathophysiology of mental illness influence diagnosis, prognosis, and decisions about treatment? How do psychiatric disorders affect consciousness and agency? Could the presumed salutary effects of neural interventions for pathological thought and behavior change one's mental states in undesirable ways? What are the ethical and social justice issues regarding access to treatment and experimental and innovative interventions for treatment-refractory conditions? What are the obligations of clinicians and researchers to patients and research subjects in psychiatry? Could the interests of society in preventing public harm override the cognitive liberty of criminal offenders with a psychiatric disorder to refuse an intervention in the brain? Would it be rational for a person with a chronic treatment-resistant disorder to request euthanasia or assisted suicide (EAS) as the only way to end his suffering? Could psychiatric disorders be prevented? If so, then how could they be prevented? I raise and discuss these questions in a comprehensive, systematic, and thematically integrated way. The book is written for a multidisciplinary audience, including psychiatrists, neurologists, neurosurgeons, philosophers, psychologists, legal theorists, and informed lay readers.

These questions fall within the domain of neuroethics. This is an interdisciplinary field at the intersection of the brain sciences, radiology, cognitive psychology, philosophy, and law. In a seminal paper, Adina Roskies distinguished between two branches of neuroethics: the ethics of neuroscience and the neuroscience of ethics (2002, pp. 21–22). The first branch generally considers the risks and potential benefits to patients and research participants whose brains are mapped or monitored by structural and functional imaging, as well as when they are altered by drugs, surgery, and electrical or magnetic stimulation. The ethics of neuroscience also considers the decisions that patients and research subjects make in receiving treatments and participating in research in light of the potential benefits and risks. In addition, this branch of neuroethics pertains to the obligations of clinicians and investigators to benefit patients and protect them and research subjects from harm. The neuroscience of ethics generally pertains to the neurobiological basis of the mental capacity for rational and moral decision-making. In particular, this branch pertains to the capacity to understand the nature of one's medical condition and make informed decisions to consent to treatment or participate in research. At a deeper level, Roskies asked whether future developments in neuroscience might cause us to revise our definition of "normal" behavior (2002, p. 22). She concluded by arguing that neuroethics should not be confined to specialists in neuroscience, philosophy, and law. It should also include public debate and broad social participation from all members of society in considering the implications of reading and changing people's brains (2002, p. 23).

While acknowledging that the ethics of neuroscience and the neuroscience of ethics "can be pursued independently to a large extent," Roskies noted that "perhaps most intriguing is to contemplate how progress in each will affect the other" (2002, p. 21). One example of overlap between the two branches of neuroethics is when a patient with a psychiatric disorder, such as schizophrenia or major depression, decides to accept or refuse an intervention in the brain or participate in research. This requires informed consent from the competent patient as an expression of his autonomy and ability to act in his own best interests. Respect for patient autonomy obligates the clinician or researcher to respect the patient's decision regarding the intervention (ethics of neuroscience). Competence and consent presuppose the cognitive and emotional capacity to weigh the potential benefits and risks of an approved or experimental intervention, the reasons for or against it, and to make an informed decision on this basis (neuroscience of ethics). This can be problematic if the disorder is moderately severe or severe and involves significant impairment in the relevant mental capacities. It may raise questions about whether the patient can meet the criteria of consent to receive therapy or participate in research.

I construe "neuroethics" broadly to include more than questions about the patient's capacity to weigh the benefits against the risks of different interventions in the brain and the obligations of clinicians and researchers to protect patients and research subjects. In addition, neuroethics pertains to how psychiatric disorders can harm people by distorting the content of their mental states, impairing their will, and altering their identities. It also pertains to how certain therapies can benefit people by restoring mental content, the will, and the self to normal functional levels. In these respects, issues in the philosophy of mind as well as normative ethical theory can influence how we assess ethical issues in psychiatry. At the same time, psychiatry can influence how we assess questions in the philosophy of mind and normative ethics. Some philosophers may question the extent to which neuroscience and psychiatry can elucidate philosophical questions and provide guidance on how to address them. They may hold that psychological explanations are sufficient and that appeals to the brain add nothing to them. Yet the use of brain imaging in psychiatric research provides evidence that neural circuits and networks mediate psychomotor, cognitive, emotional, and volitional capacities associated with the mind, the will, and identity. Although imaging has its limitations, techniques such as computed tomography (CT), magnetic resonance imaging (MRI), positron emission tomography (PET), and functional magnetic resonance imaging (fMRI) showing structural and functional abnormalities in these circuits and pathways can help to explain why these capacities become impaired in major psychiatric disorders.

One of the best examples of how impaired reasoning and decision-making is traceable to brain damage and dysfunction is the case of Phineas Gage. This man lost many of his rational and moral capacities due to damage to his ventromedial prefrontal cortex from a metal projectile that penetrated this region of his brain while he was working on the Burlington and Northern Railroad in Vermont in 1848. The changes in Gage's personality and behavior were so significant that "in the words of his friends and acquaintances, 'Gage was no longer Gage'" (Damasio, Grabowski, Frank et al., 1994, p. 1102). In addition, functional neurosurgery on awake patients with neurological and psychiatric disorders can confirm that cognitive and emotional processing is mediated by different regions in the brain. Patients' reports of their experiences from techniques that probe and modulate neural circuits validate the neurobiological basis of their mental states. They can also confirm when dysfunction at the neural level manifests in dysfunction at the mental level.

Some cognitive psychologists and neuroscientists have claimed, or suggested, that knowledge of brain structure and function and its effects on the mind can completely explain, or explain away, the psychological aspects of concepts such as free will and personal identity (Wegner, 2002; Seung, 2013). They ignore the many ways in which the mind, body, and environment influence the brain, which rejects the neuroreductionism behind these claims. Although neuroscience in general and psychiatry in particular cannot provide a complete account of the mind, they can yield a better understanding of ordered and disordered mental states. As Georg Northoff points out, neuroscience enables us to "study the unwell brain for clues about the healthy mind" (2016, p. ix). Because the brain–mind relation underlies thought, identity, and agency, the implications of psychiatry for these philosophical questions are significant (Kendler and Parnas, 2012, 2014, 2017).

Since the declaration of the 1990s as the "Decade of the Brain," much of the research in psychiatry has endeavored to explain psychiatric disorders in terms of dysfunctional neural circuits and neurotransmitters mediating motor and mental functions (Insel, 2010, p. 188). The gradual shift in focus from observed and reported symptoms in patients to the underlying neurobiology of mental illness has driven the field of biological psychiatry (Walter, 2013). In particular, this shift motivated the 2009 National Institute of Mental Health (NIMH) strategic plan that included the Research Domain Criteria (RDoC) as a research classification system for mental disorders (Insel, Cuthbert, Garvey et al., 2010; National Institute of Mental Health, 2011; Casey, Craddock, Cuthbert et al., 2013). While the RDoC focuses mainly on neural circuits, it also examines how genetics, the environment, and other processes influence brain structure and function, and how a synthesis, or "matrix," of all of these factors can result in a better understanding of how psychiatric disorders develop and persist in people. The neural circuit-based criteria of the RDoC provide a necessary framework to complement the symptom-based criteria of the fifth edition of the *Diagnostic and Statistical Manual of Mental Disorders (DSM-5)* (American Psychiatric Association, 2013) which until recently was the dominant paradigm for conceptualizing and classifying mental illness (Kendler and Parnas, 2017).

I avoid discussing mental disorders whose nosological status is ambiguous. Instead, I focus on what have been classified unambiguously as major psychiatric disorders. These include schizophrenia, major depressive disorder (MDD), bipolar disorder I and II (BD I and BD II), obsessive–compulsive disorder (OCD), generalized anxiety disorder (GAD), post-traumatic stress disorder (PTSD), and anorexia nervosa (AN). I mention other disorders as well, though I consider them to be variants of the major disorders. I focus mainly on moderately severe to severe psychiatric disorders because most of the contentious ethical questions in psychiatry arise from predicting, diagnosing, and intervening in the brains of people who are affected by them. One possible exception to this categorization is psychopathy, which I discuss in Chapter 6. Although it should not be included in the same category as other disorders I have listed in terms of symptom severity and burden of disease, psychopathy is included in the *DSM-5* as a specifier for antisocial personality disorder (p. 765). More importantly, this disorder has significant implications for the field of forensic psychiatry, particularly regarding the justification of interventions in the brains of criminal psychopaths to alter their behavior.

I do not take "mental disorder" to be a natural kind. A natural kind is defined in terms of how its properties combine in the natural world. It has an objective ontological status and is not the product of concepts we apply to the world. The criteria psychiatrists use to classify psychiatric disorders are the product of these concepts. Psychiatric nosology is not a naturalistic but an interpretive enterprise. It is objective in the sense that classification of major psychiatric disorders results from agreement among a community of researchers and clinicians in psychiatry. This is not just an empirical process but also a normative one. Psychiatrists interpret and agree, or disagree, on what data from brain imaging, overt symptoms, and other measures reveal about thought and behavior in diagnosing and treating psychiatric disorders. John Sadler points out that there are nonmoral and moral senses of normativity in psychiatry. He raises the question of whether psychiatric disorders should be considered "moral bads" warranting some form of moral judgment, or "nonmoral bads" like "medical diseases or surgical injuries" (2004, p. 221). Sadler writes, "I would like to make the, perhaps controversial, argument that mental disorders . . . should involve, substantively, non-moral evaluations in the core concepts, and such normative evaluations 'filter up' to define and constrain diagnostic criteria as well" (2004, p. 221).

The "moral bad" attribution to major psychiatric disorders has diminished over the last 50 years, thanks largely to research elucidating the processes underlying their etiology and pathophysiology. This research has helped to reduce some of the stigma attached to them (Sadler, 2009). Mental illness continues to be stigmatized to an unacceptable degree. Different interpretations of some of the causal factors of psychiatric disorders have impeded rather than promoted the elimination of stigma. Psychiatric genetics is one example. Raising ethical concerns about translating psychiatric genomics research into mental healthcare, Camilla Kong, Michael Dunn, and Michael Parker state that "the genetic essentialism that is commonly associated with the genomics revolution in health care might inadvertently exacerbate stigma toward people with mental disorders" (2017, p. 1). In contrast, in their analysis and discussion of schizophrenia, Michael Owen, Akira Sawa, and Preben Mortensen state that "a genetic diagnosis might . . . have psychological benefits for patients and their families by reducing internalized stigma and self-blame" (2016, p. 88). Each of these comments attributes too much of a causal role to genetics in psychiatric disorders. How genes express themselves in the brain and influence brain function depends on epigenetic and environmental factors. This refutes any hint of genetic essentialism in psychiatry.

The idea of a genetic diagnosis based on identifiable mutations is equally problematic. Thomas Insel points out that "the diversity and private nature of these mutations preclude a simple genetic explanation for schizophrenia," even though "these findings may yield important clues to pathophysiology" (2010, p. 188). Insel acknowledges that genetics is an important causal factor, but it is not the only causal factor in this disorder. While the genetic component is more significant in schizophrenia than in other psychiatric disorders, it is also a factor in bipolar disorder and depression. Yet the same qualifications about the causal import of psychiatric genomics in schizophrenia apply to these disorders as well.

What contributes to the persistence of stigma is a primary or exclusive focus on one dimension of mental illness. Focusing solely or mainly on the psychological dimension may facilitate the dismissive comment that psychiatric disorders are "all in the mind." The most effective way to reduce the stigma is for researchers and clinicians to educate the public that psychiatric disorders develop and persist not because of biological, psychological, or social processes operating independently of each other, but because of the interactions between all of them. This education should emphasize that therapies can take weeks, months, or even years to be effective. It should also point out that some disorders are treatment-resistant. For example, as many as 20% of depressed patients fail to respond to multiple treatments over many years (Holtzheimer and Mayberg, 2010, p. 1437, 2011, p. 2). The rate of treatment-resistance is even higher in other disorders. Knowledge of these facts could help to dispel the view that controlling symptoms and "curing" mental illness is simply a matter of taking the "right" pill. It could help to disabuse people of the attitude that, if symptoms persist, then the patient must be taking the "wrong" pill or otherwise doing something wrong. It may also help to emphasize that no two people's brains are alike. How genes and other biological factors shape brain structure and function, how the brain responds to stress, and how it responds to drugs or techniques can vary considerably from one person to the next. Ultimately, reducing stigma depends on families and colleagues of affected individuals making the necessary effort to inform themselves of the many causes and dimensions of mental illness (Thornicroft, Mehta, Clement et al., 2016).

Methodologically and structurally, *Psychiatric Neuroethics* is divided roughly into two parts. In Chapters 1 and 2, I examine and discuss different conceptions of psychiatric disorders in terms of their etiology, pathophysiology, and symptomatology and the ways in which they impair thought and behavior. In Chapters 3 through 8, I describe different interventions in the brains of people who have psychiatric disorders, as well as interventions in processes that occur before they exist, and discuss the ethical and broader philosophical questions these interventions raise. I interweave the science of psychiatry with the philosophy of psychiatry. Philosophical questions can be appropriately addressed only when they are appropriately framed by the science of the brain and mind. These questions arise from less and more invasive interventions to control and ameliorate symptoms. They become more pressing and controversial the more resistant the disorder is to treatment and the more invasive the treatments are. Most controversial is EAS for patients with treatment-resistant depression (TRD) and other disorders, where the intervention does not control but eliminates symptoms by ending the life of the person who experiences them. This underscores the need to prevent the onset of psychiatric disorders, or to slow or stop their progression at an early stage.

My discussion of the normative dimensions of psychiatry is not driven by a single ethical theory. Instead of selecting a theory and then discussing particular issues around it, I first raise the issues and then explicitly or implicitly appeal to a theory to explain why a particular course of action or policy is justifiable or unjustifiable. Questions about what to do in a particular case, or which policy to adopt, drive the application of the theory, rather than the other way around. A competent patient's right to receive or refuse treatment or participate in research is based on deontology, as is the duty of clinicians and investigators to respect competent patients' decisions and protect patients and research subjects. Concern about treatment outcomes in ameliorating symptoms and reducing side effects rests on consequentialism. Yet insofar as these outcomes are in the best interests of consenting patients, nonconsequentialism may guide ethical assessment of the key issues. Outcomes matter, but they are not the only factor that matters in evaluating an action or policy. Indeed, deontological, consequentialist, and nonconsequentialist considerations may all be relevant to a single issue.

We have to assess which theory has more weight in adjudicating competing moral claims about a course of action. In terms of the bioethical principles corresponding to the ethical theories, I frame the ethical discussion by appealing to the standard principles of autonomy, nonmaleficence, beneficence, and justice (Beauchamp and Childress, 2012, Chapters 4–7). While these principles are limited in their scope of application to ethical debates in medicine, they serve my framing purpose for psychiatric neuroethics as well as any alternatives. Much of the discussion in this book addresses how psychiatric disorders impair control of thought and behavior, and how interventions in the brain can restore it. Control is a measure of autonomy in the sense that one's motivational states and actions are one's own. Autonomy is also germane to informed consent to participate in psychiatric research. This is significant given that many interventions for psychiatric disorders are still experimental. Nonmaleficence grounds researchers' obligation to protect subjects enrolled in clinical trials from harm. Beneficence grounds clinicians' obligations to provide patients with proven therapies consistent with best practices. Justice is germane to the question of whether patients with treatment-resistant psychiatric disorders have a right to participate in clinical trials testing experimental drugs and neuromodulation techniques. It is also germane to the question of whether subjects in clinical trials testing deep brain stimulation are entitled to retain a brain implant after the conclusion of these trials. I base most of my examples on actual cases, or hypothetical variants of them. This gives substance to the principles and the ethical and broader philosophical issues better than the fanciful thought experiments that are so common in armchair philosophy.

In addition to ethical questions surrounding standard forms of psychopharmacology, I examine some questions emerging from experimental use of the psychotropic drugs ketamine, psilocybin, and 3,4-methylenedioxymethamphetamine (MDMA) for depression and PTSD. I discuss newer closed-loop forms of deep brain stimulation (DBS) as a potentially safer and more effective form of neuromodulation than open-loop DBS. I also discuss optogenetics, focused ultrasound, and temporal interference as novel neuromodulating techniques for a range of psychiatric disorders. My discussion of ethical issues arising from historical, current and emerging interventions in the brain and mind shows the evolution of psychiatric neuroethics.

In Chapter 1, I define psychiatric disorders as disorders of the brain, mind, and the person's relation to the world. The etiology, pathophysiology, and symptomatology of these disorders is influenced by interactions between the brain, mind, immune and endocrine systems, the subject's perception of the body, and how the person responds to the environment. A biopsychosocial model provides the best account of the development of these disorders and a guide for research and treatment. I discuss some of the merits and limitations of the symptom-based *DSM-5* and the more recent circuit-based RDoC and claim that they can be complementary models in a paradigm for psychiatry research and clinical practice. Noting the considerable overlap in pathophysiology between neurological and psychiatric disorders, I argue that there are sound reasons for relaxing the strict distinction between the two disciplines. However, there are distinctive features of psychiatric disorders that warrant treating them separately in some respects. I defend nonreductive materialism as the theory best able to account for the different dimensions of the brain–mind relation in psychiatry. In addition, I propose that the self in psychiatry should not be defined solely in terms of conscious mental processes but as a complex set of conscious and nonconscious processes that emerge from and are shaped by many factors inside and outside of the brain.

I discuss major psychiatric disorders as disorders of consciousness, memory, and will in Chapter 2. Schizophrenia, major depression, and OCD are disorders of consciousness in the sense that they involve disturbances in how the brain processes and integrates information about the body and external world. Anxiety, panic, some forms of depression, and PTSD are disorders of memory content. The emotionally charged representation of a memory of a traumatic or disturbing experience can cause hyperactivation in the brain's fear memory system and result in maladaptive responses to environmental stimuli. The distorted mental content in these psychopathologies impairs the capacity to consider different action plans, and to form and execute particular plans in particular actions. Dysfunctional mental states correlating with dysfunctional neural states impair the capacity for flexible behavior and adaptability to the environment. This dysfunction also impairs the capacity for insight into a psychiatric disorder and understanding the need for and motivation to seek treatment. In these respects, neural and mental dysfunction impairs free will. As disorders of consciousness, memory, and will, psychiatric disorders disable the capacity for autonomous agency.

In Chapter 3, I analyze and discuss different types of psychopharmacology. I cite the view held by some psychiatrists that drugs targeting monoamines to treat psychiatric disorders may be based on a mistaken hypothesis about the pathophysiology of these disorders. I mention recent research on the role of dysfunctional glutaminergic signaling and how novel pharmacological treatments such as ketamine and psilocybin for depression, and MDMA for PTSD, have considerable therapeutic potential. Questioning the distinction between noninvasive and invasive treatments in psychiatry, I point out that some presumably noninvasive treatments could be described as invasive because they can cause changes in the brain. This can occur in the absence of intracranial surgery. I propose that the invasive–noninvasive distinction be replaced by a distinction between less and more invasive interventions, where the degree of invasiveness corresponds to the extent of changes the intervention induces in the brain. I discuss the potential benefits and risks, as well as the limitations of electroconvulsive therapy (ECT), transcranial magnetic stimulation (TMS), and transcranial current stimulation (tCS). The indications for using TMS, tCS, and psychotropic drugs to treat psychiatric disorders support reasons for maintaining the distinction between therapy and enhancement. Placebos and neurofeedback (NFB) are distinct from the other interventions I consider because the cognitive and emotional responses of the patient to the physician or images of the patient's brain can ameliorate symptoms without psychotropic drugs or neurostimulation. While deception and potential erosion of trust are the main ethical issues in using placebos, in some cases even deceptive use of placebos can be justified in psychiatric treatment. I raise some social justice issues regarding access to and affordability of NFB. Yet this and other techniques that induce psychological responses from patients may not be effective in treating moderately severe and severe forms of psychiatric disorders. With a view to potential future therapies, I consider how the neurostimulating technique of temporal interference could potentially result in higher response rates and better control of disease progression and symptoms.

I discuss a range of ethical issues in psychiatric neurosurgery in Chapter 4. This is functional neurosurgery designed to modulate dysfunctional neural circuits mediating sensorimotor, cognitive, emotional, and volitional capacities. Because it is largely still experimental and investigative, functional psychiatric neurosurgery falls within the domain of psychiatric research. It is used for psychiatric disorders that have not responded to other interventions. After surveying the history of this practice, I assess the comparative benefits and risks of neural ablation and DBS as the two most invasive forms of neuromodulation. This includes neural ablative techniques of radiofrequency neurosurgery, Gamma Knife® radiosurgery, and high-intensity focused ultrasound. It also includes open-loop and closed-loop versions of DBS. I discuss the question of whether individuals with a severe or moderately severe psychiatric disorder have enough cognitive and emotional capacity to weigh the reasons for and against DBS and give informed consent to undergo it. This question includes consideration of whether some patients might be motivated by a therapeutic misconception to participate in a functional neurosurgery clinical trial. It also considers whether the idea of DBS as a treatment of "last resort" unduly influences their perception of risk. In addition, I discuss the obligation of investigators conducting these trials to research subjects and the medical and ethical justification for a sham control arm in psychiatric neurosurgery trials.

Social justice issues are relevant here as well. I examine the issue of fairness in patients having or lacking access to neurostimulation when it is the only intervention that can control and relieve symptoms of a psychiatric disorder. In the last section of the chapter, I describe the mechanisms of optogenetics and discuss the therapeutic potential of this novel form of neuromodulation. The ability of this technique to control gene expression in the brain and a broad range of neural activity could make it a superior form of neuromodulation to DBS. Yet the fact that optogenetics manipulates both genetic material and neural circuits and has been tested only in animal models makes it unclear what its benefit-to-risk ratio would be.

In Chapter 5, I address concerns that people with devices in their brains regulating neural and mental functions are not in control of their thoughts and actions. I argue that DBS or any other neuromodulating system that operates safely and effectively does not undermine control or agency. Rather, by restoring motor and mental capacities, DBS enables autonomous agency that has been impaired or undermined by a psychiatric disorder. There is shared control between the person and the device, and this allows enough control for autonomy and free will. Nor does neuromodulation necessarily cause substantial changes in a person's mental states and alter her identity. When it functions properly, neuromodulation does not alter but restores the mental capacities impaired by the disorder. Rather than disrupting psychological connectedness and continuity, DBS and other techniques can re-establish these relations and return the patient to her premorbid self. Nevertheless, the control a patient has with a device may entail certain expectations about operating it to maintain normal neural and mental functions. I discuss whether these expectations impose an unfair burden of control on these patients compared with people who do not need a device to maintain these functions

Extending the discussion of interventions aimed at restoring control of mental capacities in psychiatric disorders, I explore some of the implications of this desired outcome for forensic psychiatry in Chapter 6. I discuss whether pharmacological intervention in the brains of criminal psychopaths to modify and enable them to control their behavior could be justified as an alternative to continued incarceration. I consider the question of whether treatment designed to rehabilitate the offender could be forced on him against his wishes and whether it would violate his cognitive liberty. One of the key issues is weighing the interests and rights of the offender against the interests of society in preventing recidivism and protecting the public from harm.

In Chapter 7, I discuss reasons for and against euthanasia and physician-assisted suicide for patients with TRD or other psychiatric disorders. Although these actions may seem anathema to the goal of treating psychiatric patients in order to prevent suicide, there may be cases in which it would be permissible to bring about or assist in the death of a person with one of these disorders. The permissibility of these actions depends on four conditions. First, the patient must be competent enough to weigh the reasons for and against EAS. Second, the patient must make an informed and persistent request for it. Third, the suffering the patient experiences from the disorder must be unbearable and interminable. Fourth, the disorder must be resistant to all indicated treatments given to the patient over many years. A corollary to the fourth condition is that there must be a reasonable limit to the time a patient could be expected to wait for a possible treatment to relieve symptoms. When these conditions obtain, continued life may not be in the patient's best interests. He could make a rational request for a psychiatrist or other physician to end his life or assist him in ending it.

Shifting the focus from events occurring in early adulthood and adolescence to events occurring perinatally and prenatally, I discuss different ways of predicting and preventing psychiatric disorders in Chapter 8. After considering reasons for and against intervening with psychotropic drugs during the prodromal phase of disease, I discuss how the identification of biomarkers for psychiatric disorders in childhood or adolescence might predict who would be at risk of developing them. Biomarkers could indicate which interventions could reduce this risk or eliminate it altogether. I raise questions about the predictive value of biomarkers in psychiatry and discuss some of the ethical and social issues arising from how different parties might interpret them. In some cases, the identification and interpretation of biomarkers may be more harmful than beneficial to those who have them. Abnormal neuroimmune and neuroendocrine interactions may disrupt normal rates of synaptic pruning and myelination in childhood and adolescence and increase the risk of schizophrenia and other disorders. I discuss how immune-modulating drugs could reverse this process and how to balance the potential benefits against the risks of intervening in the brain in this way. I speculate on the possibility of using focused ultrasound to open the blood–brain barrier (BBB) to allow the infusion of growth factors at an early stage of pathogenesis when neurodevelopmental abnormalities may signal early neurodegeneration. This might reverse the disease process in severe disorders such as schizophrenia and change what would have been a life of mental illness into a life of mental health. I also consider noninvasive interventions such as altering the environment to prevent epigenetic factors from influencing gene expression in the brain and making a person susceptible to mental illness. This could obviate the need for psychotropic drugs or neurotrophic factors that could have permanent adverse effects in the brain. In the last section of the chapter, I explain how prenatal and perinatal events can increase the risk of developing a psychiatric disorder in the second or third decade of life. I consider different interventions before birth that might prevent people from having a disorder after birth. These interventions include not conceiving, terminating a pregnancy, or having and carrying a pregnancy to term at one time rather than another. If potential parents knew that a child they had would be at risk of developing a psychiatric disorder, then they could control to a certain extent whether they brought into existence a person who would have a disorder or a different person who would not have it.

After briefly summarizing the main points from the preceding chapters, in the Epilogue I consider whether an artificial or purely mechanistic model of the brain could lead to a better understanding of mental health and mental illness. It is doubtful that such a model could simulate the processes of a natural brain. It is also doubtful that it could simulate the complex interactions between biological, psychological, and social factors necessary to explain how psychiatric disorders develop and how they might be treated or prevented. In addition, I point out that mental illness can be as disabling and impose more of a burden on more people than physical illness. On grounds of fairness, diseases of the brain and mind should have priority over diseases of the body in the allocation of funding for research into treatment and prevention. This is necessary to relieve the burden of disease, enable functional independence for people with major psychiatric disorders and ideally eliminate this burden altogether.

# Chapter 1

# A paradigm for psychiatry

What type of disorder is a psychiatric disorder? What is it a disorder of? Are schizophrenia, unipolar and bipolar depression, and other conditions diseases of the brain? Are they diseases of the mind? Are they diseases of the brain *and* mind? If they involve both neural and mental aspects, then how does the relation between the brain and mind influence the etiology, pathophysiology, and symptomatology of these disorders? Are psychiatric disorders fundamentally distinct from neurological disorders? Do they overlap in some respects? If they overlap, then what are the diagnostic, prognostic, and ethical implications? These questions drive my discussion of different concepts and categories in this chapter in establishing a paradigm for psychiatry. The aim is not only to lay out a nosology of psychiatric disorders but also to develop a framework that can help to explain their causes and progression and guide therapeutic and preventive interventions (Kendler and Parnas, 2017).

I discuss some of the merits and limitations of the symptom-based *DSM-5* and the more recent neural circuit-based RDoC. These models should be considered complementary and together necessary to explain mental health and illness as the result of neurobiological, psychological, and environmental processes. The RDoC is the latest stage in the evolution of biological psychiatry. I trace the history of the sciences of the mind from the nineteenth-century view that neurology and psychiatry were not fundamentally different to the more recent view that they form distinct disease categories. One of the consequences of this distinction is the tendency toward a type of nosological dualism: neurological disorders are disorders of the brain; psychiatric disorders are disorders of the mind.

Following other neurologists and psychiatrists, I point out that most major disorders of these two types have both neurobiological and psychological features. This needs to be factored into assessment of the burden of diseases of the brain and mind to provide a broader diagnostic and therapeutic framework. One way of avoiding the problems associated with brain–mind dualism and a rigid distinction between neurology and psychiatry is a merging of the two disciplines into a single discipline of neuropsychiatry. Indeed, many clinical and research neuroscientists now categorize diseases of the brain and mind as neuropsychiatric disorders. However, noting that motor symptoms are more common among neurological disorders and that cognitive and emotional symptoms are more common among psychiatric disorders, I point out that these disorders fall along a spectrum of motor and mental dysfunction. In cases where the main symptoms are motor, and in cases where the main symptoms are cognitive or emotional, there may be sound neuroscientific reasons for upholding the distinction between neurology and psychiatry. In cases where motor and mental symptoms overlap at the same or different times, there may be sound neuroscientific reasons for adopting a less strict distinction.

The complementarity of the *DSM-5* and the RDoC rests on a particular conception of the brain–mind relation. The most plausible theory for understanding how neural and mental processes maintain mental health, or how dysfunction in these processes causes mental illness, is neither substance dualism nor reductive materialism but nonreductive materialism. On this view, mental states emerge from and are sustained by the brain but cannot be explained entirely in neural terms. The mind can have a causal role in the neural dysfunction of some psychiatric disorders. It can also restore some degree of normal function in these disorders through its modulating effects on neural circuits. I propose a conception of the psychiatric self. This consists of a set of continuous interacting biological, psychological, and environmental processes with effects at conscious and unconscious levels. Interactions between all of these factors shape the content of a person's mental states and the experience of being embodied and embedded in the environment. Psychiatric disorders are disorders of the self in the sense that they distort a person's perception of her relation to her body and the external world (Gillett, 2009; Fuchs, 2012; Maiese, 2016). Psychiatric disorders can also disrupt the psychological connectedness and continuity between mental states that shape the experience of persisting through time as the same person. In addition, these disorders can impair agency by impairing the affected person's cognitive, emotional, and motivational capacity for rational deliberation and decision-making. A biopsychosocial model consisting of complex interactions between the brain and genetic, immune, endocrine, psychological, and environmental factors is necessary to explain the characteristic features of these disorders (Engel, 1977). It is also necessary to explain how they develop and how they might be more effectively treated or prevented.

## *DSM* and RDoC

In 1918, the American Medico-Psychological Association (now the American Psychiatric Association) attempted to develop a standardized nosology of psychopathologies. This led to the first version of the *DSM* in 1952. Now in its fifth version, the *DSM* still classifies and distinguishes psychiatric disorders based on overt symptoms. The *DSM-5* (American Psychiatric Association, 2013) defines a "mental disorder" as "a syndrome characterized by clinically significant disturbance in an individual's cognition, emotion regulation or behavior that reflects a dysfunction in the psychological, biological or developmental processes underlying mental functioning. Mental disorders are usually associated with significant distress in social, occupational or other important activities" (*DSM-5*, p. 20; Stein, Phillips, Bolton et al., 2010). While there has been disagreement among psychiatrists about which conditions should be included or excluded from the *DSM*, the practice of basing the classification of major psychiatric disorders on a specific set of symptoms has remained constant over the last century.

I include schizophrenia, MDD, BD I and BD II, OCD, GAD, PTSD, and AN among major psychiatric disorders. This is not an exhaustive list. Most psychiatric disorders are spectrum disorders. Generally, they extend from minor temporary symptoms to major recurrent symptoms. The symptoms may progress from being mild to moderate to becoming moderately severe or severe in terms of intensity and extent of functional impairment. My focus in exploring ethical and other philosophical questions in psychiatry is on moderately severe to severe forms of these disorders. While some may not include psychopathy in this group, severe forms of it could be categorized as a major psychiatric disorder. As noted in the Introduction to this book, the *DSM-5* lists psychopathy as a specifier for antisocial personality disorder (*DSM-5*, p. 765). Unlike the *DSM*, the eleventh edition of the *International Statistical Classification of Diseases and Related Health Problems* (*ICD-11*) of the World Health Organization (2016) includes not only psychiatric disorders but also disorders of all bodily systems. Its classification of these disorders based on symptoms generally corresponds to that of the *DSM*.

The *DSM-5* lists two or more of the following symptoms for at least 1 month (unless successfully treated) for the positive subtype of schizophrenia: delusions (of grandeur, experience of alien control or false beliefs); hallucinations, disorganized speech; and disorganized or catatonic behavior (*DSM-5*, pp. 100–101; Castle and Buckley, 2015, p. 4). The development and course of symptoms distinguishes schizophrenia from schizoaffective and schizophreniform disorders. The negative subtype of schizophrenia includes blunted affect, disorganized thought, poor concentration, anhedonia (inability to experience pleasure), and avolition (inability to motivate oneself to act) that are often associated with social withdrawal.

For a diagnosis of MDD, one must have five or more of the following symptoms for a duration of 2 or more weeks: cognitive-emotional and somatic symptoms (pain), depressed mood, anhedonia, avolition, feelings of worthlessness or guilt, poor concentration, indecisiveness, appetite or weight changes, circadian rhythm/sleep disturbances, changes in psychomotor activity, fatigue, or suicidal ideation (*DSM-5*, pp. 160–161; Belmaker and Agam, 2008). Some of these symptoms overlap with the symptoms of the negative subtype of schizophrenia. Persistent depressive disorder (dysthymia) is distinct from MDD in having fewer of the characteristic symptoms (*DSM-5*, pp. 168–169). Mood-congruent and mood-incongruent psychotic features are specifiers of MDD (*DSM-5*, p. 186).

BD I is defined by a person's experience of mania and depressive symptoms. BD II is defined by the occurrence of at least one hypomanic episode and one or more depressive episodes (*DSM-5*, pp. 123–127; Strakowksi, 2014, p. 10). Mania involves euphoria or irritable mood, impulsivity, grandiosity, excessive energy, and decreased need for sleep. A manic episode lasts "at least 1 week and is present most of the day, nearly every day" (*DSM-5*, p. 124). A hypomanic episode "lasts at least 4 consecutive days" (*DSM-5*, p. 124). The main differences between mania and hypomania are that the first state involves greater severity or intensity and greater functional impairment than the second state. Although mania and hypomania are the distinctive features of BD I and BD II, respectively, depression occurs more often during the course of the illness, hence the term "bipolar depression." Depressive symptoms in BD I and BD II are the same as in MDD. This makes "depression the more disabling mood state" in BD and the main source of the affected person's functional impairment (Strakowski, 2014, p. 10; Frye, 2011). While these "mixed" states often occur at different times, in half of the cases of BD, mania and depression may occur concurrently (Strakowski, 2014, p. 9). The bipolar spectrum extends "from minor depressive symptoms or dysthymia (chronic low-grade depression) through recurrent depressive episodes that gradually progress to the addition of increasing manic symptoms (e.g. cyclothymia) through full hypomania (bipolar II disorder) and mania (bipolar 1 disorder)" (Strakowski, 2014, p. 11).

A diagnosis of GAD includes excessive anxiety and worry about events for at least 6 months, and difficulty controlling the worry. The anxiety and worry are associated with at least three of the following six mental and physical symptoms: restlessness, or a feeling of being "on edge," fatigue, difficulty concentrating, irritability, muscle tension, or sleep disturbance. These symptoms are not due to the physiological effects of substances or other medical conditions (*DSM-5*, p. 222; Stein and Sareen, 2015). There can be symptom overlap between depression and anxiety. Some psychiatrists and primary care physicians may describe this as "anxious depression" (Stein and Sareen, 2015). Symptoms may be comorbid or co-occurrent and not easily separable. There are differences between them as well. Murray Stein and Jitender Sareen point out that "persistent anhedonia . . . which is a characteristic of major depression is not a symptom of generalized anxiety disorder" (2015, p. 2060). Another difference between these disorders is that "patients with generalized anxiety disorder often describe a sense of helplessness, whereas patients with major depression may feel hopeless" (2015, p. 2060). There is more variability in the age of onset in MDD and GAD than other disorders. Some cases begin in adolescence and most begin in early adulthood, but some occur in later adulthood. MDD occurs in 2% of adults aged 55 years or older (Kok and Reynolds, 2017).

In OCD, obsessions are unwanted, intrusive thoughts. Compulsions are repetitive behaviors often performed to address anxiety associated with obsessions. They are an abnormal compensatory strategy in response to the thoughts. Obsessions include fear of contamination, persistent doubting, fear of causing harm, and superstition. Compulsions include excessive hand washing or cleaning of household items, hoarding, repeatedly checking that appliances are turned off or that doors are locked, and excessively checking writing for reassurance that it is error-free (*DSM-5*, pp. 237–238; Hirschtritt, Bloch, and Mathews, 2017, p. 1361). The *DSM-5* clearly separates OCD and GAD.

The core features of PTSD are "the persistence of intense, distressing and fearfully avoided reactions to reminders of a triggering event, alteration of mood and cognition, a pervasive sense of imminent threat, disturbed sleep and hypervigilance" (*DSM-5*, pp. 271–274; Shalev, Liberzon, and Marmar, 2017, p. 2459). The *DSM-5* and *ICD-11* add self-denigration and negative worldview to the set of symptoms characterizing PTSD. Environmental and cultural factors may have a greater role in PTSD than in other major psychiatric disorders. These include "exposure to repeated upsetting reminders" of a traumatic experience, as well as how differences across cultural groups can influence the type of exposure to and "the meaning attributed to the traumatic event" (*DSM-5*, p. 278).

In AN, the main diagnostic criteria are restriction of energy intake resulting in weight that is significantly lower than normal, intense fear of gaining weight, and disturbance in how one perceives and experiences one's body weight and shape (*DSM-5*, pp. 338–339). Distorted bodily perception results in negative self-evaluation and a lack of recognition of the seriousness of low body weight. It results in failure to recognize that one has a disease and the reasons for treatment. These symptoms make AN one of the most intractable psychiatric disorders and the disorder with the highest mortality rate.

The *DSM-5* includes a mixed features specifier to describe the coterminous occurrence of manic and depressive symptoms in bipolar depression (*DSM-5*, pp. 149–150). A complication with this and other specifiers is that there can be mixed states not only in a single disorder such as bipolar depression but also between different but often overlapping disorders such as depression and anxiety. There may also be mixed features between neurological and psychiatric disorders. As I discuss in the next section, the spectrum of states that cross or blur the traditional diagnostic boundary between neurology and psychiatry suggests revising the conception of these as distinct disciplines. One positive consequence of the mixed features specifier is that it reflects the conceptual model of clustering symptoms from different disorders, which may result in more effective treatments. I discuss this concept in Chapter 3.

Despite the prominence of the *DSM* in the last century and its focus on mental and somatic symptoms of psychiatric disorders, there is a longer history of research into the neurobiological bases of these disorders. This highlights the main shortcoming of the *DSM*. Its emphasis on symptoms fails to offer an account of the neurobiological, genetic, and other causes of these symptoms. Although the *DSM* mentions biological processes underlying mental functioning in mental disorders, it does not provide a satisfactory explanation of these processes. In the late nineteenth century, the dominant model in psychiatry was associated with Emil Kraepelin's theory that abnormal thought and behavior resulted from organic brain dysfunction (Kraepelin, 1896/1913). This was not an entirely original view and had many historical precedents. The idea that the source of mental disease is a dysfunctional brain is the main impetus for the RDoC. The general aim of this initiative is to identify brain mechanisms that can explain the etiology and pathophysiology of psychiatric disorders, provide earlier and more accurate diagnosis, and predict treatment responses and outcomes (Insel, Cuthbert, Garvey et al., 2010; Casey, Craddock, Cuthbert et al., 2013; Cuthbert and Insel, 2013).

Bruce Cuthbert and Thomas Insel spell out four principal aims of the RDoC. First, to bring together experts in clinical and basic sciences to identify the behavioral components of mental disorders amenable to neuroscientific approaches. Second, to determine variations in neural and mental functions from normal to pathological. Third, to develop reliable measures of the fundamental components of mental disorders in research and clinical settings. Fourth, to integrate genetic, neurobiological, behavioral, environmental, and experiential components of mental disorders (Cuthbert and Insel, 2013, p. 126). Highlighting its differences from the *ICD-11*, Cuthbert and Insel describe seven pillars of the RDoC. First, a strong translational research perspective. Second, a dimensional approach to psychopathology. Third, reliable measures of the components of mental disorders. Fourth, certain types of design and sampling strategies in research. Fifth, equal weight to behavioral functions and neural circuits. Sixth, solid evidence to serve as a platform for ongoing research.

Seventh, flexibility in defining disorders (Cuthbert and Insel, 2013, p. 126). Although the RDoC includes multiple causal influences in its classification of psychiatric disorders, dysfunctional brain circuits are the key component. This is confirmed by Insel's claim that schizophrenia, for example, is "a collection of neurodevelopmental disorders that involve alterations in brain circuits" (2010, p. 188). By examining how biological, behavioral, and environmental factors cause mental illness, and how knowledge of these factors can inform interventions to modulate brain dysfunction, the mainly circuit-based RDoC fills explanatory gaps left by the symptom-based *DSM*.

Neuroimaging and electrophysiology can identify dysfunctional neural circuits and dysfunctional connectivity between these circuits. Data from genetics, combined with data from neuroimaging, can confirm the presence of neurobiological signatures, or biomarkers, associated with psychiatric disorders (Insel, Cuthbert, Garvey et al., 2010; Insel and Wang, 2010; Insel, 2013; Walter, 2013, p. 4; Charney, Sklar, Buxbaum et al., 2013). These signatures can contribute to more accurate diagnosis and prediction of responses to treatment. They can also be used to guide neuromodulating techniques aimed at restoring function in neural circuits and the larger neural networks they constitute. I discuss the research and therapeutic potential and limitations of these modalities in more detail in subsequent chapters. It will be helpful to briefly explain them and their neurobiological significance here.

Dysfunctional neural circuits displayed by brain imaging can confirm the neurobiological underpinning of psychiatric disease. Researchers often use "biomarker" to designate a biological signature at an early stage of pathology. I use the term in a more general predictive, diagnostic, and prognostic sense applicable to earlier and later stages of disease. Biomarkers may be mutations detected through genetic testing and screening, abnormal proteins discovered in bodily fluids, or structural and functional features of the brain displayed by neuroimaging (Boksa, 2013). Detecting these biological signatures might enable researchers and clinicians to identify those at risk of developing a disorder when they are in a preclinical state or have prodromal symptoms. MRI, diffusion-weighted magnetic resonance imaging (dwMRI), diffusion tenor imaging (DTI), PET, fMRI, and voxel-based morphometry (VBM) can detect changes in the brain and confirm them as signatures of neural circuit dysfunction underlying psychiatric disorders.

In schizophrenia, imaging can identify a biomarker such as gray or white matter abnormalities or dysfunctional corticostriatal connectivity when a person is experiencing prepsychotic symptoms such as mild hallucinations and paranoia before a first psychotic episode (Fornito, Harrison, Goodby et al., 2013). The presence of these abnormalities could warrant early psychopharmacological treatment. Similarly, imaging can identify interhemispheric disconnectivity in bipolar patients with psychotic features (Sarrazin, Poupon, Linke et al., 2014). Based on correlations between brain dysfunction and early symptoms, these features can guide interventions to control or prevent psychosis in patients with these disorders, Identifying biomarkers could contribute to more accurate diagnosis and prognosis and more effective treatment of these and other disorders when symptoms alone are ambiguous.

Detection of biomarkers as abnormalities in neural circuits through imaging is also important for neuromodulating techniques such as DBS. Although neurosurgeons, neurologists, and psychiatrists typically administer DBS at an advanced stage of disease, imaging can enable neurosurgeons to modulate dysfunctional circuits and monitor the effects of stimulating them at an earlier stage. While recognizing and categorizing symptoms is necessary to establish a diagnosis and confirm whether a therapy is effective, this does not explain the neurobiology underlying the onset of symptoms, how they impair motor and mental functions, or why they remit or become more severe over time. This underscores the limitations of the *DSM* and the importance of detecting abnormal neurobiological signatures and mechanisms implicated in these disorders.

Some neuroscientists and psychiatrists have questioned the use of the *DSM-5* to assess indications for and responses to treatment for major psychiatric disorders. Insel claims, "symptoms alone rarely indicate the best choice of treatment" (2013, p. 4). In addressing the need to advance research in psychiatry, he spells out his rationale for moving away from the *DSM* and accepting the RDoC as a paradigm for psychiatry: "We cannot have success if we use DSM categories as the 'gold standard.' The diagnostic system has to be based on the emerging research data, not on the current symptom-based categories. Imagine deciding that ECGs ( = electrocardiograms) were not useful because many patients with chest pain did not have ECG changes. That is what we have been doing for decades when we reject a biomarker because it does not detect a DSM category. We need to begin collecting the genetic, imaging, physiological and cognitive data to see how all the data—not just the symptoms—cluster and how these clusters relate to treatment response" (2013, p. 4).

Despite Insel's claims, the RDoC may not adequately emphasize the extent to which neuroimmune and neuroendocrine interactions and psychosocial stress can adversely affect neural circuits, neurotransmitters, and the mental states they mediate. Cytokines released in response to infection may result in elevated levels of inflammatory biomarkers in the blood. These in turn may lead to inflammatory changes in the brain and alterations of neural circuits and cause or exacerbate mood disturbances and cognitive and volitional impairment in depression (Miller and Raison, 2016). Neuropathology in some psychiatric disorders may be traced to prenatal events. Maternal antibodies produced in response to infection during pregnancy can activate immune processes that can trigger an inflammatory reaction in the fetal brain and alter its development. Another limitation of circuit-level explanations is that they may not adequately account for how psychosocial factors influence people's stress response to environmental stimuli or the variability of these responses and their effects in the brain. Chronic psychosocial stress can cause dysregulation in the hypothalamic–pituitary–adrenal (HPA) axis, causing high circulating levels of norepinephrine (noradrenaline) and cortisol that can impair normal prefrontal–limbic connectivity and cognitive-emotional processing (Southwick, Vythilingam, and Charney, 2005; Hohne, Poidinger, Merz et al., 2014; Miller and Raison, 2016). This impairment can become more severe from subsequent atrophy in the prefrontal cortex (PFC) and hippocampus resulting from the long-term effects of stress hormones in these brain regions (Sapolsky, 2000; Sorrells, Caso, Munhoz et al., 2009).

Circuit-level explanations of these disorders can elucidate their biological aspects more than their psychological aspects. As the examples of the neural and mental effects of stress-induced responses to stimuli illustrate, focusing primarily on neural circuits cannot account for the causal role of an affected person's mental states in MDD and GAD. It cannot explain how the mind influences the brain in a top-down manner, just as the brain influences the mind in a bottom-up manner. Nor can identifying dysfunctional neural circuits fully account for the phenomenology of experiencing anhedonia, anxiety, delusions, or hallucinations (Kendler, 2016). These subjective aspects of the disorders are essential for knowing how they affect people. They are also essential for confirming diagnoses and responses to treatments. Psychiatric disorders are disorders of brain–mind and mind–brain interactions and accordingly require a model that includes both neurobiological and psychological features. It is questionable whether the "behavioral" and "experiential" components in the fourth aim of the RDoC can fully capture the psychological features of mental disorders. While the identification of more biomarkers and associations between dysfunctional neural circuits and dysfunctional mental states will lead to a better understanding of many aspects of psychiatric disorders, it will not provide a complete explanation of them.

By focusing mainly on dysfunctional neural circuits as the main source of psychiatric disorders, the RDoC does not satisfactorily explain how biological and nonbiological factors, and the interactions between them, influence these circuits. It does not adequately account for how systems other than the central nervous system (CNS), as well as the environment, interact with the CNS in causing neural and mental dysfunction. In its current form, the RDoC may be too limited as a theoretical model to provide a complete understanding of why psychiatric disorders develop, how they progress, and how different treatments might control them. A paradigm that includes the *DSM-5* and the RDoC as complementary components of an explanatory framework for psychiatric disorders will best guide research and clinical practice in psychiatry. This hybrid paradigm may provide a more satisfactory model for explaining the etiology, pathophysiology, and symptomatology of psychiatric disorders than one based on the *DSM* or RDoC alone (Glannon, 2015a). Such a paradigm could fully integrate biological, psychological, and social factors into its classification of mental illness. Due to the multifactorial etiology of psychiatric disorders and the heterogeneity of symptoms, examining them in terms of neural circuits will not replace but supplement and refine other criteria for predicting, diagnosing, and monitoring treatment responses to them.

## Biological psychiatry

Although the psychological properties of the person are at the core of psychiatric diagnosis as reflected in the *DSM*, in many respects the history of psychiatry has been the history of *biological* psychiatry. Many practitioners of psychotherapy and psychoanalysis tend to separate the psyche from brain science. Yet the father of psychoanalysis, Sigmund Freud, attempted to formulate a scientific psychology of the mind in his *Project for a Scientific Psychology* (Freud, 1895). Freud's attempt to link neural mechanisms to psychodynamic concepts was unsuccessful because, at the time, he and other researchers had only limited knowledge of the neurobiological underpinning of the psyche (Northoff, 2011, p. 1). This was an obstacle to Freud's and Kraepelin's aim to trace psychopathology to an organic source in the brain.

Henrik Walter describes three eras, or waves, in the evolution of biological psychiatry and its importance for psychiatric nosology (Walter, 2013; see also Trimble and George, 2010; Kendler and Parnas, 2012, 2017). The first wave of biological psychiatry was in the second half of the nineteenth century. It was characterized "by the ambition to uncover the relation between mind and brain by doing systematic research linking neuropathology and mental disorder and using the experimental method in animals and humans" (Walter 2013, p. 1). Walter cites Wilhelm Griesinger as being particularly influential in establishing the theory that mental disorders were disorders of the brain (2013, p. 1).

The second wave of biological psychiatry began in the second half of the twentieth century. It was driven by the discovery that psychiatric disorders, particularly schizophrenia, had a genetic component, and that genetics and neurotransmitter imbalance were the main components of an explanatory model for these disorders (Walter, 2013, p. 1). Beginning around 1950, this was the era in which antipsychotic and antidepressant medications were introduced into psychiatric treatment. There was significant opposition to this development by the antipsychiatry movement in the 1960s. This movement was driven by Thomas Szasz's declaration that "mental illness is a myth" (1961, p. 1). Szasz and other proponents of this view did much to discredit psychopharmacology and ECT at the time. Indeed, the antipsychiatry movement generated a misperception of ECT that many people continue to hold today. It has also contributed to one aspect of the stigma associated with mental illness and suffering by people affected by it in suggesting that it is an imagined condition. Antipsychiatry promoted the view that people with so-called mental illness were weak-willed and failed to take responsibility for controlling their thoughts and behaviors. Combined with the reported experiences from psychiatric patients, neuroimaging and other neurobiological measures of brain dysfunction have refuted Szasz's unfounded and professionally irresponsible claim and confirmed the reality of mental illness.

The third wave of biological psychiatry began in the last part of the twentieth century, and it continues to evolve in the twenty-first century. A landmark in this phase was Eric Kandel's 1998 paper, "A New Intellectual Framework for Psychiatry" (Kandel, 1998). Kandel argued that psychiatry demanded "a greater knowledge of the structure and functioning of the brain than is currently available in most training programs" (1998, p. 457). He argued that, "the analysis of the interaction between social and biological determinants of behavior, can best be studied by also having a full understanding of the biological components of behavior" (1998, p. 457). Walter mentions progress in the molecular neurosciences and neuroimaging as the key components of this wave (2013, p. 2). Neuroimaging has enabled the development and application of neuromodulating techniques such as DBS. Electrophysiological and imaging techniques can record brain activity and guide and monitor the effects of neurostimulation. The RDoC is a manifestation of this third wave of biological psychiatry. Walter describes the upshot of it as follows: "According to the third wave of biological psychiatry, mental disorders are relatively stable prototypical, dysfunctional patterns of experience and behavior that can be explained by dysfunctional neural systems at different levels" (2013, p. 2). He adds: "As with any understanding of disease in general, the notion of a 'dysfunction' inevitably involves normative judgments of what is regarded as normal, functional, healthy on the one hand, and as abnormal, dysfunctional, pathological on the other hand" (2013, p. 2).

"Normative" does not imply anything about moral judgments associated with disease classification. It does not imply that there is something morally "bad" about mental illness. Rather, it reflects the fact that classifying a mental or neural condition as a disease is the result of an interpretive process. It is the result of psychiatrists reaching consensus on defining normal mental function and what counts as deviation from a standard functional level. Consensus can be difficult to reach in conditions excluded from or added to different versions of the *DSM*, such as disruptive mood dysregulation disorder added to the *DSM-5*. These conditions generate questions about the sense in which they are mental disorders and the extent of functional impairment they cause. Psychiatric disease classification involves more than the empirical process of collecting genetic, epigenetic, and imaging data. It also involves discussion among psychiatrists in assessing this data in light of patients' behavior. There is less disagreement regarding major psychiatric disorders than in mild or moderate disorders. The more severe the disorder is and the greater the functional impairment it causes, the less controversial is a psychiatric diagnosis. Functional impairment in thought and behavior should be the main diagnostic criterion for these disorders.

A more specific respect in which psychiatric nosology can be normative is the interpretation of neuroimaging used to confirm a diagnosis or predict disease progression of and treatment responses to psychiatric disorders. Structural imaging in the form of CT, MRI, or VBM can reveal volume reductions in gray and white matter correlating with certain symptoms. Functional imaging in the form of PET, fMRI, or DTI can reveal dysfunctional connectivity in circuits correlating with other symptoms. Imaging displaying neural circuit dysfunction seems to confirm the hypothesis that psychiatric disorders are neural circuit disorders. Yet there can be differences in how researchers interpret neuroimaging data and how they draw inferences from this data to form and confirm hypotheses about the neurobiological basis of psychopathology. Judgments about the meaning of a single scan of a particular patient or the statistical significance of series of scans of a population of patients may be fraught with considerable uncertainty because of inherent limitations of brain imaging as an accurate measure of brain function. These limitations should make us circumspect in making claims about the relation between the brain and thought and action. Interpreting data from brain imaging and drawing inferences from this data to make judgments about behavior have been especially controversial in forensic psychiatry (Jones, Wagner, Faigman et al., 2013).

The imaging technique that may have the greatest potential for more accurate diagnosis and prediction of responses to treatment for psychiatric disorders is fMRI. This modality has its limitations, however. The blood oxygenation level-dependent (BOLD) signal in this technique measures hemodynamic changes, not changes in neural activity (Roskies, 2013a, 2013b). Blood flow usually lags several seconds behind the neural activity that produces it. It is not a direct measure of this activity. There are also problems with the signal-to-noise ratio in fMRI. This is a measure of how much relevant information (signal) is corrupted by junk information (noise). The ratio is too low in a single scan for it to have neurophysiological value. For this reason, images from fMRI have to be averaged over many brains from many studies to have any statistical significance. In addition, the fMRI signal cannot distinguish between excitatory and inhibitory neural activity. This makes it difficult to know whether brain activity indirectly displayed by scans has an enabling or disabling effect on cognitive, emotional, and volitional capacities at the mental level.

Images from PET or fMRI scans are not "snapshots" of events or processes occurring in the brain. They are described more accurately as scientific constructs than real-time indices of neural activity (Illes and Racine, 2005). There is an inferential distance between images of metabolism and blood flow and what actually occurs at the neural level (Roskies, 2008, 2013a). There is also the issue of task dependency, focusing on local neural activity associated with the performance of a specific cognitive task. This can limit the validity of generalized claims about global neural activity (Bell and Racine, 2009). It is also significant for the RDoC and psychiatry, since mental illness often correlates with brain dysfunction involving not just a localized node of a neural circuit but dysfunction in distributed neural networks. Even if imaging could provide an accurate account of brain activity, there would be an additional inferential distance between this activity and thought and behavior. Although structural and functional neuroimaging may show correlations between neural activity and behavior, correlation is not causation. The absence of a causal connection between the brain and behavior indicates that the former cannot completely account for the latter.

In addition, there are questions about the accuracy of imaging. A recent meta-analysis showed a false-positive rate of up to 70% among researchers interpreting data from fMRI results (Eklund, Nichols, and Knutsson, 2016). The authors point out that spatial autocorrelation in statistical analyses of imaging data can lead investigators to "find" brain activity where it does not exist. The review also reinforces skepticism about the claim that brain function or dysfunction alone can provide a satisfactory explanation of the content of a person's thought and how it influences her behavior. Another review of imaging data is more pertinent to psychiatry. A meta-analysis of fMRI and PET studies to assess the neurobiological basis of cognitive and emotional processing in unipolar depression found inconsistencies across individual experiments investigating aberrant brain activity (Muller, Cieslik, Serbanescu et al., 2017). These problems were attributed to different inclusion and exclusion criteria, differences in experimental design, and different statistical inferences drawn from imaging data. Both meta-analyses illustrate the limitations in identifying a precise neurobiological underpinning of depression and other mental illnesses at earlier and even later disease stages. Some forms of imaging may provide more accurate information than others regarding early changes in the brain as indications of psychopathology. Yet all neuroimaging involves at least some inferential distance between brain activity and imaging data, on the one hand, and brain activity and pathological thought and behavior, on the other. For all of these reasons, neuroimaging remains a largely experimental modality in diagnosing, monitoring treatment responses, and assessing the risk of psychiatric disorders. According to Helen Mayberg, "with some exceptions, neuroimaging is still a research tool, not ready for use in clinical psychiatry" (Mayberg, 2014, p. 31; see also Farah and Gillihan, 2012).

Another significant feature of biological psychiatry is that cultural differences are important but not critical to diagnosing psychiatric disorders. Combining psychiatric and anthropological observations, Arthur Kleinman has pointed out that there is a cultural dimension to some of these disorders. "Certain of these disorders—e.g., depression and anxiety disorders—have particularly high rates in situations of uprooting, refugee status, and forced acculturation" (Kleinman, 1988, p. 2). While most psychiatric disorders begin earlier in life, those mentioned by Kleinman may also occur later in life. When they occur later, cultural influences are one aspect of the role of the social and natural environment in their development. These influences are particularly pertinent to difficulty in adapting to changing environmental circumstances. Culture may also reflect how people report their symptoms. People with depression in Western cultures may report more cognitive and emotional symptoms, while those in Eastern and Middle Eastern cultures may report more somatic symptoms (Kleinman, 1988, Chapter 2). How patients report their symptoms may reflect different cultural narratives of disease. But all psychiatric disorders have the common feature of disordered thought and behavior. Walter writes, "It is now widely acknowledged that cultural differences and social factors play important roles in the expression of symptoms, e.g., in the content of delusions. But it is also clear that for certain prototypical diseases (e.g., schizophrenia, BD, depression, and some anxiety disorders) there are invariant patterns in experience and behavior despite eminent cultural differences" (2013, p. 4).

One controversial hypothesis is that there may be evolutionary reasons for psychiatric disorders, specifically depression. Some psychiatrists and psychologists have claimed that there may be a survival advantage to depression. It may have developed as an adaptive mechanism to alert us to projects or situations in which a desired goal is unattainable. The content of beliefs and emotions associated with depression enables us to withdraw from these situations, modify our goals and expectations, and thereby prevent psychological harm from failure to attain or meet them (Nesse, 2000; Wrosch and Miller, 2009). Mild depressive symptoms could be interpreted in this way. However, many people lack the awareness and insight to recognize these situations before symptoms develop. Once they develop, they can impair the cognitive and emotional capacity to be aware of these situations and take steps to alter or withdraw from them. The idea that depression or other psychiatric disorders provide a survival advantage presupposes that individuals have considerable control over their immediate environment. Yet it is often the experience of losing control over the environment, and the reaction to this experience, that triggers the cascade of neurobiological and psychological events resulting in depression. The adaptive hypothesis may be plausible for mild psychiatric disorders. But the degree of functional impairment in moderately severe and severe disorders makes them maladaptive rather than adaptive (Friedman, 2012).

## Psychiatry, neurology, neuropsychiatry

At the beginning of this chapter, I raised the question of how to categorize psychiatric disorders. A typical response would involve distinguishing between psychiatry and neurology. Many people inside and outside of medicine hold the view that psychiatric disorders are disorders of the mind and neurological disorders are disorders of the brain. The neurobiological thesis that neural functions generate and sustain mental functions has refuted substance dualism about the relation between the brain and the mind. However, it has not refuted a disciplinary dualism about the relation between neurology and psychiatry. According to George Graham, a mental disorder is a disability, incapacity, or impairment of mental faculties that can result in harmful consequences for the subject (2013, pp. 19–44). The "mental" in mental disorders refers to consciousness and intentionality. These two features are awareness of one's self and surroundings and the content of a person's desires, beliefs, emotions, and action plans. This content consists of the actual and possible situations to which these mental states are directed. In mental disorders, there is a disturbance in this content and the phenomenology of these states.

It is unclear whether these features alone distinguish psychiatric disorders from neurological disorders. Epileptic seizures, for example, involve disturbance in consciousness and intentionality. Similar disturbance occurs in hemispatial neglect, where there is reduced awareness of stimuli on one side of space in some patients following a stroke in the right cerebral hemisphere. Regarding the presumed differences between psychiatry and neurology, Graham argues that mental disorders such as schizophrenia and depression have psychological features that distinguish them from proper neurological (brain) disorders such as stroke, Parkinson's disease (PD), and Alzheimer's disease. Neurological disorders are caused by mechanical processes in the brain that are not amenable to psychological treatment (Graham, 2011, pp. 53–70). It is questionable whether a strict distinction between "mental" disorders and "pure brain" disorders is accurate and can be sustained. A comment by Walter appears to support a rejection of such a distinction: "In fact, many proponents of biological psychiatry now accept an interplay of neurobiological and psychological (mental) factors" (2013, p. 7). This might suggest collapsing psychiatric and neurological disorders into a single category of neuropsychiatric disorders.

A position statement by the Berlin School of Mind and Brain clarifies the connection between brain dysfunction and mental dysfunction and the goals of psychiatric research embodied in the RDoC. On the topic of "Brain Disorders and Mental Dysfunction," the statement reads, "Mind and brain are bound to each other in a tight knot—in good, but also in bad times. When there is something wrong with your mind, researchers observe a changed brain; if there is something wrong with your brain, you experience mental symptoms. This existence of this knot is a trivial truth—but to untie the knot is an ongoing experimental and conceptual challenge, a challenge that forces historically distinct disciplines together" (Berlin School of Mind and Brain, 2016). These "distinct disciplines" may be psychiatry and psychology. They may also be psychiatry and neurology. All three of these disciplines are related to radiology, where imaging can display functional and dysfunctional neural circuits. They are also related to functional neurosurgery, which can modulate these circuits when they are dysfunctional.

More importantly, the statement from the Berlin School suggests that neurology and psychiatry may not be conceptually distinct. It has only been in the last century that research and clinical neuroscientists have distinguished them. The evolution of neuroscience in general and biological psychiatry in particular has not contributed to dualist thinking about brain and mind as distinct substances. Yet it has contributed to dualist thinking about the two main disciplines of neuroscience. This mode of thinking is now gradually changing to one in which an increasing number of researchers are advocating a return to a more unified conceptual framework of diseases of the brain. The basic idea is that we cannot explain mental processes apart from neural processes, or neural processes apart from mental processes.

This questions the presumed distinction between psychiatric disorders as disorders of the mind and neurological disorders as disorders of the brain. If brain and mind influence each other, if both major neurological and psychiatric disorders are traceable to dysfunctional neural circuits and neurotransmitters, and if the same or similar symptoms occur in both types of disorders, then there is no compelling reason for maintaining a strict distinction between them. To be sure, there are sound neuroscientific reasons for considering dystonia as a neurological disorder impairing movement. There are also sound neuroscientific reasons for considering major depression as a psychiatric disorder impairing cognition, mood, and motivation. We can characterize these functions as roughly along a spectrum, with motor functions at one end and mental functions at the other. Yet many disorders of the brain and mind involve disturbances in both motor and mental functions. It is in the extensive middle region of this spectrum where motor and mental functions can overlap. At a particular time, neurobiological features and symptoms may indicate either a neurological or a psychiatric disorder. Over an extended period, however, psychomotor as well as cognitive, emotional, or volitional impairment may be present.

The commonalities between neurological and psychiatric disorders in how they disrupt thought and behavior suggest a merging of them into a single category of neuropsychiatric disorders. Biological psychiatry supports this position in the sense that both types of disorder have a common neurobiological underpinning. Despite differences between motor dysfunction and mental dysfunction, and the fact that motor or mental impairment may be the only or main symptom, all of these symptoms are traceable to dysfunctional neural circuits and neurotransmission. Adam Zeman outlines four types of overlap between neurology and psychiatry: "neurological disorder can present with psychological symptoms; psychological [psychiatric] disorder can present with neurological symptoms; neurological disorder can cause a psychological reaction; psychological disorder can cause a neurological reaction" (2014, p. 140). The third and fourth categories refer to reactive symptoms that are secondary to the symptoms of a primary disorder. Only the first two categories are pertinent to the argument for collapsing neurological and psychiatric disorders into one diagnostic category. Still, the overlap between them is considerable.

Some researchers have cited differences in brain imaging data from patients with neurological and psychiatric disorders to uphold the distinction between these two disease types (Crossley, Scott, Ellison-Wright et al., 2015; David and Nicholson, 2015). This may weaken the case for collapsing them into one category. Yet the overlap between them supports the position that, even if a distinction should remain, it should be less strict than it has been in the last 50 or more years. There are three reasons for adopting this position.

First, many disorders occurring along the neuropsychiatric spectrum may have not only motor or mental symptoms but a combination of both. These symptoms may be co-occurrent or appear at different disease stages. For example, the main symptoms of PD with its classification as a movement disorder are traceable to neural degeneration in the basal ganglia. Yet in some cases, cognitive and emotional symptoms may precede motor symptoms. Indeed, up to 36% of patients with PD have some evidence of cognitive impairment at disease onset (Foltynie, Brayne, Robbins et al., 2004). Approximately 40% of these patients develop depression over time (Mollenhauer and Weintraub, 2017). Depression can be a causal risk factor for, or an early prodromal symptom of, PD up to 10 years before diagnosis (Gustafson, Nordstrom, and Nordstrom, 2015). One explanation for the connection between PD and MDD involves altered expression of the p11 protein in both disorders (Mollenhauer and Weintraub, 2017). This may be linked to changes in particular features of neurotransmission. Serotonin dysregulation associated with mood disturbance and impaired cognition can inhibit dopamine release in the striatum and result in motor dysfunction (Gustafson, Nordstrom, and Nordstrom, 2015).

Another explanation for the connection between PD and MDD pertains to neural circuits. Close proximity of motor, associative, and limbic circuits in the basal ganglia suggests that dysregulation in one of these circuits may cause dysregulation in the other two (Castrioto, Llommee, Moro et al., 2014). Approximately 30% of ischemic stroke patients develop depression (Anderson, 2016; Ferro, Caeiro, and Figueira, 2016). Damage to neural tissue from ischemia in prefrontal and limbic regions can disrupt connectivity between them and interfere with cognitive-emotional processing. One could describe depression in these cases as a secondary disorder resulting from the primary event of a cerebrovascular accident. Nevertheless, the long-term neuroanatomical and neurophysiological effects in brain regions mediating cognition and emotion in some stroke patients may be similar to the effects in patients with TRD.

Trauma or psychosocial stress can trigger psychogenic movement disorders (PMDs). This suggests that dysfunctional cognitive-emotional processing may play a causal role in their pathogenesis. Some studies have shown that suggestion in the form of placebos can effectively treat PMDs in many cases (Shamy 2010; Rommelfanger, 2013). Other studies have confirmed the release of endogenous dopamine in the striatum of patients with PD in response to biochemically inert pills and sham surgery (de la Fuente Fernandez and Stoessl, 2002; Lidstone, Schulzer, Sossi et al., 2010; Ko, Feigin, Mattis et al., 2014). These studies indicate that at least some types of neurological (movement) disorders may be amenable to psychological treatment. Catatonia is characterized as a subtype of schizophrenia in the *DSM-IV-TR*. Yet the *DSM-5* and most psychiatrists now categorize it as a type of movement, or psychomotor, disorder (*DSM-5*, p. 119; Castle and Buckley, 2015, p. 9). Avolitional syndrome may appear in both the negative subtype of schizophrenia and a subtype of depression. This syndrome is both a volitional and movement disorder. Insofar as anhedonia impairs the ability to form and execute action plans, it is a disorder of emotional, volitional, and motor capacities. These considerations weaken the view that neurology is a discipline that investigates motor functions, and psychiatry a discipline that investigates mental functions.

Second, there is a link between late-life depression and cognitive decline associated with dementia (Steffans, 2017). What Kraepelin described as *dementia praecox* (Kraepelin, 1896/1913) is comparable to the modern classification of schizophrenia because both disorders have a similar chronic neuropathology (Hafner, 2004). There is, then, a connection between schizophrenia and dementia. Progressive changes in the brain associated with a psychiatric disorder earlier in life may result in reduced brain volume and cognitive decline later in life. Dementia may be the best example of a disorder that is both neurological and psychiatric because it involves motor, cognitive, emotional, and volitional impairments. This goes some way toward explaining the increasing number of geriatric psychiatrists treating patients with Alzheimer's disease and other dementias.

Third, as the preceding paragraph indicates, some neurodevelopmental disorders earlier in life become neurodegenerative disorders later in life. One example is atrophy in the PFC and hippocampus associated with chronic excess levels of stress hormones in depression and anxiety. Moreover, because of its degenerative effects on the brain, some researchers have raised the question of whether schizophrenia should be categorized as a neurodevelopmental or neurodegenerative disorder (Keshavan, Kennedy, and Murray, 2004; Owen, Sawa, and Mortensen, 2016, p. 94). The distinction between psychiatric (neurodevelopmental) and neurological (neurodegenerative) disorders becomes blurred in many cases when one considers the pathogenesis and progression of diseases of the brain and mind, not at one stage of life, but over the course of the person's life as a whole. This is not the case in all neurological or psychiatric disorders, as I have pointed out. But the extent of overlap in motor and mental symptoms, and the common global changes in brain structure and function associated with both disorder types justifies relaxing the distinction between them.

The comment from the Berlin School of Mind and Brain about forcing "historically distinct disciplines together" suggests a return to the era when neurology and psychiatry were conceived of as two dimensions of a unified discipline of neuropsychiatry. Before these disciplines were divided during the middle of the twentieth century, many prominent researchers in the sciences of the mind believed in a unified conception of them. For example, echoing earlier views of Hippocrates (400 BCE/1981) on "the sacred disease" of epilepsy and Sir Thomas Willis (1681) on neuroanatomy, in the nineteenth century Paul Broca claimed that "the great regions of the mind correspond to the great regions of the brain" (1861, p. 55). This was not a reductionist claim. Rather, Broca was acknowledging that brain and mind are inseparable and have complementary roles in mediating motor and mental functions.

In a recent editorial, Michael Fitzgerald writes that "the separation of neurology from psychiatry has led to a separation of the brain from the mind—the physical from the mental—which has been unhelpful for both disciplines" (2015, p. 106). In light of the influence of biological psychiatry, this comment may not be an accurate account of current research and treatment in psychiatry, which is not based entirely on psychological processes. Fitzgerald's comment is more about categorical than substance dualism and directed at an underestimation of the extent of mind–brain interaction in disorders of thought and behavior. Fitzgerald also claims that, if they were considered as "two equal partners, then both disciplines would enrich each other enormously" (2015, p. 106). In addition, he claims, "neurology and psychiatry are simply two 'sides of the same coin.' Certainly in the area of neural plasticity, neurology and psychiatry overlap" (2015, p. 106). This last point is pertinent to my discussion in Chapter 8 of the possibility of infusing growth factors in the brains of people with disorders that may be both neurodevelopmental and neurodegenerative.

Zeman expresses a similar view: "The argument that 'neurology is psychiatry, and vice versa,' doesn't make any assumptions about the nature of matter or mind and, in particular, is not 'mind-denying.' Rather, it insists that to understand and manage disorders of the brain, we need to take into account experience, behavior and physiology at all times, This is a practical message, usefully encapsulated in the concept of biopsychosocial medicine: every disorder—indeed every moment of healthy functioning—has biological, psychological and social dimensions. Doctors ignore any one of these at their peril" (2014, p. 143). Despite the considerable overlap between psychiatric and neurological disorders, and despite a common neurobiological underpinning between them, psychological and social factors generally have a greater role in the etiology of major depression, anxiety, and some other psychiatric disorders than PD and other neurological disorders. The biopsychosocial model is more relevant to psychiatry than to neurology. The differences between them may be of degree rather than kind. Apart from what neuroimaging might show, however, the differences between them are significant.

Psychiatric disorders generally have more deleterious effects on the content and integrity of an affected person's mental states. The disturbed phenomenology of having major depression or schizophrenia is very different from that of PD. With exceptions like PMDs and psychogenic amnesia, psychosocial stress also appears to have a greater causal role in the development of psychiatric disorders than in neurological disorders. Moreover, not only biological but also psychological and environmental factors in these disorders can have disabling effects on free will. The capacity to reason and translate intentions into actions requires not only motor but also cognitive, emotional, and volitional capacities. Some or all of these capacities are impaired to a greater degree in psychiatric disorders. Psychosocial factors can shape the disturbed mental content and impaired mental capacities of these disorders, and thus they cannot be divorced from the contexts in which an affected person lives and acts. The cognitive and emotional aspects of psychiatric disorders are also more significant than the motor aspects of neurological disorders in the disruption of the psychological connectedness and continuity necessary for personal identity. Accordingly, distinguishing between psychiatric and neurological disorders to some degree seems warranted.

Nevertheless, the similarities between neurology and psychiatry have important practical implications for both the ethics of neuroscience and the neuroscience of ethics. Temporally extended clustering of motor and mental symptoms and identification of common neurobiological dysfunction may lead to a better understanding of how motor and mental capacities become impaired. It also helps to monitor how short- and long-term positive and negative effects of interventions to treat mental illness can benefit or harm people who suffer from it. This same sort of clustering can also provide a more informed assessment of a patient's cognitive and emotional capacity to consent to treatment or research. Although PD is associated with motor rather than cognitive dysfunction, a person at a more or even less advanced stage of the disease may not have sufficient cognitive capacity to meet the requirement of consent to undergo DBS. The disease may have affected not only the motor circuit of the basal ganglia but also associative and limbic circuits. A patient's or research subject's capacity for reasoning and decision-making may be impaired in addition to her impaired capacity for movement. The fact that both overt motor symptoms and subtle cognitive symptoms, or vice versa, may be present at the same time or at different times underscores the need to monitor disorders of the brain and mind over longer periods of a person's life. This can allow timely interventions to better control disease progression and reduce the extent of disrupted thought and behavior. What matters for the patient is not whether a disease fits into a specific diagnostic category but how it affects her physical and psychological abilities.

## The brain–mind relation

Structural and functional brain imaging provides the best evidence for the claim that dysfunctional mental states in major psychiatric disorders are associated with dysfunctional neural states. As I pointed out in my discussion of biological psychiatry, however, imaging is limited in this regard. Correlations between brain dysfunction displayed by imaging and mental dysfunction displayed by a person's behavior do not prove that the first directly causes the second. Despite its limitations, by confirming these correlations neuroimaging can elucidate different aspects of the brain–mind relation for psychiatry. Imaging is also critical for psychiatric therapy by indicating which treatments are appropriate and by monitoring responses to them in the brain.

My use of the hyphenated terms "brain–mind" and "mind–brain" does not indicate an identity relation and the idea that the mind is just the brain. This idea fails to account for the interconnected but different ways in which neural and psychological processes maintain or disturb mental health. It also fails to account for what goes awry in these processes in mental illness. The most appropriate conception of this relation for psychiatry is one in which brain and mind are functionally interdependent, mutually influencing systems. This is the "tight knot" mentioned in the Berlin School's policy statement. Neurons, synapses, and neural networks enable an organism to form representations of the body and the environment. The content and intentionality of desires, beliefs, and emotions enable a person to form more accurate representations of the world than what neural networks can provide on their own.

In major psychiatric disorders, there is a disruption of normal integrated information processing in the brain. There is a distorted representation of the world to the organism at an unconscious level. This corresponds to the distorted mental content of an affected person at a conscious level. Ordinarily, internal constraints in the brain ensure that neural circuits are neither overactive nor underactive in their information processing function. The content of mental states provides further constraints by ensuring a more refined representation of the world so that the brain responds appropriately to stimuli. Neural and mental functions balance each other in a series of re-entrant loops. These loops form a process of circular causation that promotes the ability to adapt to the natural and social environment. Both neural and mental functions are crucial for this adaptability. A normally functioning brain and mind enable a person to experience a harmonious relation with the world. A dysfunctional brain and mind can cause a person to experience a disrupted relation to the world. Although brain function and dysfunction generate positive and negative experiences in persons, these experiences are not located in the brain. Also, while the brain constructs a representation of the environment in which the subject has these experiences, the environment is not located in the brain either. Appeal to brain systems alone cannot provide a complete account of how the world influences the person and how the person interacts with the world.

Biological psychiatry in general and the RDoC in particular support a materialist theory of mind that explains mental phenomena in terms of their neural correlates. To some, a materialist theory of mind might suggest that mental diseases are just diseases of the brain (Fuchs, 2012). There are reductive and nonreductive versions of materialism, however (Baker, 2009). According to reductive materialism, phenomena at one level can be completely explained in terms of more basic elements at a different level. On this view, normal and abnormal mental states are nothing more than products of brain function and dysfunction. According to nonreductive materialism, the brain necessarily generates and sustains mental states but cannot account for all of their properties (Northoff, 2014b, pp. 101–102; Baker, 2013, Part II). Mental phenomena are partly but not completely explained in terms of their neural correlates. Brain-level systems are necessary but not sufficient to account for the content of a person's ordered or disordered mental states. This content is influenced not only by the brain but also by the person's bodily systems and the natural and social environment in which the person exists and acts. The person's mental states are both embodied and embedded (Maiese, 2016; Walter, 2013; Northoff, 2015, pp.102–103).

Northoff describes subjects' experience of these internal and external factors as "neurophenomenology" (2015, p. 103). "Unlike in reductive neurophilosophy [reductive materialism], neurophenomenology takes the phenomenal features of experience, like subjectivity, intentionality and the sense of self, seriously, and does not eliminate them by declaring them to be illusory" (p. 103). "Reductive neurophilosophy ultimately eliminates the first-person perspective and its phenomenal features in favor of the third-person perspective and a purely neuronal account" (p. 103). Northoff further claims, "Neurophenomenology can be considered a first step toward the future development of a non-reductive neurophilosophy that includes phenomenal features in a non-reductive way. Moreover, neurophenomenology presupposes a *brain-based* rather than *brain-reductive* stance . . . in its account of the mind" (p. 103, emphasis added). All of this is consistent with a nonreductive materialism whereby mental states emerge from and necessarily depend on neural processes but whose properties cannot be fully accounted for by what occurs in the brain.

Mechanistic explanations of the mind are a modified version of reductive materialism. These explanations identify the physical parts (e.g., systems, cells, and molecules) and processes (e.g., activation, firing, and phosphorylation) that realize organism-level functions (Craver, 2007; Bechtel, 2008). They are an advance over computational theories of the brain–mind relation because they focus on more than just informational input and behavioral output (Teufel and Fletcher, 2016). Yet by focusing only on neural parts and processes, mechanistic explanations provide at best an incomplete account of psychiatric disorders and the experience of people who have them. They are too limited to explain the extent to which biological, psychological, and social factors influence brain function and dysfunction, and the role of these factors in diagnosis, prognosis, and treatment. Mechanistic explanations emphasize bottom-up causation in which lower-level *physical* parts and processes realize higher-level *physical* functions. They fail to capture bidirectional bottom-up and top-down causal connections between physical and *psychological* events in brain–mind and mind–brain interactions. They also fail to capture how bodily systems other than the CNS and how a person responds to the environment can influence the activity of neural circuits and networks and their effects on mental content. Mechanistic models from cognitive psychology and cognitive science fail to include all of the dimensions necessary to understand healthy and diseased brains and the relevance of these interacting dimensions for psychiatric research and practice.

It may appear that the RDoC is moving psychiatry in the direction of reductionist biological psychiatry. This is not an accurate claim, since the RDoC examines how genetics and the environment influence neuroanatomy and neurophysiology. Although it focuses on neural circuits, it does not focus exclusively on them. In this respect, the RDoC is not entirely neurocentric. Nevertheless, the RDoC does not adequately consider the subjective character of experience for people who have psychiatric disorders. This is its main limitation as a paradigm for psychiatry.

Some might appeal to the theory of supervenience to test the ontological claim that mental disorders are brain disorders. According to this theory, there cannot be a change in a property of a system at one level without a corresponding change in a property of that system at a different level. The system at issue is a human organism and the levels are mental (mind) and physical (brain). A change at the mental level "supervenes" on a change at the neural level. Conditions involving the first type of change supervene on conditions involving the second type of change. This involves not only the question of ontological reduction but also explanatory reduction in the sense that mental disorders can be explained entirely in terms of brain dysfunction.

Analyzing diagnostic criteria of certain mental disorders, Charles Olbert and Gary Gala argue that "at least some mental disorders fail to supervene upon brain disorders" and conclude that "at least some mental disorders are not and cannot be (merely) brain disorders" (Olbert and Gala, 2015, p. 203). Some mild or moderate mental disorders might not have detectable neural correlates. Yet in major and especially severe forms of psychiatric disorders, evidence of brain abnormalities corresponding to psychomotor, cognitive, emotional, and volitional impairment confirm that they *are* brain disorders. The limitations of brain imaging and evidence that factors outside of the brain influence neural structure and function do not support a strict distinction between two types of disorder—one mental or psychological, the other physical or neurobiological. Correlations between observable brain abnormalities and the characteristic symptoms of schizophrenia, MDD, BD I, BD II, OCD, and other major disorders are sufficient to establish that they have a neurobiological underpinning. One can make this claim even though psychiatrists and neuroscientists do not know the exact nature of the relations between neural and mental processes.

Although there is variability in the imaging data between psychiatric patients, structural neuroimaging studies of patients with major depression have indicated volume changes in the amygdala, hippocampus, anterior cingulate, and ventromedial and prefrontal cortices (Mayberg, 2009). Functional neuroimaging of patients with this same disorder has indicated abnormalities in resting-state blood flow and glucose metabolism and disrupted connectivity between frontal, limbic/paralimbic, and subcortical regions (Mayberg, 2009; Northoff, 2014a, pp. 391 ff.). While major psychiatric disorders are brain disorders, the causal role of processes outside of the brain in their development and persistence indicates that they are *not solely* brain disorders. This qualified claim about mental disorders being brain disorders avoids ontological and explanatory reductionism in psychiatry. While this claim is compatible with Olbert and Gala's use of "merely" in the passage cited in the preceding paragraph, it also supports the position that there is a neural basis of all major psychiatric disorders.

A more problematic feature of using supervenience to explain psychiatric disorders is that it typically refers to local changes in properties of different levels of a system. Olbert and Gala take "supervenience" to "refer to a relationship of mental disorders to local brain disorders rather than the global physical state of the world" (2015, p. 207). "Global" can also apply to the brain. Indeed, "global" more accurately captures the scope of neural and mental dysfunction than "local." Most psychiatric disorders involve dysfunctional connectivity between neural networks impairing not one but many mental capacities. The dysfunction tends to be distributed across different brain regions rather than circumscribed to a single region. As Walter notes, "in brain science, the paradigm of locationist thinking is substituted increasingly by thinking in functional systems and brain connectivity patterns" (Walter, 2013, p. 2; see also Buckholtz and Meyer-Lindenberg, 2012).

Psychiatric disorders are multifactorial disorders resulting from different types of adverse interactions between genes, neurons, immune and endocrine systems, and the person's responses to the environment. Major psychiatric disorders involve disturbed homeostasis. This refers to the innate capacity of the organism to regulate and maintain equilibrium among its internal systems (Cannon, 1932; Fuster, 2013, p. 19, note 17). This equilibrium enables the organism to adapt to and survive in the environment by counteracting any threatening influences on it. Homeostasis requires bidirectional communication between central nervous, immune, and endocrine systems in balancing the demands of the internal and external milieu (Cacioppo and Berntson, 2011). The fight-or-flight (or freeze) response is an example of the body's reaction to threats to the organism. A disturbance in one of these systems can result in disturbances in other systems, disrupting normal brain–mind interaction and in some cases resulting in major psychiatric disorders. For example, a hyperactive response from microglia to infection can cause inflammation in the brain that can adversely affect brain development. This is one hypothesis for the genesis of schizophrenia emerging in adolescence or early adulthood. A chronic heightened fear response to stimuli can cause dysregulation in the HPA axis. This can result in dysfunctional connectivity between prefrontal and limbic regions and impaired cognition, emotion, sleep, and other disturbances characteristic of depression and anxiety. The mind can play a critical role in this second situation in the sense that the person's perception of stimuli as threatening is one of the triggers in this cascade of adverse neurophysiological events.

Explaining psychiatric disorders at a brain-systems level and in terms of neuroimmune and neuroendocrine interaction is necessary but not sufficient for understanding their etiology and progression. Although dysfunctional neural circuits and neurotransmitters underlie these disorders, it is not brains but people who have them. Persons are constituted by their brains and bodies, but they are not identical to them (Johnston, 1992; Baker, 2000; Bennett and Hacker, 2003, pp. 68–107, 355–377). The conscious and unconscious mental states that emerge from the brain and define persons are influenced by a dynamic and interacting set of factors both inside and outside of the brain. Our brains alone do not determine everything about who we are and how we experience the world (cf. Churchland, 2013). These considerations suggest that nonreductive materialism is a more plausible theory than reductive materialism for explaining the mind–brain relation in psychiatry and a more helpful theoretical model for diagnosing and treating psychiatric disorders.

Todd Feinberg's conception of the mind as a process that emerges from the brain in a nested hierarchy of neural and mental events supports nonreductive materialism (Feinberg, 2001, pp. 129–131, 2009). Higher-level processes associated with conscious and unconscious mental states are compositionally dependent on, or nested within, lower-level processes associated with neural circuits. There is bidirectional interaction between these processes. Feinberg's related concept of constraint can explain how interacting neural and mental processes promote homeostasis within an organism and its adaptability to the external world. Constraint refers to the control that one level of a system exerts over a different level of the same system. The system at issue is a human organism, and the relevant levels are brain and mind, or neural and mental events and processes. Constraint operates in both bottom-up and top-down directions as neural and mental processes mutually influence each other. Neural functions constrain mental functions to ensure that a person accurately perceives and interprets information from the environment. Mental functions constrain neural functions to ensure that they are neither overactive nor underactive. Beliefs or emotions with heightened emotional content can over-activate the limbic fear system, disable prefrontal cortical constraint on this system, and lead to depression, anxiety, or panic disorders. Disabled constraints on the content of auditory or visual perceptions and beliefs from dysfunctional frontal–temporal–parietal connectivity can result in the hallucinations and delusions found in the positive subtype of schizophrenia.

Proponents of nonreductive materialism hold that mental properties are part of the material world. They also hold that mental events can be causally efficacious without being reducible to material events (Baker, 2009). Critics of this position argue that if mental events are not reducible to physical or material events, then they are epiphenomenal (Kim, 1998, 2010, Chapter 7). Mental events are the effects of material causes but cannot cause any material (physical) events. If mental states and events are not reducible to their neural correlates and are epiphenomenal, then presumably they have no causal influence in the development of psychiatric disorders. Nor do mental states and events have any causal influence in patients' responses to therapies.

There are many examples in psychiatry, and some in neurology, where mental states and events can disrupt or modulate neural function. Trauma or chronic psychosocial stress can disrupt prefrontal–limbic connections mediating cognitive-emotional processing and result in major depression and generalized anxiety. These same processes can result in PMDs. In OCD, excessive conscious reflection on motor tasks ordinarily performed as a matter of course may have disruptive effects on frontal–limbic–striatal pathways and impair psychomotor, cognitive, and affective functions.

Mental states and events can be part of a therapeutic process as well. In cognitive behavioral therapy (CBT), patients with anxiety, depression, or OCD can be trained to reframe and alter the content of their beliefs in a way that can rewire prefrontal–limbic pathways mediating some aspects of thought and behavior. Studies have shown that CBT can modulate function in these pathways and result in significant improvement of symptoms (Goldapple, Segal, Garson et al., 2004; Beauregard, 2007). In a study testing NFB, psychological responses to brain activity displayed by electroencephalography (EEG) and fMRI improved mood and motivation in some subjects with depression (Linden, Habes, Johnston et al., 2012). Commenting on this effect of mind–brain interaction, the study's lead author, David Linden, writes that NFB involves "a holistic approach that overcomes bio-psychological dualisms" (Linden, Habes, Johnston et al., 2012, p. 9). In these cases, bottom-up adverse effects of neural dysfunction on the mind can be controlled or reversed to some degree by top-down mental modulating effects on the brain.

## The psychiatric self

David Hume claimed that, while we have sensory impressions, there is no idea of a persisting self that has these impressions. This is his "bundle" theory, an ontological thesis according to which a person just consists of a collection of properties or relations. In Hume's own words: "There is no impression, constant and variable. Pain and pleasure, grief and joy, passions and sensations succeed each other and never all exist at the same time. It cannot, therefore, be from any of these impressions, or form any other, that the idea of a self is derived, and consequently there is no such idea" (1888/1978, Book 1, Part IV, Sec. VI).

Some contemporary philosophers have adopted Hume's position and argued that there is no persisting substance identifiable as a "self" (Parfit, 1984, Part III; Metzinger, 2003). If this is true, then there may be no basis for the view held by many psychiatrists and philosophers that disruption of the self and its relation to the world is a core feature of psychiatric disorders. If there is no real self, then there is no entity whose integrity could be threatened by schizophrenia, major depression, or other forms of mental illness. The presumed relation between an entity and the world cannot be disrupted if there is no such entity. Michelle Maiese makes a case for the ontological status of the self: "The sense of self is not merely a useful fiction or illusion, nor is it an accidental or extrinsic feature of our conscious lives. Instead, the sense of self is a necessary structural component of consciousness among living creatures like us, one which is bound up with our active endeavors to stay alive as we interact with our surroundings" (2016, p. 51; see also Zahavi, 2003; Sadler, 2004; Gillett, 2009; Browne, 2018, pp. 5–19). One of the main features of psychiatric disorders is a disturbance of the integrity of the self and its connection to others and the world.

Philosophers arguing against the idea of a persisting self tend to ignore the influence of unconscious neural, mental, and bodily processes on conscious experience. There are conscious and nonconscious dimensions to the self (Damasio, 2010, Part III). Properties that emerge at the mental level are the product of a holistic system involving interactions between the brain, body, and the external world. The influence of these three dimensions on the mind is not intermittent but constant. Psychiatric disorders involve a disruption of the unity and integrity of psychological properties because of dysfunctional neural processes that ordinarily generate and sustain these properties. The potential for disruption of conscious experience in people at risk of developing a disorder from genetic mutations, psychosocial stress, or other factors is always present. This is the case even during periods when this potential is not actualized. A person may be susceptible to mental illness when she is asymptomatic or presymptomatic, as well as through relapsing and remitting periods if she has a disorder. There is a self that persists through these changes. A person with a psychiatric disorder or who is at risk of having one is an enduring subject constantly experiencing, or susceptible to experiencing, psychomotor, cognitive, emotional, and volitional impairment. This self is present in both mental health and mental illness, depending on interaction among factors inside and outside of the brain. The idea that psychiatric disorders divide the conscious self and disrupt the feeling of being connected to the world, as well as how interventions can restore the integrity of the self, presupposes a dynamic substrate that includes biological, psychological, and environmental processes.

Neuroendocrine and neuroimmune interactions form an organism's external and internal surveillance system necessary for homeostasis. Ordinarily, interactions between central nervous, immune, and endocrine systems influence the content of a person's mental states to enable him to respond appropriately to the environment. Yet a maladaptive response to the internal or external milieu can cause chronic neuroendocrine and neuroimmune miscommunication and disturbances in cognitive and emotional aspects of the conscious self. The dysfunctional neural and bodily processes resulting in these disturbances may be present before symptoms appear. They are present during the prodromal phase of illness and later if the illness becomes full-blown.

Immunologists often discuss the concept of an "immune self" (Clark, 2008). This refers to the combined action of the innate and adaptive arms of the immune system in responding to pathogens that pose a threat to the organism. The system attacks what it identifies as "not-self" to protect what it identifies as "self." Particularly important in this process is the capacity of the adaptive arm to develop an immunologic memory of antigens (Clark, 2008, pp. 29 ff.; Talbot, Foster, and Woolf, 2016, p. 421). Antigenic memory enables the system to recognize and kill microbes through the combined action of antibodies, complement, and macrophages. Sebastien Talbot, Simmie Foster, and Clifford Woolf explain how the immune and nervous systems combine to form "a holistic, coordinated defense system" (2016, p. 421). This allows "living organisms to identify and react to environmental danger" that would threaten homeostasis and the survival of the organism. They note that "neuroimmune interactions occur in many situations, including in response to injury, infection, or autoimmune-mediated damage of neurons themselves, and the microglial-related pathology" (2016, p. 422). The environment may be internal or external to the body. An overactive immune response to a pathogen can damage neural tissue and cause dysfunction in neural circuits mediating cognition, emotion, and volition. Cytokines and microglia are two critical components of the immune system's protective role for the organism. Hyperactive responses and inflammation from these proteins and cells have been implicated in major depression and schizophrenia.

Cytokines released in response to infection can be psychoactive and contribute to or exacerbate depressive symptoms. An immune memory of the pathogen can trigger cytokine release each time the pathogen enters the organism and cause repeated release of inflammatory cytokines. Even a person whose depression is under control may still be susceptible to relapse and a return of symptoms because of the potential of these proteins to cause neural and mental dysfunction (Miller and Raison, 2016). These processes may predispose a person to anxiety in addition to depression. The correlation a patient may draw between influenza and a possible relapse of depression from recalling a flu-induced depressive episode can cause fearful anticipation and avoidance of activities during the flu season. This is an example of the "freeze" response I added to the "fight-or-flight" response symptomatic of anxiety and panic disorders. Immune functions and their interaction with the brain can influence thought and behavior in adaptive or maladaptive ways.

Microglia are the immune system's guardians against infection and tissue damage in the brain. Under normal circumstances, these cells ensure neural integrity by protecting the brain from pathogenic threats. Yet a hyperactive microglial response to a pathogen can result in an adverse inflammatory neural environment that can disrupt this integrity and result in neural and mental dysfunction. Like cytokines, microglia are components of the immune system's surveillance system promoting the survival of the organism (Talbot, Foster, and Woolf, 2016). This surveillance is always active. Like endocrine processes, immune processes contribute to homeostasis and adaptability when they are neither hyperactive nor hypoactive. When they lose this balance, immune processes can disrupt neural and mental processes and result in psychopathology.

The psychiatric self is a continuous and unified set of biological and psychological processes interacting at unconscious and conscious levels. These processes, and environmental influences on them, operate throughout the lifetime of the person. They affect whether a person's thought and behavior is adaptive or maladaptive and whether she experiences mental health or mental illness. In major psychiatric disorders, dysfunction in these processes results in a disordered self.

Some phenomenologists describe the self as "embodied, embedded and enacted" (Walter, 2013, p. 3). A disordered or divided self in psychiatric disorders results from disturbances in one or more of these three dimensions. Embodiment figures prominently in many phenomenological accounts and the philosophy of mind in general (Rowlands, 2010). Citing the work of Gallagher (2005) and Kiverstein and Clark (2009) on how the body shapes the mind, Maiese argues that human consciousness and cognition are *essentially* embodied (2016, pp. 2, 8). To say that cognition is essentially embodied is to say that there is a "unique, non-trivial and cognitively limiting role for the body in the determination of mental states" (Kiverstein and Clark, 2009, p. 2). The body's role in cognition depends on proprioceptive and somatosensory processing in the brain and its relation to the body. Still, the phenomenological model does not adequately explain what goes wrong at the neural level when one's experience as an embodied self becomes a psychopathology. This experience is traceable to dysregulated neural mechanisms mediating body perception.

AN is a case in point. This involves a pathologically distorted perception of the body resulting in a life-threatening eating disorder. People affected by this psychiatric disorder would not deny that they are essentially embodied. Rather, the psychopathology is associated with an abnormal perception of *how* they are embodied. AN may be included in a class of disorders that Feinberg describes as "neuropathologies of the self" (2011). These are "a continuum of disorders of self and identity that occur in the presence of identifiable brain pathology" (Feinberg, 2011, p. 75). A greater degree of brain pathology corresponds to a greater degree of psychopathology. Brain imaging may help to elucidate how disrupted somatosensory and proprioceptive processing correlates with the experience of disturbed embodiment. This experience is linked to dysfunctional connectivity between primary somatosensory and frontoparietal areas of the brain. These areas are involved in processing proprioceptive and interoceptive bodily information underlying own-body representations (Blanke, 2012; Bauer, Diaz, Concha et al., 2014). Alina Coman and coauthors provide a more specific description of brain dysfunction in AN: "At present, the aetiology and pathophysiology of AN are not completely known, yet genetic and neuroimaging studies are revealing greater insight into the underlying neural correlates which might be involved in the aetiology of AN. To date, neuroimaging, especially fMRI studies, suggest alteration on the dorsolateral prefrontal cortex area (DLPFC), insula, parietal and anterior cingulate cortex, all of which are areas involved in emotional processing, processing of reward and body perception" (Coman, Skarderud, Reas et al., 2014, p. 1). In addition, VBM imaging studies have shown reduced brain structure in reward and somatosensory regions of people affected by AN (Titova, Hjorth, Schioth et al., 2013).

Northoff identifies neural dysfunction underlying schizophrenia and depression and explains why this dysfunction is critical for understanding the psychopathology of these and other major psychiatric disorders. His account underscores the shortcomings of phenomenological and cognitive science models for psychiatry in failing to provide a satisfactory account of what goes wrong in the brains of people with the psychomotor, cognitive, emotional, and volitional impairment characteristic of these disorders. Northoff raises two key questions regarding the self in psychiatry: "How do psychiatric patients experience their own selves, and how is the subjective self altered in their experience of contents originating either in themselves (as thoughts) or in the environment (as mental imagery and perceptions)?" (2015, p. 87). He responds to these questions by spelling out what he calls a "neurophenomenal approach," which "aims to link the phenomenology of psychopathology with underlying neural processes" (2015, p. 86). This "approach aims to directly link those phenomenal features of our consciousness and its experiencing self to the neural mechanisms of our brain" (2015, p. 87). Northoff focuses on abnormalities in resting-state activity of the brain's midline region as the main source of the disordered self. He draws from studies showing "that a subcortical-cortical-paralimbic network is central in mediating self and consciousness" (2015, p. 95). Dysfunction in this network disrupts the psychological content and continuity of the conscious self.

Northoff points out that, in depression, there is "increased self- and body focus, and decreased environment focus" (2014a, p. 405, 2015, p. 83) corresponding to disturbances in cognition, mood, and volition. In schizophrenia, delusions, hallucinations, and other cognitive symptoms are products of "abnormality in self-specificity" (Northoff, 2015, p. 106). There is resting-state hyperactivity in the anterior midline network in depression (2015, p. 99). There is resting-state hyperactivity in anterior and posterior sections of this network in schizophrenia (2015, p. 105). In both disorders, the brain is impaired in its capacity to filter, process, and encode information from environmental stimuli as well as from the body (2015, p. 106). At the level of the conscious mind, this impairment results in abnormalities in the experience of self (2014a, p. 392).

He distinguishes his *neurophenomenal* approach from *neurocognitive* and *neurophenomenological* approaches to the disordered self in depression and schizophrenia (Northoff, 2015, pp. 86–88, 2014b, pp. 102–103). Neurocognitive models are unsatisfactory in explaining these disorders because, by focusing on how psychological dysfunction mediates the link between neural and phenomenal features of the self, they fail to appreciate the extent to which neural dysfunction can directly affect these features. This criticism can be applied more generally to cognitive science models for psychiatry. By focusing on simulation and computation, these models do not provide an adequate account of how neural circuit and neurotransmitter dysfunction results in mental dysfunction and the person's experience of it. Neurophenomenological models are also unsatisfactory because they focus on the experience of a disordered self without considering the neural mechanisms underlying its development. Each of these approaches fails to adequately explain what goes wrong at the brain-systems level in psychiatric disorders. Consistent with nonreductive materialism, what it is like to experience an ordered or disordered self is not reducible to neural function or dysfunction. Yet it cannot be explained independently of neural function or dysfunction either (Feinberg, 2009).

Northoff concludes his analysis as follows: "For clinicians, the neurophenomenal approach will make possible the detection of direct causal linkages between neuronal and phenomenal features of psychiatric symptoms" (2015, p. 109). He acknowledges that, "the exact neural mechanisms underlying the self in general and its abnormal changes in psychiatric disorders remain unclear." Yet he also says that, "future investigations will reveal the neural mechanisms underlying psychopathological experience and may then yield diagnostic and therapeutic markers that allow for new modes of diagnostic assessment and intervention" (2015, p. 108). If psychiatric research could yield a better understanding of why neural mechanisms are dysfunctional in psychiatric disorders and how to modulate them, then this could reduce the incidence of treatment-resistance among major psychiatric disorders and ameliorate disabling symptoms. Ideally, this understanding could lead to interventions that could prevent them. In the remaining chapters, I discuss how abnormalities in neural circuits and networks, in addition to those in the resting-state of the midline region, can result in psychiatric disorders. I also discuss how different interventions in these circuits and networks might restore normal brain and mental functions.

Combined with motor and mental impairment, disturbances in the experience of the conscious self are the primary burden of mental illness.

People who experience disruption in the continuity of their mental states and a distortion of mental content during and after the onset of symptoms will not identify with these changes. They will reject them as alien to their identities and welcome symptom relief and a return to their premorbid selves. There may be exceptions to this attitude, however. In some cases, hypomanic or manic states of BD may provide a creative advantage to people who would not have it otherwise. At the same time, these states and the more frequent and more disabling depressed periods can result in significant functional impairment, self-harm, and harm to others (Strakowski, 2014, p. 7). On balance, the negative effects of these states on different dimensions of a person's life seem to outweigh any positive effects of painting, writing fiction or poetry, or any other creative endeavor. Even if it enables creativity, the personal costs of mania or hypomania seem too high.

The twentieth-century poet Robert Lowell is one example of someone whose creativity may be attributed at least in part to BD. While he may have identified with the mania-influenced poetry, he most likely did not identify with the mania-influenced mental suffering. Which pattern of thought and behavior defined his real self? Did his true self disappear with the onset of his mental illness? Was the mania that influenced his poetry a different dimension of his true self that was unrealized before his illness and realized after its onset? There may not be straightforward answers to these questions in this or other cases of the same type.

In a review of Kay Redfield Jamison's book, *Robert Lowell, Setting the River on Fire* (2017), Jed Myers raises an intriguing question: "If poem creation, or any artistic fervor fueled by manic escalation, is a kind of medicine itself (however weak it proves as the tidal wave builds and breaks), shouldn't we, physicians and society, be working with rather than against these creative thrusts?" (2017, p. 989). Noting how drugs such as lithium can dampen these thrusts, Myers further writes, "I wonder also if some clinicians, some of the time, could find ways to work closely enough with their patients with bipolar disorder to give their creative advantages some play. Can collaborative titration of medications allow some poems to be written that otherwise would not be?" (2017, p. 989). Perhaps the right dose of lithium or a different drug could allow this "play" without also unleashing irrational, self-destructive behavior. Yet controlling manic or hypomanic states in this way would require a high level of precision medicine in psychopharmacology, a high-maintenance doctor–patient relationship, and a better understanding of the connections between the patient's brain, mind, and behavior. It may be possible to achieve a controlled state of hypomania in striking a balance between moderate creativity and moderate psychopathology. This may require novel drugs with mechanisms of action different from those of existing drugs for BD. However, any treatment plan enabling the expression of creative potential would have to ensure that the patient retained functional independence in other dimensions of his life. Only in this way would the benefit of such an approach outweigh any harm.

## Conclusion

Psychiatric disorders are disorders of the brain and mind associated with dysfunctional neural circuits and neurotransmitters and dysfunctional psychomotor, cognitive, emotional, and volitional processing. They are also disorders of a person's interaction with other persons and the world (Gillett, 2009; Fuchs, 2012). People with healthy brains and minds display flexible thought and behavior in meeting the demands of and adapting to the environment. Diseases of the brain and mind cause those affected by them to lose or become impaired in this capacity. Brain–mind interaction consists in a circular causal process of bottom-up and top-down re-entrant loops operating at both neural and mental levels. Nonreductive materialism best explains this interaction and the idea that neural and mental processes are interdependent and mutually influence each other. These processes are shaped by how genes are expressed in the brain, how epigenetic mechanisms influence this expression, how the CNS interacts with immune and endocrine systems, and how the person responds to the natural and social environment. Ordinarily, all of these factors interact in a balanced way to maintain homeostasis in the organism. In psychiatric disorders, there is disruption in equilibrium between the internal and external milieu, between the central nervous and other bodily systems, and between the person and the environment. This results in the dysfunctional thought and behavior of schizophrenia, major depression, BD, OCD, and other psychopathologies.

The psychiatric self is a continuous and unified set of biological and psychological processes interacting at unconscious and conscious levels. People affected by psychiatric disorders experience the effects of dysfunction in these processes and have disordered selves. There is significant overlap between psychiatric and neurological disorders. But there are unique subjective features and a broader range of mental and motor dysfunction in schizophrenia, major depression and other forms of mental illness that distinguish them from PD and other movement disorders. The characteristic features of psychiatric disorders are more germane to philosophical questions about free will, personal identity, and the respects in which people can be harmed than the features of neurological disorders.

The *DSM* alone is inadequate to explain major psychiatric disorders because it focuses on symptoms without accounting for the neural circuit and neurotransmitter dysfunction underlying symptoms. Nor does it account for the causes of these disorders. The RDoC alone is also inadequate because it pays too little attention to the psychology of the people affected by these disorders and factors outside of the brain that influence this psychology. Combining the *DSM* and RDoC as complementary components of a model including biological, psychological, and social factors can provide a more satisfactory account of the etiology, pathophysiology, and symptomatology of psychiatric disorders. This paradigm can serve as a foundation for psychiatry research and potentially result in safer and more effective interventions to treat or prevent mental illness.

Brain–mind interaction provides the neurobiological and psychological underpinning of consciousness and memory and their role in agency. Neurobiological and psychological dysfunction can disrupt information processing in the brain. It can impair the capacity for normal recall of experiences and the capacity to choose and act freely. While in general terms major psychiatric disorders are disorders of the brain–mind relation, in specific terms they are disorders of consciousness, memory, and the will. This is the focus of Chapter 2.

# Chapter 2

# Disorders of consciousness, memory, and will

Psychiatric disorders involve different types and degrees of neural dysfunction resulting in impaired thought and behavior. They can distort the content of a person's desires, beliefs, and emotions. This distortion can interfere with the capacity to translate these mental states into actions. The neural dysfunction in these disorders causes disruption in the brain's ability to process information internally from the body and externally from the world. Because consciousness consists in the integration of information in the brain and mind, and psychiatric disorders involve disruption of this information, they can be described as disorders of consciousness. The hallucinations and delusions of persons with the positive subtype of schizophrenia is one example of this disruption and the distorted content of their beliefs. What Northoff describes as "increased self-and body-focus" and "decreased environment-focus" in depression and "abnormality in self-specificity" (2014, p. 391, 2015, pp. 93, 106) in schizophrenia are manifestations of dysfunctional information processing in the brain. Some of this information is in the form of memories. A disturbing or traumatic experience can trigger the formation and retention of an emotionally charged memory of the experience that results in maladaptive behavior. Pathological fear memories in anxiety, panic, and PTSD are disorders of the emotional memory system. The emotionally charged content of these memories can disrupt the processing of information about the world. The representation of the memory in the brain distorts one's perception of current and future events as threats to one's self. This can disable the capacity to form and execute action plans.

The will is a complex set of psychomotor, cognitive, emotional, and volitional capacities. The will is free when a person is able to exercise these capacities in acting or refraining from acting. Cognitive-emotional capacity is necessary to recognize and respond to reasons for and against certain actions, deliberate, and form plans, or intentions, to act. Volitional capacity is necessary to translate plans into actions. Motor capacity is necessary to perform voluntary bodily movements corresponding to the actions. The ability to form and execute different action plans is an indication of flexible behavior in adapting to the demands of the environment. Agency and the motor and mental capacities that enable it are mediated by interconnected neural networks that include, but are not limited to, cortical (PFC), limbic (anterior cingulate cortex), and subcortical (striatum and cerebellum) regions. Major psychiatric disorders can impair some or all of these capacities and thereby impair the capacity for flexible and adaptive behavior. This impairment comes in degrees, depending on the severity of the disorder and the extent to which it disables the relevant motor and mental capacities.

All major psychiatric disorders are disorders of consciousness and will because they all involve disruption of the information processing necessary for awareness of one's self and autonomous agency. More precisely, because the capacity to process information is necessary to deliberate and choose between different courses of action, at a mental-systems level, psychiatric disorders are *primarily* disorders of consciousness and *secondarily* disorders of will. This corresponds to describing them at a brain-systems level as disorders of neural circuits and neurotransmitters.

In this chapter, I explain the respects in which psychiatric disorders interfere with the capacity to perceive the world accurately and respond to it appropriately in forming and executing action plans. My analysis and discussion of these disorders as disturbances in neural and mental processing shows how psychiatry can elucidate philosophical questions about consciousness, agency, and free will. Explaining schizophrenia, major depression, OCD, and disorders of the fear memory system in these terms can give us a clearer sense of how the normal brain enables and how the abnormal brain disables thought and behavior. The unwell brain can give us clues to the healthy (and unhealthy) mind.

## Disorders of consciousness

Three main theories have been proposed to explain the mechanisms of the neural correlates of conscious mental states. Neural synchronization theory claims that consciousness arises from the synchronization of dynamic and fluctuating rhythms of neural activity in different regions of the brain. This synchronization of large assemblies of neurons occurs against a background of electrical oscillations that are active across neural networks (Crick and Koch, 2003). The global neuronal workspace theory says that consciousness arises from neural activity distributed across the entire brain. A key component of this theory is the prefrontal–parietal network and how it responds to stimuli inside and outside the brain (Dehaene and Changeux, 2011). The information integration theory says that consciousness is generated and sustained by integrated information in thalamocortical and corticocortical networks. As the degree of integrated information in these networks increases, consciousness emerges. As the degree of integrated information decreases, consciousness fades (Tononi and Koch, 2008).

What these three theories have in common is the idea that consciousness is a graded property. The neural correlates of consciousness are neither fully on nor fully off but maintain a resting potential prior to their inhibitory or excitatory action. As an emergent property, neither consciousness nor the information in terms of which neuroscientists define it is identical to neural circuits and networks. All three neuroscientific theories of consciousness overlap in relevant respects and together provide a framework for understanding psychiatric disorders as disorders of consciousness. They are all consistent with accounts of dysfunctional neural connectivity as the immediate cause of motor and mental symptoms in psychiatric disorders. Dysfunctional neural circuits can transform the brain's resting potential into processes that are excessively inhibitory or excitatory, causing dysregulation in the neural mechanisms that mediate movement, cognition, emotion, and motivation. They adversely affect not only one's experience but also how one acts in response to this experience.

Ned Block divides consciousness into "phenomenal consciousness" and "access consciousness" (1995, p. 227, 2007). He defines the first as "experience," and says, "The phenomenally conscious aspect of a state is what it is like to be in that state" (1995, p. 227). Access consciousness consists in information processing and its "availability for use in reasoning and rationally guiding speech and action" (1995, p. 227). In severe mental illness, phenomenal consciousness and access consciousness may both be dysfunctional to varying degrees. The disordered content of experience can result in disordered behavioral responses to it. This can impair the capacity for effective agency because it distorts one's perception of the world and one's relation to it. Because consciousness arises from the activity of distributed neural networks rather than particular nodes within neural circuits, disorders of consciousness are "global" rather than "local" and require attention to dysfunction that extends across these networks (Bayne and Hohwy, 2014). They may include corticolimbic, corticothalamic, corticostriatal, and corticocortical connections and thus multiple neural pathways.

The neuroethics literature on disorders of consciousness has focused almost exclusively on post-coma chronic disorders. These include the vegetative state (VS), or unresponsive wakeful state, and the minimally conscious state (MCS) (Giacino, Ashwal, Childs et al., 2002; Fins, 2005, 2015; Owen, Coleman, Boly et al., 2006; Owen, 2008; Bernat, 2010; Laureys, Celesia, Cohadon, et al. 2010). Patients in the VS have sleep–wake cycles but no awareness of self or surroundings. Patients in the MCS have intermittent periods and incomplete levels of awareness. The ethical questions surrounding these states generally concentrate on whether life-sustaining interventions such as artificial nutrition and hydration should continue or end, and which pharmacological or neuro-surgical interventions might promote functional recovery.

This literature ignores other disorders of consciousness, such as hemispatial neglect following stroke, encephalopathy, delirium, epilepsy, and dementia. These neurological disorders affect many more people than the VS and MCS. In particular, epilepsy is more significant for the connection between phenom-enal and access consciousness and the motor and cognitive components of agency than chronic post-coma conditions. In the MCS, patients have persist-ent severely limited cognitive and motor functions. One of the key questions regarding agency is whether they have enough of these functions to perform the mental act of communicating wishes about treatment. In contrast, epileptic seizures involve a sudden and drastic change from complete awareness to a temporary state of complete loss of awareness. The loss of both phenomenal and access consciousness results in a complete loss of behavior control. The sudden shift from a conscious to an unconscious state involves a more complex set of ethical, legal, and social issues than the chronic condition of unrespon-sive or minimally conscious patients. For example, motor vehicle registries may not issue or revoke a driver's license to a person with epilepsy because of the risk of harm from a grand mal or petit mal seizure while operating a vehicle to the driver, pedestrians, and other drivers. This has to be weighed against the right of people affected by this disorder not to be discriminated against and have their activities limited because of a medical condition. Epilepsy also involves questions about responsibility for consequences of involuntary actions occurring during seizures. Despite the loss of control, a person may be respon-sible for a consequence of the action based on the capacity to foresee the prob-ability of this loss while fully conscious at an earlier time.

The neuroethics literature also ignores the fact that psychiatric disorders are disorders of consciousness. Northoff has explained that, as disorders of resting-state midline activity in the brain, schizophrenia and major de-pression are "disorders of the *organization* or *form* of consciousness" (2014, p. 393, emphasis added). They are distinct from disorders of the *level, degree,* or *state* of consciousness, as in the VS and MCS. The differences between these two types of disorders reflect differences in how dysfunction in neural circuitry and neurotransmission disrupt normal integration of information in the brain. Disturbances in the organization of this information and corre-sponding disturbances in thought and behavior affect many more people than the number affected by disturbances in the level of this information. Given the magnitude of this burden and limited health resources, research into the underlying mechanisms of psychiatric disorders of consciousness and development of more effective therapies for them in principle should have priority over research into the mechanisms of and possible therapies for post-coma disorders of consciousness.

Other questions about distributive justice generated by the first type of disorders also deserve more attention than those generated by the second. These include fairness in opportunities for participation in research, protection of research subjects, and availability of and access to treatment. Response rates to psychotropic drugs or other interventions for patients with major psychiatric disorders are often less than optimal. Yet they are much higher than response rates to interventions for patients in the MCS. To be sure, the number of minimally conscious patients is much lower than the number of psychiatric patients. Yet the fact that the number of people in the second group is much greater than the number of people in the first group indicates that the second should receive priority in allocating medical resources for research and treatment. Some might argue that priority should be given to post-coma disorders because people who have them are worse off than people with psychiatric disorders. They might claim that the number of people affected by a disorder is not the main ethical issue. Rather, what makes them worse off is the condition they have. Still, priority in allocating scarce medical resources to the worse off is not absolute but conditional on outcomes of the allocation (Rawls, 1971; Nagel, 1991). Overall, the outcomes of experimental treatment for post-coma disorders of consciousness have not been positive, which underscores the point about conditional priority (Luaute, Maucort-Boulch, Tell et al., 2010; Magrassi, Maggione, Pistarini et al., 2016).

There are also questions about the meaning of "worse off." While minimally conscious patients are worse off than psychiatric patients in the sense that they have more limited motor and mental functions, psychiatric patients have a level of awareness than can cause them to experience frustration from having symptoms they do not want to have and thus suffer from their illness. Some MCS patients with a relatively high level of awareness may suffer from knowing that they are functionally dependent on others (*W v. M*, 2011). Arguably, though, the degree of suffering in patients with psychiatric disorders is greater because of the higher level of awareness and experience of their disorder. In this respect, they are worse off than minimally conscious patients. In addition, psychiatric disorders involve more complex assessment than the MCS regarding whether patients have the cognitive and volitional capacity to seek treatment or participate in research. Varying degrees of these capacities in different patients may or may not determine whether they meet or fail to meet criteria of informed consent. Even minimally conscious patients with higher levels of awareness likely lack the requisite degree of these capacities for consent to treatment or research. These differences illustrate how the ethics of neuroscience intersects with the neuroscience of ethics in different disorders of consciousness.

Referring to the positive subtype of schizophrenia, Stanislas Dehaene states that it "drastically alters the conscious integration of knowledge into a coherent belief network, leading to delusions and confusions . . . Yet remarkably, their implicit unconscious memories may remain completely intact" (2014, p. 254). As I will explain shortly, unconscious procedural memory is critical for behavior control in the performance of basic motor and cognitive tasks. Too much activity at the conscious level can interfere with the normal function of nonconscious procedural memory and undermine control. Relying on the global workspace theory of consciousness, Dehaene claims "Schizophrenics' main problem seems to lie in the global integration of incoming information into a coherent whole" (2014, p. 255). This is consistent with earlier claims by psychiatrists such as Kraepelin, who described schizophrenia as a "disunity of consciousness" (an "orchestra without a conductor") based on clinical observation of his patients (Kraepelin, 1896/1913, p. 668, cited by Northoff, 2015, p. 85). The integration problem at the mental level correlates with white matter abnormalities and abnormal connectivity between the PFC and auditory and visual cortices.

Dehaene further points out that "diffusion tensor imaging reveals massive anomalies on the long-distance bundles of axons that link cortical regions. The fibers of the corpus callosum, which interconnect the two hemispheres, are particularly impaired, as are the connections that link the prefrontal cortex with distant regions of the cortex, hippocampus and thalamus. The outcome is a severe disruption of resting-state connectivity: during quiet rest, in schizophrenic patients, the prefrontal cortex loses its status as a major interconnected hub, and activations are much less integrated into a functional whole than in normal controls" (2014, p. 256). These functional brain abnormalities are associated with neurotransmission disruption in dopamine D2 and glutamate $N$-methyl-D-aspartate receptors (NMDARs) (2014, p. 256). At a brain-systems level, normal function of these neurotransmitters is critical for synaptic connectivity within the PFC and its projections to other brain regions. At a mental-systems level, this function is critical for cognitive-emotional processing, reasoning, and decision-making.

Dehaene's account of the information integration problem in schizophrenia is consistent with Northoff's account of abnormal resting-state activity and functional connectivity in the anterior cortical midline structures in people with schizophrenia (Northoff, 2014a, p. 393). It is also consistent with research showing disruption of integrated information processing in cortical association networks in psychotic ("positive") schizophrenia and BD. In one neuroimaging study, the brains of individuals with psychotic illness, compared with those of healthy controls, showed reductions in functional connectivity across several brain networks and especially within the frontoparietal control network (Baker, Holmes, Masters et al., 2014). Northoff asserts that, "the occurrence of abnormal contents and an abnormal self in phenomenal consciousness in schizophrenia can ultimately be traced back to their resting state activity's abnormal self-specific and preintentional organization and its subsequent carryover and transfer to any kind of stimulus-induced activity and its associated phenomenal states, i.e., consciousness" (2014a, p. 397). In addition, he writes, "Usually, auditory and visual cortices gate and control the incoming information by inhibiting it if there is too much input at the same time. These filtering mechanisms seem to be deficient in individuals with the positive subtype of schizophrenia. They can no longer filter and gate the incoming inputs and are easily flooded with sensory information" (2016, p. 155).

Schizophrenic patients' difficulty in filtering information impairs their ability to reason and make decisions in response to sensory inputs from environmental stimuli. The auditory and visual hallucinations and delusions in schizophrenia may be the most severe form of disordered consciousness. Failed inhibitory mechanisms at the neural level can result in impeded action at the mental and bodily level. Free will in the form of uninhibited or unconstrained action requires some degree of neural inhibition, where brain regions such as the PFC inhibit other regions to prevent hyperactivity in neural circuits causing different forms of psychopathology. This point requires an explanation of differences between inhibition and constraint at neural and mental levels, which I will give in the last section of this chapter.

It is also worth repeating Northoff's point that resting-state hyperactivity in the midline network correlates with the depressed person feeling disconnected or disengaged from the natural and social environment. The person ceases to interact with it, or decreases this interaction in a significant reduction in goal-directed activity. In normal agency, the content of the goals of action are actual states of affairs the agent intends to alter, or possible states of affairs she intends to bring about. When the person withdraws from and loses interest in the world, there is little or no motivation to try to have an impact on it. This can preclude the possibility of meaningful action. The scope of agency diminishes to the inner world of the person. Because choice is essential to free will, the person's perception of limited choices means that she has lost some degree of free will. The problem is not weakness of will, where one acts on a weaker reason for a particular action rather than a stronger reason for a different action. Instead, a disordered brain and mind impair the person's capacity to consider different courses of action as open possibilities for her.

In MDD, an increase in self-focus often includes an increase in body-focus. This may go some way toward explaining reports of muscle and joint pain and other somatic symptoms of some people with depression. The *incidence* of patients with depression reporting somatic symptoms may be higher in some cultures than in others (Kleinman, 1988). There may be differences in how they report these symptoms as well. Still, the *fact* that some of these patients have these symptoms is traceable to a neurobiological source. This aligns with Walter's point, cited in Chapter 1, that the neurobiology of psychiatric disorders is consistent across all cultures. This may not be a sufficient explanation for these reports; but it is a necessary explanation. Northoff explains that somatic symptoms are due to abnormal processing of interoceptive stimuli from one's body and exteroceptive stimuli from the environment (2014a, p. 403). As in schizophrenia, this abnormality can impair agency by impairing the cognitive-emotional–volitional capacity to initiate and carry out action plans. It can lead to the decreased agency symptomatic of anhedonia and avolitional syndrome (Spence, 2009, pp. 239–262). Abnormalities in how the brain represents the body and the world to the subject can cause or reinforce inflexible behavior. This can interfere with the person's ability to respond to changing circumstances.

Disturbances in the relation of the self to the world occur in both positive and negative subtypes of schizophrenia. In the positive subtype, this disturbance results from distortion of information about the world in psychotic hallucinations and delusions. The negative subtype overlaps with the subtype of depression involving anhedonia, avolition, flat affect, and impeded initiative. By undermining or weakening the desire to act, these symptoms may involve a more excessive focus on the self than psychotic symptoms. In this regard, they may be more disruptive to the person's relation to the world. Distortion of neural and mental information interferes with free will by diminishing the person's ability to exercise flexible behavior in successfully navigating the natural and social environment. In AN, the pathology associated with a severe eating disorder results from abnormal processing of reward and body perception. This alters the person's perception of her own body. Instead of a disrupted relation between the embodied subject and the world, in AN there is a disrupted relation between the subject and her body. The distorted perception of the body involves a type of delusional state in which the affected person fails to recognize the pathology and reasons to seek and adhere to treatment. In all of these disorders, there is brain dysfunction manifesting in dysfunctional mental states and maladaptive and pathological behavior. The inability to process information accurately impairs the ability to deliberate about, respond to, and act on reasons for different courses of action. To use Block's distinction, disrupted phenomenal consciousness can result in disrupted access consciousness. These disruptions can impair voluntary and effective agency.

The grand mal and petit mal seizures in epilepsy illustrate the connection between consciousness and agency. Disruption in the ability to process information can impair the ability to perform intended actions. Because seizures are intermittent rather than constant in causing loss of awareness, they can impair the will by thwarting the execution of action plans formed during periods of intact consciousness. This can occur even in brief moments of "absence" during a petit mal seizure. These episodes can disrupt the continuity of the desires, beliefs, intentions, and actions that constitute agency. They thwart the realization of intentions in states of affairs the subject wants to bring about (Boly, Phillips, Tshibanda et al., 2008). When they occur, seizures disrupt not only access consciousness but also the more fundamental phenomenal consciousness in being aware of oneself and one's circumstances. This is necessary for any form of voluntary agency.

The main difference between epilepsy and schizophrenia and depression is that in the second and third disorders there is a continuous rather than transient or intermittent disturbance of the person's self-awareness and awareness of her relation to the world. Except in severe cases of epilepsy, seizures impair or undermine agency by disrupting phenomenal and access consciousness at particular times. In schizophrenia and major depression, neural circuit dysfunction can impair or undermine agency by disrupting phenomenal and access consciousness over time. All of these disorders interfere with goal-directed behavior. The interference is more acutely debilitating in epilepsy when seizures occur. But it can be more chronically debilitating in psychiatric disorders with chronically distorted mental content. The extent to which these disorders are treatable can influence assessments of their effects on agency.

Although neuroimaging can detect dysfunction in the neural networks mediating consciousness, it is not a material property of the brain but a psychological property or process that emerges from the brain when it reaches a certain level of complexity. Together with unconscious biological mechanisms, consciousness promotes homeostasis in human organisms by enabling the subject to discriminate between threatening and benign stimuli and adapt to the natural and social environment. Psychiatric disorders are disorders not only in the sense that they involve dysfunction in the neural correlates of consciousness but also in the sense that this dysfunction impairs this adaptive ability. The distorted awareness at the core of this impairment results from but is not identical to dysfunctional connectivity between neural circuits and networks. The normal and abnormal neural correlates of consciousness cannot completely account for the phenomenology of ordered and disordered consciousness.

What it is like to have experience in mental health and mental illness depends not only on brain function or dysfunction but also on the context in which the subject has this experience. Josef Parnas describes schizophrenia as a disorder of consciousness, not in the way it disrupts information in the brain, but in the way it affects one's experience (2003, p. 236). The feeling of being disengaged from the world that is an early sign of the disorder can undermine the motivation to interact with the world (Parnas, 2003, p. 223). Similarly, Kai Vogeley defines consciousness "as the integrated internal representation of the outer world and the organism in this world. This representation is based on actual experiences, perceptions and memories providing reflected responses to the needs of our environment" (Vogeley, 2003, pp. 361–362). Psychiatric disorders characterized by psychosis, particularly schizophrenia, are disorders of consciousness in the sense that they involve a disruption in this internal representation. As the comments by Parnas and Vogeley emphasize, what matters in diagnosing and treating psychiatric disorders is not so much that they involve distorted information processing in the brain. What matters more is how this distortion adversely affects people's experience. A critical research question for psychiatry is how interventions in the brain might restore normal information processing to improve the quality of this experience.

Some cognitive psychologists have questioned the extent to which consciousness is involved in agency. For example, John Bargh and Ezequiel Morsella claim that unconscious perceptual, evaluative, and motivational systems grounded in priming and automaticity largely guide behavior. "Actions of an unconscious mind precede the arrival of a conscious mind—these actions precede reflection" (Bargh and Morsella, 2008, p. 73). Consciousness is more of a passive conduit of information than an active force of control (Wegner, 2002; Morsella, Godwin, Jantz et al., 2015). David Oakley and Peter Halligan reiterate this view in a recent article, claiming "All psychological processing and psychological products are the products of fast efficient non-conscious systems" (Oakly and Halligan, 2017, p. 1). Although these psychologists do not always identify which brain regions correspond to conscious and unconscious mental processes, the suggestion is that there is a rough correlation between conscious processes and cortical brain activity, on the one hand, and unconscious processes and subcortical brain activity, on the other. The general claim is not that consciousness has no role in our behavior. Rather, it has a much more limited role that what we assume. Still, this is an oversimplified and misleading dualistic conception of human thought and behavior. Conscious and unconscious processes in the brain and mind do not operate independently of each other or in just one direction—from unconscious to conscious—but interdependently and bidirectionally. Both unconscious and conscious processes and the interacting cortical and subcortical neural networks that mediate them are necessary for behavior control. Instead of a dualistic "either . . . or" model, a "both . . . and" model is more accurate in explaining the causal role of psychological and neurobiological processes in our thought and behavior.

The idea that unconscious neural and mental processes regulate some of our thought and behavior does not undermine the conviction that we have some conscious control of it. On the contrary, these processes are necessary to maintain optimal levels of sensorimotor, cognitive, emotional, and volitional capacities underlying our deliberation, decisions, and actions. More generally, unconscious processes are necessary to maintain homeostasis in the organism. Antonio Damasio spells out a key feature of the interconnections between unconscious and conscious dimensions of human organisms: "The reality of nonconscious processing and the fact that it can exert control over one's behavior are not in question . . . nonconscious processes are, in substantial part and various ways, under *conscious* control" (2010, p. 285). Moreover, "consciousness came of age by first restraining part of the nonconscious executives and then exploring them mercilessly to carry out preplanned, predecided actions. Nonconscious processes became a suitable and convenient means to execute behavior and give consciousness more time for further analysis and planning" (2010, p. 286).

Yet devoting too much time to analysis and planning can impair behavior control. Being overly conscious could increase the perceived need to process large amounts of information and interfere with the ability to deliberate and decide which actions to perform. It could overload the brain and mind and disable agency either by causing inaction or by causing one to perform unwanted actions. Inhibiting mechanisms in the PFC mediating conscious reflection are necessary to prevent hyperactivity in the reward system and pathologies such as impulse control disorders. Beyond a certain point, though, reflection can impede rather than promote voluntary action. OCD is a good example of how being too conscious can interfere with the motor and mental capacities necessary to act freely. We perform many motor skills and cognitive tasks automatically. This reduces cognitive load and allows the conscious mind to attend to more demanding tasks. A division of neural and mental labor ensures that a person is not overwhelmed by too much information entering and remaining in her field of awareness. In schizophrenia, this division collapses in the breakdown of the brain's information-filtering mechanism.

Behavior control requires a balance between complementary rather than competing reflective and nonreflective processes. This balance is enabled by the constraining mechanisms operating at cortical and subcortical levels in the brain. It involves a circular causal process of brain–mind interaction that regulates input from the environment and a person's response to it. In OCD, this process becomes stuck in a continuous cycle that runs from obsessions to compulsions and then back again. This results in the loss of flexible thought and behavior.

Too much conscious reflection can lead to pathologies of excessive self-focus, including not just OCD but anxiety, depression, and schizophrenia as well. Too little conscious reflection can result in behavior that is overly automatic and equally at odds with control. An excess or deficit of awareness and reflection can undermine the capacity for effectively deliberating and deciding between different courses of action. It can undermine not only the ability to make rational decisions but also the normative aspect of agency that makes us candidates for attributions of responsibility, praise, and blame.

In a study of patients with OCD, a group of psychiatry researchers concluded that people without the disorder "are able to process procedural strategies outside of awareness, whereas in patients with OCD there instead appears to be an intrusion of information and emotion into consciousness" (Stein, Goodman, and Rauch, 2000, p. 343; Goodman, Grice, Lapidus et al., 2014). This intrusion is associated with a dysfunctional information filtering mechanism in a frontal–thalamic–striatal–frontal circuit (Figee, Luigjes, Smolders et al., 2013; DeRidder, Vanneste, Gillett et al., 2016). When it functions normally, this circuit limits the amount of information that is accessible to consciousness. It keeps a substantial amount of this information outside of awareness. This mechanism goes awry in OCD. People with this disorder engage in excessive rumination about their perceptions, thoughts, and actions. The obsessions and compulsions are symptomatic of trying to have too much conscious control of their actions, which instead impedes their ability to act freely. Trying too hard to have control over one's behavior undermines control. Hyper-reflectivity interferes with unconscious processes that ordinarily enable one to perform motor skills and cognitive tasks without having to think about performing them. Too much reflection and rumination causes one to lose "trust" in procedural memory of unconscious motor plans in performing basic actions as a matter of course (Van den Hout and Kindt, 2003). This is not a sign of impaired procedural memory as such but of excessive awareness that overrides this form of nondeclarative memory.

Noting this effect on procedural memory, Sanneke de Haan, Erik Rietveld, and Damiaan Denys state that "many OCD patients are insecure about whether they have done something, or have done something correctly" (2015, p. 95). Among these patients, "too much conscious control disturbs the flow of action" (2015, p. 95). Commenting further on the relation between awareness and control, de Haan, Rietveld, and Denys make the following points: "To feel free, one needs to find the proper balance between deliberation and conscious control, on the one hand, and spontaneous unreflective action, on the other. In other words, being free also requires losing control. Moreover, our unreflective habits or abilities are just as much a part of who we are as our conscious deliberation is. To appreciate the importance of our habits, one only needs to keep in mind that spontaneous actions are informed. They are not mere reflexes or instincts but flexible and context-sensitive, and it has taken time to turn them into habits" (2015, p. 97). Conscious learning becomes unconscious habit.

The interaction of conscious and unconscious processing in OCD raises questions about the view that nonconscious brain systems drive all forms of psychological processing. Oakley and Halligan state: "All 'contents of consciousness' are generated by and within non-conscious brain systems in the form of a continuous self-referential personal narrative that is not directed or influenced in any way by the 'experience of consciousness'" (2017, p. 1). The obsessions and compulsions that are the content of consciousness in OCD have dysregulating causal effects on the brain systems that ordinarily produce normal mental content. Excessive conscious reflection causally contributes to dysregulation in the unconscious frontal–thalamic–striatal–frontal circuit implicated in the disorder. The brain systems behind the disordered content do not become or remain dysfunctional entirely for neurobiological or mechanistic reasons. How the disorder develops, how it persists, and how CBT or other therapies can modulate neural dysfunction and relieve symptoms involve at least some psychogenic processes with conscious content. Beliefs and other conscious states can have chronic destabilizing effects on unconscious brain mechanisms. Purely neurobiological or mechanistic models cannot explain why what Oakley and Halligan describe as "fast efficient non-conscious systems" become and remain so inefficient in OCD and other psychiatric disorders.

Without a balance between automatic and reflective processes in brain–mind interaction, the subject can feel overwhelmed by having to attend consciously to too many motor and cognitive tasks. Thomas Fuchs points out that, making implicit motor and cognitive functions explicit can impair them by disrupting their natural flow (Fuchs, 2011). He writes, "Self-centeredness and hyper-reflection are . . . on the one hand, the result of the illness [OCD], but on the other hand, they often additionally contribute to it" (2011, p. 239). This is one way of describing compulsions as an attempt to compensate for or neutralize obsessions in OCD. In some respects, it also describes delusions as a maladaptive compensatory strategy to make sense of abnormal cognitive and emotional states in psychotic depression. The altered phenomenology in these disorders can have a disabling effect on agency by disrupting the natural flow of unconscious and conscious events that ordinarily lead to actions.

De Haan, Rietveld, and Denys summarize their account of OCD as a disorder of consciousness: "We suggest that there is an optimal level of conscious control. Beyond a certain point, the desire for and exercise of conscious control becomes pathological and results in loss of control of one's behavior . . . For OCD patients, the challenge lies in lessening their conscious control and learning to trust, to rely on their abilities and their surroundings instead" (2015, p. 99). "Lessening control" of conscious processes is a more appropriate description of the role of consciousness in mental health than "losing control" of these processes. Our ability to act in the world and realize our considered desires and intentions requires an optimal level of conscious deliberation and decision-making. An excess or deficit of this capacity can result in psychopathology.

## Disorders of memory content

Anxiety, some forms of depression, panic, phobia, and PTSD can be characterized as disorders of the fear memory system. Unlike disorders of memory *capacity*, such as anterograde and retrograde amnesia, they are disorders of memory *content* (Kopelman, 2002; Fradera and Kopelman, 2009). The problem is not an inability to remember experiences but an inability to forget them. More precisely, the problem is a persistent and, in many cases, intractable emotionally charged representation of a disturbing or traumatic experience. Disorders of memory content constitute a significant percentage of psychiatric disorders. They include the conditions I have described, as well as addiction. This involves disruption of mechanisms of learning and memory in pursuing rewards and the cues that predict them (Hyman, 2005). Among what Daniel Schacter calls the "seven sins of memory," these disorders correspond to the "sin" of persistence (2001, Chapter 7). They are involuntary sins, however, because whether these memories develop and persist is beyond our conscious control.

One partial explanation for the psychopathology of these disorders is that the memory consolidates in the amygdala of the brain's fear memory system through the action of norepinephrine and glucocorticoids released in response to the experience (Parsons and Ressler, 2013). The memory becomes entrenched in the amygdala from the combined effects of this physiological response and the subject learning to link an aversive stimulus with a conditioned stimulus. The emotional representation of the memory persists in the person's brain, imbuing his perception of actual and possible events as threatening and resulting in some degree of mental and motor paralysis.

Endel Tulving has commented, "To remember an event means to be consciously aware now of something that happened on an earlier occasion" (1985, p. 1). Episodic memory is one of the cognitive dimensions of consciousness. Advancing Tulving's research, Daniel Schacter and Donna Rose Addis have argued that the main purpose of episodic memory is not to accurately recall the past but to use it to anticipate and project ourselves into the future (Schacter and Addis, 2007; Schacter, Addis, Hassabis et al., 2012). In its more subjective form of autobiographical memory, episodic memory enables us to experience what Tulving has called "mental time travel" (Tulving, 2002). This includes not only the ability to project ourselves backward to experienced events but also to imagine the future as a mirror image of the past. This ability is critical for goal-directed behavior. The persistence of a fear memory that has no adaptive purpose can cause fearful anticipation of the future. It can disable the cognitive, emotional, and volitional capacities necessary to deliberate about possible courses of action and to initiate and carry out action plans. It can impede flexible behavior by impeding the capacity for agency.

The disproportionate role of a fear memory in the content of consciousness in anxiety, depression, panic, phobia, and PTSD may cause more mental paralysis and impair agency more than other psychiatric disorders, even OCD. Unlike the hyperactive "fight-or-flight" response associated with some types of anxiety and depression, disorders of memory content often involve a "freeze" response to stimuli because of the affected person's conditioned fear learning. In severe cases, the memory makes the person unable to even consider action plans, much less form and execute them. Disorders of memory content can also disrupt identity. The outsized influence of a traumatic or disturbing memory can alter the contour and flow of a person's experience of persisting through time. By repeatedly drawing the person back to the event that triggered the psychopathological process, these disorders involve another form of stuck thinking in need of release or liberation.

The type of memory dysfunction in the disorders I have mentioned is different from the type of memory dysfunction in OCD. In the latter, the subject loses trust or confidence in performing tasks ordinarily regulated by unconscious procedural memory. In the former, the disorder is associated with both unconscious conditioning and a negative, emotionally charged, conscious episodic memory that dominates the content of the person's mind. The persistent memory may inhibit him to the point where he may withdraw from social interaction. In severe cases, the mental paralysis may make him unable to leave his home. The memory causes hyperactivation of the amygdala in the fear memory system, which can distort the processing and interpretation of information from the world. It causes the affected person to perceive future events as threats and with fearful anticipation. This is one explanation for the excessive worry symptomatic of GAD.

An example of this worry illustrates its disabling effects on agency. A person with anxious depression may have a persistent memory of a relapse of mood disturbances following an episode of flu. If she is aware of the possible deleterious effects of neuroimmune interactions, she may attribute the relapse to the effects of inflammatory cytokines in the brain released in response to the flu. The memory may cause her to avoid situations in which she believes she would again contract the flu and experience another relapse. Fear in anticipating this situation causes her to withdraw from social interaction and significantly limits her activity. In a different situation, unpleasant memories of one or more social interactions may contribute to social anxiety disorder, a subtype of GAD characterized by "an intense fear of social situations in which a person anticipates being evaluated negatively" by others (*DSM-5*, pp. 202–203; Leichsenring and Leweke, 2017). Panic disorder is a more severe form of anxiety disorder. It involves a difference of degree rather than kind, with a more heightened emotional response to fear-inducing stimuli associated with a memory. Whereas panic disorder has a more acutely disabling effect on agency, anxiety disorder has a more chronically disabling effect.

There is more extensive hyperactivation of the fear memory system in PTSD than in other psychiatric disorders of memory content. PTSD involves more persistent, emotionally heightened, and intractable memories than GAD. There is also greater dysfunction in prefrontal and other cognition- and emotion-mediating brain regions. In addition to causing a greater degree of suffering from the characteristic psychological symptoms, this results in more chronically disabling effects on agency. Approximately 20–30% of people who have experienced trauma also experience life-long PTSD (Parsons and Ressler, 2013). It is the fourth most common psychiatric diagnosis. In anxiety, panic, and especially PTSD, the stress of a traumatic experience can cause epigenetic changes in the brain, altering gene expression and disrupting normal fear processing in the amygdala (Shalev, Liberzon, and Marmar, 2017).

These changes involve DNA methylation and other mechanisms regulating transcription and translation factors necessary for encoding, consolidating, and storing memories. They are features of a pathogenic process that interferes with the normal transition from episodic memory formation in the hippocampus to long-term episodic memory storage in the neocortex. Instead, high chronic circulating levels of norepinephrine and glucocorticoids, combined with long-term potentiation and protein synthesis, embed the emotional information constituting the memory trace in the amygdala (Sillivan, Vaissiere, and Miller, 2015; Van Marle, 2015; Zannas, Provencal, and Binder, 2015). This overstimulates the fear memory system. It disrupts normal cognitive-emotional processing mediated by a pathway linking the limbic system to the PFC. This is turn interferes with the normal function of the PFC to inhibit emotional functions mediated by the limbic system. The emotionally charged content of the memory disrupts the brain's ability to process information internally from the body and externally from the environment. In PTSD, these pathological processes cause the characteristic symptoms of intrusion of the traumatic memory as flashbacks, nightmares, social avoidance, and hyperarousal (Shalev, Liberzon, and Marmar, 2017).

Joseph LeDoux distinguishes nonconscious from conscious aspects of fear (LeDoux, 2015, pp. 184–191). The first aspect pertains to the body's ability to detect threats to the organism and respond appropriately to them. This involves activation of the amygdala circuit in the limbic system. The second aspect is a product of cognitive systems in the neocortex. These systems project to and from the amygdala circuit in processing fear at nonconscious and conscious levels. There is a cognitive representation of the memory in the neocortex and an emotional representation of it in the amygdala. The source of the psychopathology in disorders of memory content is not the cognitive representation of the memory but the emotionally charged representation of it in the fear memory system. Erasing the memories causing or causally contributing to psychiatric disorders could prevent the intrusion of uncontrollable flashbacks of traumatic experiences in consciousness and fearful anticipation of the future. It would do this by removing the neural source of these psychopathologies. Although it is speculative, memory erasure would be one way of treating some of these disorders. I explore interventions that might erase pathological fear memories in the next two chapters.

## Disorders of the will

In discussing how psychiatric disorders involve abnormalities of consciousness and memory, I have indicated how they can impair agency. I have used "agency" in the broad sense of the mental and physical capacity to translate desires, beliefs, and intentions into voluntary actions. This capacity is a manifestation of adaptive behavior. Still, the more fine-grained concept of free will provides a more helpful framework for explaining the respects in which these disorders impair thought and behavior. This requires a more detailed account of the connections between an affected person's neural and mental states and her actions. In the introduction to this chapter, I stated that the will is a complex set of psychomotor cognitive, emotional, and volitional capacities. The will is free when a person is able to exercise these capacities in forming and executing action plans. In this section, I further explain how psychiatric disorders can interfere with these capacities and impair the will to varying degrees. I argue that autonomy and insight are necessary for a person to have control over her mental states and actions and thus have free will. I also discuss how different psychiatric disorders can undermine autonomy and insight.

Dirk De Ridder and coauthors define free will as "the ability to select for or against a course of action in order to fulfill a desire, without extrinsic or intrinsic constraints that compel the choice" (De Ridder, Vanneste, Gillett, et al., 2016, p. 239). This involves what they describe as "flexible behavior," which is "based on two functions: 1) the ability to predict future outcomes; and 2) the ability to cancel them when they are unlikely to accomplish valuable results and replace them by alternative behavioral strategies" (2016, p. 242). Psychiatric disorders impair these functions by impairing the motor and mental capacities on which they rest. Although the phrase does not appear in the *DSM-5*, the *DSM-IV-TR* mentions an "important loss of freedom" as one of the defining features of mental disorders (American Psychiatric Association, 2000, p. xxxi). This "freedom" consists in the ability to select between courses of action. Insofar as major psychiatric disorders impair or undermine this ability, they can impair or undermine free will and thus are disorders of the will (Meynen, 2010, 2012, 2015).

Forming and executing action plans is a conscious mental process explained in psychological terms. Yet the ability to perform these mental functions depends on normal brain functions. Moderately severe and severe psychiatric disorders involve abnormalities in brain structure or in functional connectivity between neural circuits and networks mediating motor and mental capacities. This impedes flexible thought, behavior, and adaptability to the environment. The affected person becomes stuck in a pattern of inflexible behavior and has difficulty breaking out of it because of deficits in these capacities. I have described how brain abnormalities in some psychiatric disorders can disrupt the content of conscious mental states and impede agency. In Chapter 1, I explained how dysfunction in frontal, parietal, and limbic regions can result in abnormal processing of emotion, reward, and body perception in AN. This may account for the cognitive and volitional impairments in this eating disorder and the difficulty or inability of an affected person to control her thought and behavior. It will be helpful to cite more examples.

Many people with schizophrenia have deficits in executive (cognitive and volitional) functions correlating with abnormal neuroanatomy (Insel, 2010, p. 189; Malloy-Diniz, Marques de Miranda, and Grassi-Oliveira, 2017). MRI showing reduced gray matter volume in the prefrontal area of the brain that ordinarily regulates these functions is one component of an explanation for these deficits. In the subtype of MDD characterized by anhedonia and avolition, fMRI and PET have confirmed a mesolimbic hypodopaminergic state caused by dysfunction in a frontal–limbic–striatal–frontal circuit (Schlaepfer, Bewernick, Kayser et al., 2014). This dysfunction impairs psychomotor and volitional capacities necessary to initiate and complete actions. In one of the first major studies of depression, imaging displaying a similar dysfunctional frontal–limbic–striatal–frontal circuit involving the subcallosal cingulate gyrus, insula, anterior cingulate cortex, and ventral striatum confirmed a neural basis for disrupted cognitive-emotional processing in a different subtype of the disorder (Mayberg, Lozano, Voon et al., 2005). Recent studies using fiber photometry and optogenetics on rats have shown that hyperactivity in a pathway involving the lateral habenula disrupts the motivation to exert effort in both aversive and appetitive contexts. Hyperactivity in this region could account for the decreased motivation in humans with major depression (Proulx, Aronson, Milivojevic et al., 2018).

Regarding the positive subtype of schizophrenia characterized by hallucinations and delusions, functional imaging has shown a hyperdopaminergic state in mesolimbic tracts and dysfunction in a cortical–thalamic–striatal–cortical circuit (Baker, Holmes, Masters et al., 2014; Castle and Buckley, 2015, pp. 43–45). In the cortical component of this circuit, there is pronounced dysfunctional connectivity in a frontal–parietal pathway associated with auditory and visual hallucinations. This dysfunction is associated with abnormalities in filtering and gating sensory information and severe impairment in the psychomotor, cognitive, and volitional processes involved in reasoning and decision-making (Northoff, 2014a, pp. 391 ff., 2016, p. 155; Javitt and Freedman, 2015). In the negative subtype of schizophrenia, functional imaging has indicated a hypodopaminergic state in mesocortical tracts and dysfunction in a frontal–thalamic–striatal circuit. This may manifest in the anhedonia and avolition characteristic of the subtype of depression I just described.

In BD, functional abnormalities in another circuit can result in the mixed states of mania (and hypomania) and depression (Strakowski, 2014, p. 34). Although the depressive states are more frequent in this disorder than manic or hypomanic states, the latter are a greater impediment to cognitive, emotional, and volitional components of the will. Among other behavior manifestations in BD, hyperactivation of the mesolimbic dopamine system and dysregulated dopaminergic processing can interfere with the normal inhibitory effect of the prefrontal region on this system (Ashok,

Marques, Jauhar et al., 2017). Uninhibited striatal activity during a manic phase can result in impulsive behavior.

OCD may be the most frequently cited psychiatric disorder that impairs free will. This may be because it involves neural circuit dysfunction affecting all four of the component capacities of the will. Earlier, I discussed how this disorder interferes with agency through its disruptive effects on consciousness. Dysfunction at the conscious mental level corresponds to dysfunction at the unconscious neural level. De Ridder and coauthors explain that, "in obsessive compulsive disorder, there is a structural hyper-connectivity between the thalamus, the orbitofrontal cortex and the anterior cingulate cortex (ACC) as confirmed by volume enlargement in the internal capsule" (De Ridder, Vanneste, Gillett et al., 2016, p. 240) indicated by MRI. Other investigators have used functional imaging to identify hyperconnectivity in a frontal–thalamic–striatal–frontal circuit (Melloni, Urbistondo, Sedeno et al., 2012; Figee, Luigjes, Smolders et al., 2013). The information received by the thalamus about the organism's relation to the external milieu is distorted by a faulty filtering mechanism. This distorts information processing in the other brain regions to which the thalamus projects. Hyperconnectivity in this circuit may at least partly explain the continuous cycle of obsessions and compulsions in OCD. An inflexible pattern of thought corresponds to a dysregulated pattern of neural activity. These behaviors, particularly the affected person's perceived need for the compulsions to control the obsessions, interfere with his ability to perform basic motor and cognitive tasks voluntarily. Ordinarily, this involves performing these tasks without having to think about them, or with only a minimal level of awareness. The neural disturbance makes one excessively aware of acting and thereby inhibits the freedom to act.

Explaining free will in terms of the ability to form and execute, or cancel, action plans based on brain–mind interaction is more plausible than most traditional philosophical explanations. Standard philosophical accounts of free will typically rest on the question of causal determinism. This is the thesis that natural laws and events in the past jointly determine the course of all future events (Van Inwagen, 1983; Strawson, 2010). If causal determinism is true, then this rules out the ability to choose between different actions. An action a person performs at a particular time is the only action she could have performed at that time. Insofar as free will presupposes alternative possibilities of action, causal determinism appears to rule out free will. Philosophers divide roughly into three groups in interpreting the upshot of causal determinism. Hard incompatibilists believe that causal determinism is true and that we lack free will (James, 1956, pp. 145 ff.). Libertarian incompatibilists believe that we have free will and that causal determinism is false (Kane, 1996). Compatibilists believe that we have free will when we act on considered desires and intentions without coercion, compulsion, or constraint (Frankfurt, 1988, Chapter 1; Fischer, 1994; Dennett, 2015).

Compatibilism is traceable to Aristotle's account of voluntariness in the *Nicomachean Ethics* (Aristotle, 1984, Volume II). He specifies two necessary negative conditions for voluntary action: one must not be forced to act; and one must not be ignorant of the circumstances of action. The first of these can be described as the metaphysical, or freedom-relevant, condition, and the second as the epistemic, or knowledge-relevant, condition. The metaphysical condition corresponds roughly to the sensorimotor and volitional capacities of the will, and the epistemic condition corresponds roughly to the cognitive and emotional capacities of the will. Following Aristotle, we can assume that a person is able to act freely unless there is behavioral and neurobiological evidence to the contrary. Although the Aristotelian model can serve as a framework for assessing free will in psychiatric disorders, the exclusion of constraint from the compatibilist freedom-relevant condition needs to be qualified in light of certain features of the brain–mind relation. I will do this in the next section of this chapter.

For the compatibilist, causal determinism does not threaten free will because laws of nature and events in the past do not directly affect whether or how we act. If the control necessary for free will consists in an executive capacity to form and carry out action plans, then the appropriate model for assessing whether one has this control is not an external one involving natural laws and the past but an internal one involving the brain–mind relation and how this influences deliberation, decision-making, and acting. Nevertheless, some might claim that the presumed determinism of the external world applies to the internal neural and mental world as well (Roskies, 2006, 2010). But there is no conclusive empirical evidence for the claim that global brain activity is completely determined by events occurring at the level of neurons, synapses, and neurotransmitters. Nor is there conclusive empirical evidence for the claim that this activity is indeterminate. Oscillations in neural activity and fluctuations in functional connectivity in brain regions associated with reasoning and decision-making suggest that the connections between brain states and mental states are probabilistic rather than deterministic. Neuroscientists Harald Atmanspacher and Stefan Rotter note: "The intricate relations between determinacy and stochasticity raise strong doubts concerning inferences from neurobiological descriptions to ontological statements about the extent of determinism in the brain" (2012, p. 98). They further state: "Our bottom line is that pretentious claims as to deterministic or indeterministic brain activity are unfounded, and so are the consequences drawn from them" (2012, p. 99).

What matters in assessing free will in psychiatry is not whether causal determinism is true or false. Instead, what matters is how brain function enables and brain dysfunction disables the sensorimotor, cognitive, emotional, and volitional capacities necessary to form and translate intentions into actions, or to cancel these intentions and refrain from acting. Whether or to what extent a person has or lacks free will depends on how the interaction of neural and mental processes promotes flexible thought, behavior, and adaptability to the natural and social environment. This is a more plausible conception of the will than one based on natural laws and the past. It more accurately captures the idea of a person's control of how she reasons, decides, and acts. A real-life example supports this claim. A former student of mine with a history of major depression suffering from severely impeded initiative told me that, during the lowest troughs of the disorder, she experienced "psychic paralysis" and had "no free will." She was reporting a lived experience of avolition. Neural and mental dysfunction provide a much more plausible explanation of her experience than a combination of natural laws and events in the remote past. This case is just one example of how the actual thought and behavior of real people with psychiatric disorders can tell us more about free will than armchair theorizing using thought experiments and imaginary people.

An internal conception of free will in terms of how the brain mediates motor and mental functions, and how much control a person has over these functions, is also more plausible than a conception adopted by some who use a phenomenological approach to psychiatry. Matthew Ratcliffe claims that " 'agency,' or 'free will,' does not consist in an 'internal' feeling but . . . is instead embedded in the experienced world, in the form of certain kinds of possibility that the world offers. Hence a change in how the world appears can also be a change in the feeling of being able to act" (2015, p, 12). On this view, psychiatric disorders impair free will by disrupting the relation of the subject to the external world. An impairment in the ability to act is symptomatic of a disordered self. Radcliffe's view supports Northoff's account of major depression as a state in which an excessive focus on the self causes the subject to feel detached from the world (Northoff, 2014a, p. 391; 2016, p. 109). Significantly, though, Northoff explains that this feeling of detachment correlates with hyperactivity in the brain's midline network, as revealed by functional neuroimaging.

What it is like to experience detachment is not reducible to neurobiology. Yet a satisfactory account of this experience requires a neurobiological explanation in addition to a psychological one. Social contextual factors can influence how one perceives options for action and cause a person to feel constrained from acting or compelled to act against his wishes. Chronic psychosocial stress associated with these factors may alter brain structure and function and interfere with motor and mental capacities. Events and processes inside and outside the brain can shape these capacities and thus whether, or to what extent, one has free will. The critical point here is that in moderately severe and severe psychiatric disorders, disruption of the relation between the subject and the world is the *effect* rather than the *cause* of dysfunction at neural and mental levels. The main source of disruption in the ability to voluntarily perform or refrain from performing actions is not external but internal to the subject. How the world appears to the subject depends on the internal neural and mental representation of the world. It is not the world but dysfunction of the subject's brain and mind that distorts this representation and impairs the capacity for voluntary action.

## Two types of constraint

I have used "inhibit" and "constrain" to describe how some regions of the brain interact with others in regulating neural and mental activity. A breakdown in inhibiting or constraining mechanisms can result in different psychopathologies. For example, in impulse control disorders, dysfunctional inhibitory mechanisms in the PFC allow hyperactivity in the mesolimbic dopamine reward system. These mechanisms may be disabled in addiction as well. In anxiety, panic disorder, and some subtypes of depression, dysfunctional inhibitory mechanisms in the PFC can allow hyperactivity in the amygdala and the brain's fear system. These pathological processes may operate in both top-down and bottom-up directions. Dysfunctional constraining mechanisms in the ventral striatum and cerebellum may allow hyperactivity in the PFC associated with excessive conscious reflection and rumination in OCD.

Intuitively, any form of inhibition or constraint on conscious motivational states would seem to impair or undermine behavior control. It suggests limitations that conflict with the concepts of control, autonomous agency, and free will. Indeed, most compatibilist defenses of free will claim that constraint, together with coercion and compulsion, is one of the conditions that preclude control. Moreover, recall that according to De Ridder and coauthors, free will requires the "absence of extrinsic or intrinsic constraints" (De Ridder, Vanneste, Gillett et al., 2016, p. 239) in choosing between different courses of action. Despite sounding counterintuitive, some degree of constraint from some neural circuits on other circuits and on cognitive, emotional, and volitional functions is necessary for persons to control their thought and behavior. Although inhibition at the mental level may impair free will, inhibition at the neural level is necessary for it.

Sean Spence states, "The human capacity for volition, for voluntary control, or the apparent expression of 'willed' actions, is subject to multiple constraints" (2009, p. 363). These constraints operate at the neural circuit level and enable this volitional capacity. This process is consistent with Feinberg's conception of constraint as bidirectional control that neural functions exert over mental functions, and vice versa. Constraint in the brain consists in a circular causal series of re-entrant loops extending from anterior and posterior regions of the cortex to limbic regions such as the amygdala and anterior cingulate and the subcortical regions of the striatum and cerebellum, which then project back to the cortex. While higher-level cortical and mid-level limbic regions are typically associated with cognitive and emotional functions and lower-level subcortical regions with motor functions, regions such as the cerebellum in this level also have a role in coordinating action plans. The combined activity of these regions ensures a balance between excitatory and inhibitory mechanisms in the brain. It ensures that neural and mental processes are neither overactive nor underactive. Mental states also have a role in re-establishing and maintaining this balance. CBT, for example, shows that beliefs can have modulating effects on hyperactive cortical and limbic functions.

Balanced neural and mental interaction suggests the idea of optimal levels of neural and mental functions in ensuring behavior control. Spence adds that, "if the human agent possesses any freedom at all, then it is a freedom that is expressed under optimal conditions, be they structural, neurochemical, interpersonal or situational" (2009, p. 378). These conditions are optimal in the balanced sense I have described in promoting the flexible, adaptive thought and behavior associated with free will. Interpersonal and situational factors constitute what Spence calls "the human response space" (2009, p. 361) for agency. Neural processes shape the limits of this space. However, there is enough room within it for cognitive, emotional, and volitional maneuvering. This enables us to be the authors of at least some of our actions and construct meaning from them. Our actions are not predetermined by events in the brain or the world. Spence claims, "An action creates a new event in the world. Michelangelo's hands created images that had not existed previously. Charlie Parker's fingers improvised new melodies. Before these movements were made, there were 'gaps,' potential spaces for action" (2009, p. 60). The "interpersonal" and "situational" factors that Spence includes among the optimal conditions for the human response space are reflections of the environment in which the person lives and acts. In this and other respects, focusing on the brain alone cannot provide a complete explanation of free will. Nevertheless, understanding the neurobiological underpinning of the mind, and how this underpinning disrupts the mind when it is dysfunctional, is necessary to understand how psychiatric disorders can disable the will.

As neural functions mediate mental functions, we need to distinguish constraints operating at neural and mental levels. Constraint at the first level is necessary for freedom from constraint or compulsion at the second level. It is the second type of constraint that impedes free will. Unregulated or unconstrained hyperactivity in one or more nodes of a frontal–thalamic–striatal–frontal circuit that mediate cognitive and motor functions can cause a person with OCD to feel compelled to perform undesired actions and inhibited in performing desired actions. Unregulated hyperactivity in limbic regions that mediate fear processing can cause a person with GAD to feel constrained from performing actions he ordinarily would perform. Unregulated hyperactivity in the reward system can compel a person with an addiction, impulse control disorder, hypomania, or mania to act differently than she would if this system were functioning normally. Constraining mechanisms in neurotransmission and neural circuit function that prevent hyperactive and hypoactive neural and mental activity are necessary for persons to control how they form their motivational states and translate them into actions.

## Autonomy

The ability to deliberate and choose between different courses of action is necessary but not sufficient for the will to be free. A person with psychotic hallucinations or delusions may retain some ability to form and execute action plans. Yet the control of thought and behavior we associate with free will is lacking or impaired in these cases because the hallucinations and delusions are false beliefs about the world and the relation of the self to the world. In these disorders, neural processes fail to constrain mental processes and result in a reduction or loss of this control. The mental states leading to actions must be autonomous for these actions to be products of a will that is free.

Personal autonomy is the capacity for self-determination or self-regulation (from the Greek *autos* = self + *nomos* = law). It consists of two general capacities: competency and authenticity (Dworkin, 1988; Frankfurt, 1988a, 1988c, 1988d; Taylor, 1992; Mele, 1995). The first capacity involves the cognitive and emotional ability to reflect critically on one's desires, beliefs, and intentions that issue in actions. The second capacity involves the cognitive and emotional ability to identify with or endorse (or reject) these mental states following this critical reflection. The process of reflecting on and identifying with one's mental states and the actions that result from them is what makes them one's *own*. They are authentic in the sense that they constitute one's true self (Taylor, 1992).

The psychiatric self is the product of biological, psychological, and environmental factors. The psychological dimension of the self is the one most pertinent to personal autonomy. Mental states with which one does not identify following the critical reflective process, as well as the actions in which they issue, are "alien" to the subject. Autonomy is necessary to control the motor and mental springs of one's actions. Autonomy thus involves more than the ability to perform bodily movements. It also involves the independence and authorship of the mental states that move us to act, as well as how they move us to act. In order to have free will and act freely, we must not just be agents, but autonomous agents. Harry Frankfurt includes an autonomy condition in his hierarchical conception of free will. He defends a conception of free will as a capacity consisting in a general second-order desire to have particular first-order desires move one to perform particular actions (Frankfurt, 1988a, 1988c). To act freely, each conscious action must align with a rational disposition to perform actions of a certain type. This is one way of defining autonomous agency. While Frankfurt does not explicitly include this in his conception of free will, to be free, one's actions must follow from beliefs that accurately reflect external states of affairs in the different contexts in which one acts.

I have just outlined a procedural account of autonomy that does not consider the agent's values or moral attitudes. These are an essential part of a substantive account of autonomy, where one's motivational states and actions reflect "normative competence" in identifying good and bad, right and wrong behavior (Wolf, 1990). The more basic procedural account of autonomy consisting in basic mental competency and authenticity is sufficient for an explanation of the role of self-regulation in free will for psychiatry. We only need to assess how the agent's mental states result in action or inaction, and how psychiatric disorders influence this process, to assess whether a person with a psychiatric disorder has free will. We do not need to consider how values or normative attitudes might influence actions to judge whether an agent is autonomous. Focusing on the motor and mental capacities that enable agency is sufficient for determining whether or to what extent a person can control his behavior. Accordingly, I rely on a procedural account of autonomy in discussing the question of control.

As I pointed out in my discussion of consciousness, there are limits to the reflective capacity necessary for autonomy. Too much reflection on one's motivational states can result in mental paralysis and undermine autonomous agency. Autonomy requires some degree of automatic behavior. It requires a balance between conscious and unconscious processes in exercising motor and mental capacities in actions. Yet striking this balance may not be enough for these actions to be voluntary. Even when it operates at an optimal level, the reflective process may be the product of pathological mechanisms that distort information about the world, the self, and the relation between them. This may distort the content of the motivational states that lead to action. Insight is also necessary to ensure that the relevant information is accurate and that one's actions are truly free.

## Insight

One measure of how much autonomy or control a person with a psychiatric disorder has of her thought and behavior is whether or to what extent she has insight into her condition. Insight, or self-awareness, is "the ability to recognize and describe one's own (and others') behaviors, cognitions and mental states. Dysfunctional insight characterizes various neuropsychiatric disorders" (Goldstein, Craig, Bechara et al., 2009, p. 372; Blakemore, Wolpert, and Frith, 2002; Cooney and Gazzaniga, 2003). "Impaired awareness in these disorders can take the form of failure to recognize an illness, denial of illness, compromised control of action and unawareness of the patient's social incompetence. Although seemingly disparate, the signs and symptoms of impaired awareness in these disorders have been organized into coherent theoretical networks. These models primarily highlight internal representations of the actual, desired and predicted states of our own body and external world" (Goldstein, Craig, Bechara et al., 2009, p. 372). In psychiatric disorders, "abnormalities in self-awareness and behavioral control can be attributed to an underlying neural dysfunction. These commonalities could include a dissociation between self-report and behavior" (Goldstein, Craig, Bechara et al., 2009, p. 372). One important aspect of insight is interoception, "defined as the sense of the physiological condition of the entire body, or as a generalized homeostatic sensory capacity that underpins a conscious representation of how we feel" (Goldstein, Craig, Bechara et al., 2009, p. 373). Many people with major psychiatric disorders have distorted interoception and thus limited insight into their condition and their relation to the world.

Like other cognitive capacities and the more general idea of behavior control, insight is not an all-or-nothing capacity but one that comes in degrees. There is an inverse relation between cognitive impairment and insight. Generally, the more cognitively impaired one is, the less insight one has. Psychiatric disorders with psychosis involve greater cognitive impairment, less insight, less control of thought and behavior, and more diminished free will. These include the positive subtype of schizophrenia, BD, and a subtype of depression. Insight should be included in the knowledge-relevant condition of voluntary action and free will. In psychiatric disorders, the insight condition should include not only knowledge of the circumstances in which a person acts but also his under-standing of the disorder and self-knowledge.

How much insight an affected person has depends on whether the disorder is ego-dystonic or ego-syntonic. This distinction derives from psychoanalysis and is pertinent to psychiatric disorders as well (Freud, 1914; Fenichel, 1946). Ego-dystonic conditions are those in which the subject experiences internal conflict or perceives incongruity between the mental states he has and the mental states he wants to have. They may also involve incongruity between the mental states one has and those one recalls having before the onset of the illness. The subject does not identify with the symptoms of the disorder but rejects and wants to rid himself of them. In contrast, ego-syntonic conditions are those in which the subject experiences no such internal conflict and does not perceive incon-gruity between his actual mental states and those he had before the onset of the illness. Individuals with ego-syntonic disorders are not distressed by their abnormal perceptions and thoughts or the mental and bodily strategies they develop to respond to them. The denial symptomatic of lack of insight into AN, for example, can preclude internal mental conflict and characterize it an as ego-syntonic disorder. Contrary to what intuitions might suggest, lack of internal conflict does not mean that the person can reason and act freely. If her beliefs do not align with the actual state of her body and the world, then her actions based on these beliefs are not voluntary. They fail to meet the Aristotelian epistemic condition of voluntariness.

Similar dysfunction underlies the "double bookkeeping" of some persons with delusional beliefs (Bleuler, 1911/1950, pp. 127–130; Sass, 2014). This phe-nomenon can occur in two forms. In one form, the person lives in two worlds at the same time: the world of imagined voices or visions or delusions; and the world as perceived by others. Both worlds seem equally real to the subject, and he remains unbothered by the discrepancy or inconsistency between them. In the other form, the person develops false beliefs as a reaction or compensatory strategy to try to make sense of abnormal perceptions and beliefs. They are a maladaptive response to the abnormal mental states. This strategy is similar in some respects to the compulsions that patients with OCD develop in a failed attempt to counteract and neutralize obsessions. Instead, they sustain and may even exacerbate them. In delusional disorders and OCD, strategies intended to control a psychopathology introduce a second psychopathology. These processes are a manifestation of failed stabilization of default mechanisms in the brain (Northoff, 2016, p. 157). They are examples of a breakdown of neural constraints on mental processing. The mind is doing double cognitive duty, but there is distortion in both cognitive processes. The person perceives no incon-gruity and experiences no internal conflict between the abnormal perceptions and the false beliefs he constructs in response to them. In these respects, psychotic disorders can be characterized as ego-syntonic disorders. Insight and the presence or absence of internal conflict or incongruity in one's mental states are measures of how much control a person with a disorder has over his mental states and actions. They may be influenced by the symptoms of the disorder and how they alter his perception of himself and his relation to the world.

The less insight one has into one's disorder and the more ego-syntonic it is, the less autonomous one's thought and behavior are. Consequently, the less free will one has. Increased cognitive impairment correlates with decreased capacity for insight. The cognitive impairment in hallucinations and delusions can preclude insight by distorting the content of one's beliefs. Severe AN is a good example of an ego-syntonic disorder. The affected person is cognitively impaired to such a degree that she lacks insight into her disorder and loses behavior control. There is a distortion in the processing of reward and body perception, causing her to fail to recognize the pathology of her body. Ego-syntonic psychiatric disorders in which the person has little or no insight into her condition weaken or undermine free will. The cognitive impairment interferes with her capacity to know what is in her best interests and to reason and act in accord with these interests. It can interfere with the cognitive and volitional capacity to recognize the severity of the condition and to seek and adhere to treatment. This lack of insight is one possible explanation for the high mortality rate in AN relative to other psychiatric disorders.

There are two categories of delusions: delusions as disorders of experience, or "alien control"; and delusions as false beliefs (Walter and Spitzer, 2003, p. 436; Frith, 1996). Although both types of delusions can undermine control, I am focusing on the second category. My use of "alien" in my discussion of autonomy does not imply anything about real or imaginary external agents controlling one's thoughts, which may occur in auditory hallucinations. Rather, it means that the mental states that lead to actions are not the states one would want to have or would have in the absence of a psychiatric disorder. Like patients with AN, the lack of incongruity between beliefs and the actual state of the world in people with delusional disorders does not mean that these beliefs are autonomous. Nor does it mean that the actions that result from them are free. On the contrary, double bookkeeping or other cognitive strategies they might devise are more likely symptomatic of an ego-syntonic disorder and lack of insight. In that case, their mental states and actions are the mark of impaired autonomy and will. They too fail to meet the epistemic condition of voluntariness. Delusions are irrational or false beliefs about oneself or the world (Bortolotti, 2009; Gerrans, 2014). Irrational beliefs as such do not necessarily impair the cognitive component of the will. They can impair it when there is a large discrepancy between belief content and the actual state of the world.

As with other aspects of belief, this discrepancy and its effects on the will can be a matter of degree. Beliefs whose content does not align with the natural and social environment are not the sort of mental states one would endorse and retain following critical reflection. Indeed, delusions may very well preclude this critical capacity. Delusional individuals may appear to voluntarily form and carry out intentions in actions. Their motivational states and actions are not autonomous, though, if they reflect a distortion of information about the self and its relation to the world. As false beliefs, delusions can interfere with the deliberative process through which one comes to identify beliefs, desires, and intentions as the authentic springs of one's actions.

There is a question about whether OCD precludes the capacity for insight and how much control people with this disorder retain over their thought and behavior. This question may be difficult to answer because OCD typically does not involve the denial characteristic of some psychotic disorders and AN. The *DSM-5* removed "the requirement that individuals have insight into their obsessions, that is, recognizing that they are a 'product of his or her own mind,' and the addition of a specifier to distinguish among good or fair, poor or absent insight" (Hirschtritt, Bloch, and Mathews, 2017, p. 1358). According to the *DSM-5*, "For individuals whose obsessive-compulsive and related disorder symptoms warrant the "with absent insight/delusional beliefs" specifier, these symptoms should not be diagnosed as a psychotic disorder" (2013, p. 236). These specifiers are consistent with my claim that insight can be a matter of degree. How much insight one has or retains depends on the severity of the condition. It depends on the extent to which it interferes with one's cognitive capacity for self-awareness and accurate beliefs about their condition and the natural and social environment. Many, if not most, individuals with OCD are aware of their obsessions and experience them as unwanted thoughts. Given a choice, an affected person would choose not to have rather than retain them. This suggests retention of some capacity to consider alternative courses of action to improve their condition and thus some degree of insight and free will.

Gerben Meynen points out that people with OCD feel alienated from their behavior. They do not consider it their own and want to change it (2010, 2012, 2015). Commenting on the attitudes of his OCD patients undergoing DBS, psychiatrist Michael Schurmann states, "Patients don't see their obsessions as part of their personality. They see them as something imposed on them, as something they yearn to be rid of" (cited in Abbott, 2005, p. 18). These are indications of insight into an ego-dystonic disorder and some degree of control of thought and behavior. Awareness that the obsessions and compulsions are not their own, and the internal mental conflict and distress these mental states cause, can motivate them to seek and adhere to treatment. Unlike patients with psychosis, many OCD patients retain a degree of cognitive and volitional control of how they think and act despite the disabling symptoms. They have enough insight into the disorder to recognize the need for treatment that may restore a greater degree of this control. They are impaired but not entirely lacking in free will.

Among disorders with psychotic features, one must not overgeneralize the implications of these features for free will. One must not overlook differences among people who have these disorders. Not all people with delusions completely lack insight and control of their thought and behavior. Even when the content of a person's mental states does not align with external events, misalignment between one's mind and these events may occur to varying degrees. Psychoses may wax and wane over different periods of a person's life. Even when some cognitive impairment persists, waning periods may involve enough cognitive capacity for some degree of insight. Depending on the extent of the delusions and alignment or misalignment, an affected person's ability to control her actions may be impaired but not absent.

Some accounts of mathematician John Nash's life with paranoid schizophrenia suggest that he retained some insight into his condition and some control of his behavior. In a March 2002 interview with Mike Wallace on the CBS program "60 Minutes," in response to the question of why his condition seemed to improve beyond a certain point, he said that he "became disillusioned with the delusions" (Nash, 2002). This indicates some degree of insight and recognition of reasons for seeking and adhering to treatment. It also indicates that Nash retained a sense of humor, which may also be a sign of some insight. Although the disorder limited his cognitive capacity, he retained enough of it for some degree of autonomous agency and ability to perform cognitive tasks associated with his research. An explanation for the fact that Nash retained some of his cognitive capacities is that he probably had a less severe form of the disease. The disruption of information in his brain and the resulting hallucinations and delusions were not so chronically debilitating as to completely undermine control of his thought and behavior.

Although in many cases schizophrenia progresses from first-episode psychosis to a chronic disease that becomes difficult to manage, Nash's condition appeared to improve. At least it appeared not to progress beyond a certain dysfunctional level. This enabled him to return to limited academic work. While Nash's mental effort may have influenced his improvement, it was not entirely the result of this effort or sheer will power. It was more likely the result of the disorder being less severe than other cases and his response to antipsychotic medication and social circumstances. If it had been more severe, then Nash and those treating and caring for him might not have been able to promote the degree of recovery he experienced. Nash's ability to control his condition could be attributed to a comprehensive set of interventions, including medication, support from family and colleagues, and teaching and mentoring a small group of students. Research indicates that this comprehensive approach to treating schizophrenia can be effective in controlling the disease and improving the quality of life for those who have it (Kane, Robinson, Schooler et al., 2015). The approach is most effective immediately after a first-episode psychosis. Nash's case suggests that it could be effective in a range of psychotic disorders. I will say more about this treatment model in Chapter 3.

One hypothesis is that Nash's schizophrenia may have played some role in his influential work in mathematics (Nutt, 2015). This may have some intuitive plausibility when considering that schizophrenia causes an increased focus on the self and a corresponding decreased focus on the environment. This could have enhanced his ability to focus intensively on the mathematics behind his major contribution to game theory, for which he was awarded the Nobel Memorial Prize in Economic Sciences in 1994. A more plausible account is that Nash's creative work preceded his first psychotic episode at age 30 in 1959 and that the illness interfered with his cognitive capacities thereafter. The fact that he had completed his doctoral dissertation before then supports this account.

Similar questions about the connection between creativity and productivity and psychiatric disorders have arisen regarding artists during manic episodes of BD. One example of this is the painting of Vincent Van Gogh. Although some researchers have identified temporal lobe epilepsy as the main illness in the last two years of his life, this was preceded by episodes of reactive and bipolar depression (Blumer, 2002). Enhanced creativity and productivity have also been associated with hypergraphia resulting from seizure activity in temporal lobe/insular epilepsy. Some commentators attribute Fyodor Dostoevsky's prolific literary output and insight into the human condition to "ecstatic epilepsy" (Morgan, 1990; Geschwind and Picard, 2016). Yet, in these cases artistic creativity or writing productivity is part of a psychopathology (Flaherty, 2005, 2011). Any positive aspects of these creative states cannot be separated from the harmful effects on the artist's or writer's life. The quality of the writing from hypergraphia does not necessarily align with its quantity, either. In this regard, Dostoevsky's case is notably different from other cases of this neuropsychiatric condition and is the exception rather than the rule. In BD, the harm from the more frequent depressed episodes outweighs any benefits of creativity during less frequent manic episodes. Indeed, harm to oneself and others resulting from irrational behavior during manic episodes can outweigh any benefit from them.

Any presumed insight into different aspects of the human condition in mania, hypomania, or ecstatic epilepsy may correspond to a lack of insight into the fact that a brain disorder is largely driving the creative impulse. Like these other disorders, the debilitating cognitive, emotional, and physical effects and lost productivity of schizophrenia in Nash's life far outweighed any presumed positive effect it might have had on his early work in mathematics. The lifetime mental burden of what is in every sense a psychopathology is much greater than any benefit that might come from it. All psychiatric disorders involve a significant loss of free will. The degree of this loss depends on the type and severity of the disorder. It also depends on whether and to what extent the disorder responds to treatment.

Recall the discussion of Robert Lowell's bipolarity in Chapter 1. His life seemed to illustrate differences between a nonmanic normal self and a manic creative self. For Lowell and others with this disorder, manic episodes can preclude insight into their disabling effects on the person's mind and life. This lack of insight and the functional disability from other aspects of mania impaired Lowell's capacity to control his thought and behavior and thus impaired his free will. Myers makes the constructive suggestion of a "more attuned engagement" and "collaborative titration of medication" that might have given the "creative advantages [of BD] some play" (2017, p. 989). Yet this would presuppose that some of Lowell's rational capacities were intact. It would require striking a delicate balance between excitatory activity in the reward circuitry of the mesolimbic dopamine system and inhibitory activity in the prefrontal region. This balance might preempt uncontrolled mania or hypomania and thus allow the patient to retain some degree of free will while finding meaning in exercising his creativity. Such a controlled mild euphoria would require close monitoring from the treating psychiatrist.

A plan of action that, as Myers describes it, "incurs some risks but keeps close watch" might control mania and enable some expression of creative impulses. It could enable the patient to plan and complete projects that would be meaningful to him. Still, how much free will such a patient had would depend not only on his ability to exercise creative potential but also on how the neural and mental processes behind this potential affected his capacity to think and act in other dimensions of his life. If the disorder caused the person to be more functionally disabled than enabled, then it is questionable whether the value associated with a creative endeavor could compensate for the disvalue of the other aspects of the disorder.

## Conclusion

Major psychiatric disorders including schizophrenia, major depression, OCD, BD, and AN are disorders of consciousness in the sense that they involve disturbances of information processing in the brain and mind. These disturbances result from dysfunctional connectivity in neural circuits and dysfunctional neurotransmission. They can disrupt how the brain and mind filter information from the body and the external world. This disruption in turn can impair sensorimotor, cognitive, emotional, and volitional capacities that constitute the will. They can alter the content of a person's desires and beliefs and constrain them from performing actions they want to perform or compel them to perform actions they do not want to perform. Psychiatric disorders can impair the capacity to initiate and execute action plans. They can impair the capacity for flexible, adaptive behavior. In many or most of these disorders, there is an increased focus on the self and a decreased focus on the environment and others. The subject tends to reduce his agency and limits or ceases his interaction with others and the world. Anxiety, panic, PTSD, and a subtype of depression are disorders of memory content associated with hyperactivity in the fear memory system. They are also disorders of the will because fearful anticipation of events can have a paralyzing effect on motivation and action. They can interfere with autonomous agency but interfering with the capacity to critically reflect on these states and identify them as one's own. In all of these respects, psychiatric disorders are disorders of consciousness, memory, and will.

How much control an affected person retains over her thought and behavior depends on the extent to which the disorder impairs the relevant motor and mental capacities. One way of measuring the degree of autonomy an affected person has is how much insight she has into the disorder and whether it is ego-dystonic or ego-syntonic. Insight, autonomy, and free will are all matters of degree depending on the severity of a psychiatric disorder. Some people with these disorders may retain these capacities to a greater or lesser extent than others. Having a psychiatric disorder as such does not necessarily undermine autonomy or free will. The case of John Nash may very well be the exception rather than the rule for people with psychoses. Nevertheless, it is an example of how moderately severe disorders may allow some capacity for some patients to control their mental states and actions. This control requires an equilibrium of conscious and unconscious processes. Too little conscious reflection can result in behavior that is largely automatic and at odds with the idea of autonomous agency. Too much conscious reflection can upset the balance between actions we ordinarily perform as a matter of course and actions requiring conscious mental effort. Excessive rumination can impose a cognitive load on the agent that can significantly impair agency. OCD is a good example of how this imbalance can result in a psychopathology.

Psychotropic drugs, ECT, TMS, CBT, placebos, and other interventions have been given to patients with psychiatric disorders to ameliorate symptoms and improve their quality of life. When they are effective, they can restore some degree of normal conscious processing and control of thought and behavior. There is considerable variability in the safety and efficacy of these interventions. For some patients, these interventions may relieve symptoms and may result in disease remission. Many patients may have a positive response to a drug or technique but fall short of a complete remission. For other patients, none of these interventions induces a therapeutic response and their condition remains treatment-resistant. Interventions in the brain for psychiatric disorders may have both beneficial and harmful effects, prompting ethical questions about how to weigh the trade-offs in assessing whether to initiate, continue, or discontinue them. I discuss some of the medical and ethical issues surrounding less invasive and noninvasive treatments for these disorders and then more invasive treatments in the next three chapters.

## Chapter 3

# Treating psychiatric disorders: Less invasive and noninvasive interventions

Psychotropic drugs have been first-line treatment for major psychiatric disorders since the reported use of lithium for mania in 1949. This was followed by the introduction of chlorpromazine in 1952, imipramine in 1957, haloperidol in 1958, and diazepam in 1963. Most of these drugs were antipsychotics or antidepressants prescribed mainly for schizophrenia and unipolar and bipolar depression. Pharmacological treatment was and largely still is based on neurotransmitter imbalance as the explanatory model for psychiatric disorders (Walter, 2013, p. 1). Lithium can downregulate hyperdopaminergic activity associated with mania in BD I. Among other antipsychotic drugs, the typical haloperidol and the atypical clozapine also act as dopamine receptor antagonists in treating positive symptoms in schizophrenia. Introduced in the 1980s, selective serotonin reuptake inhibitors (SSRIs) such as sertraline and paroxetine block the reuptake of serotonin in the synaptic cleft and can improve mood and cognition in some patients with major depression. Serotonin and norepinephrine reuptake inhibitors (SNRIs) such as venlafaxine can modulate levels of two neurotransmitters with similar therapeutic effects. These more recent antidepressant drugs avoid many of the side effects of the older tricyclics such as imipramine and monoamine oxidase inhibitors. Not all patients with these disorders respond to these drugs, however. Many respond with some symptom relief only to experience serious side effects. Some fail to respond altogether. Variable responses may be due to differences in how genetic, epigenetic, and other biological and environmental factors influence people's brains.

At a deeper level, the overall suboptimal response rates to psychotropic drugs may be due to a mistaken hypothesis about the dysfunctional neurotransmitter system underlying these disorders. Most psychotropic drugs target the monoamines dopamine, serotonin, epinephrine, and norepinephrine. Recent research suggests that targeting other neurotransmitter systems may result in higher responses rates to psychotropic drugs. The glutamate-targeting drug ketamine may be superior to existing monoamine-targeting drugs in treating depression. More controversial is the experimental use of psilocybin to treat depression and anxiety. Even when existing or novel psychotropic drugs control some psychiatric symptoms, they may also induce or exacerbate others. CBT has been effective in controlling symptoms in major depression and generalized anxiety, especially in combination with antidepressant and anxiolytic drugs. However, pharmacotherapy and psychotherapy are limited in treating the most severe psychiatric disorders. In moderate disorders, psychotropic drugs may not be any more effective than placebos. This may be due not just to biochemical limitations of the drugs but also to the brain's innate ability to adjust to change and maintain or restore homeostasis. The limited efficacy of pharmacotherapy and psychotherapy underscores the importance of different forms of neuromodulation to treat psychiatric disorders.

In this chapter, I analyze and discuss ethical issues arising from the use of drugs and some neuromodulating techniques to restore some degree of normal neural and mental function in psychiatric disorders. The general focus is on weighing the potential benefit again the risk of harm from these interventions in the brain and mind. I point out some of the neurophysiological challenges in using psychotropic drugs and that more promising psychopharmacology may result from targeting neurotransmitters other than the monoamines. A more serious problem is a significant decrease in investment by the pharmaceutical industry in developing potentially safer and more effective drugs for depression, schizophrenia, and other disorders. I raise questions about the conceptual distinction between invasive and noninvasive treatments and argue that this distinction may not be very helpful in clarifying the risks of different interventions in the brain.

I discuss ethical issues associated with ECT. Despite a negative public perception of this technique, it can be a relatively safe and effective treatment for some patients with severe mood disorders in unipolar and bipolar depression. Some patients undergoing ECT experience retrograde amnesia. As with all other brain interventions, though, the risk of amnesia must be weighed not only against the potential benefit but also against the risk of psychic and physical harm from continuing to live with an untreated disorder. On balance, the benefits outweigh the risks and thus the technique is medically and morally justified.

Then I consider TMS and tCS. The main ethical concern with these techniques is that they can be used outside of clinical and research settings without adequate monitoring or regulation. Misuse of them could result in undesirable effects causing more harm than benefit. Moreover, the fact that the current they transmit does not penetrate deeper regions of the brain raises questions about their efficacy in treating major psychiatric disorders. The novel technique of temporal interference (TI) may overcome this obstacle and modulate subcortical structures associated with neural and mental dysfunction. I explain the circumstances in which placebos can be ethically justified in clinical psychiatry without undermining trust or respect for patient autonomy. In addition, I discuss EEG- and fMRI-based NFB for depression and anxiety and show how this technique can benefit patients by modulating brain function and ameliorating anxiety, cognition, and mood. It can also benefit them through the realization that the technique enables their own mental effort to produce salutary effects in their brains and minds. At a health systems level, NFB may be the most cost-effective treatment for depression and anxiety. These less invasive and noninvasive treatments may be able to fill the therapeutic vacuum when psychopharmacology is ineffective or unavailable to patients.

## Psychopharmacology

Establishing an accurate diagnosis is crucial to controlling psychiatric disorders and optimizing treatment outcomes. This is especially crucial in BD. Patients with this disorder experience depression (32% of the time) more often than mania (9%) or mixed symptoms (6%) (Strakowski, 2014, p. 12). Although most of the functional impairment is associated with depression, the fact that patients can move from manic to depressive symptoms presents challenges for drug selection. Pharmacological treatment for bipolar affective disorder is based on the dopamine hypothesis and the idea that dopamine dysregulation underlies the manic and depressive symptoms. The challenge in selecting drug therapy for BD is that these different symptoms are associated with different types of dopamine dysregulation. Manic and hypomanic episodes are associated with hyperdopaminergic activity, while depressive episodes are associated with hypodopaminergic activity (Ashok, Marques, Jauhar et al., 2017).

Antidepressants targeting serotonin receptors that are effective in treating anxiety and mood disturbances in unipolar depression may be ineffective for bipolar depression. This class of drugs may increase the risk of and precipitate mania in BD I (Strakowski, 2014, p. 59). They may also increase the rate of mood cycling in some individuals with this disorder. This risk is greater with the older tricyclics and less with the newer SSRIs. The anticonvulsant lamotrigine is more effective in preventing depression but not hypomania or mania. Atypical antipsychotics can treat mania but not depression. Antipsychotics may have extrapyramidal side effects from hypersensitization of dopamine receptors. These effects may include movement disorders such as tardive dyskinesia and metabolic and cardiovascular abnormalities. Lithium has been the standard therapy for BD for years because it can prevent both manic and depressive episodes and decrease suicidality (Strakowski, 2014, p. 61). Lithium also decreases the risk of relapse of mania and depression, and this risk decreases over time (2014, p. 63). It is most effective when initiated after a first manic episode (Post, 2018). Lithium is not without its physiological risks. For example, it is known to cause nephropathy in some patients. Some antidepressant drugs have been associated with suicidal ideation in some patients. On balance, though, the side effects of newer-generation antidepressants are not as serious as the effects of older-generation antidepressants.

With the possible exception of clozapine, there is no convincing evidence that the newer atypical antipsychotics are more effective in treating positive symptoms in schizophrenia than the older typical antipsychotics (e.g., chlorpromazine). Significantly, the newer atypical class of these drugs (e.g., clozapine, olanzapine, and quetiapine) is less likely to cause debilitating extrapyramidal side effects at standard doses. Still, clozapine carries a high risk of weight gain and associated diseases of diabetes and hyperlipidemia. These side effects and diseases increase the burden on people already burdened by schizophrenia. They often lead to nonadherence and relapse of psychotic symptoms. The metabolic and cardiovascular risk factors from continued use of antipsychotic drugs are the strongest contributor to the 10- to 20-year reduction in life expectancy among people with schizophrenia (Owen, Sawa, and Mortensen, 2016, p. 92).

The main goal of pharmacological research is to develop newer-generation drugs that will control positive symptoms without the serious side effects. This would reduce the probability of nonadherence and increase the probability of controlling the disease. The benefit–risk calculus for patients taking antipsychotic drugs is far from optimal. Taking the drugs may control psychiatric disease but cause other diseases entailing a shortened life expectancy. Not taking the drugs means failure to control psychotic symptoms and the probability of an even shorter life expectancy due to suicide or other forms of self-harm. Ideally, a class of drugs could be developed to control both positive and negative symptoms in schizophrenia and restore sensorimotor, cognitive, emotional, and volitional capacities to normal levels. Like the mixed manic and depressive states in BD, however, this would be challenging because schizophrenia involves dysfunction in different neural pathways underlying different motor and mental capacities. This is illustrated by the fact that, with the possible exception of lithium for BD, many drugs treat some symptoms but not others associated with the same disease. In some cases, treating existing symptoms may create new ones. Pharmacotherapy can be a zero-sum game in terms of symptom control.

Even if psychotropic drugs had higher response rates and fewer side effects, they would continue to be necessary but not sufficient for controlling the progression of severe psychiatric disorders. Like other disorders, schizophrenia has not only a neurobiological dimension but psychological and social dimensions as well. This is consistent with the biopsychosocial model for understanding and treating psychiatric disorders. This model provides a conceptual framework for a comprehensive, four-part therapeutic strategy for schizophrenia. It emphasizes early intervention at first-episode psychosis and includes antipsychotic medication, psychotherapy, social and professional support to continue work or school, and education of family members to increase their understanding of the disease. The three interventions other than medication may allow drug doses to be maintained at low levels and thereby mitigate or reduce the risk of side effects, nonadherence, and relapse. They might also allow a patient to benefit from amelioration of symptoms without a complete response from the drugs, since they would not be the only treatment modality. The combination of all four interventions can help affected individuals to build and sustain social relationships and manage symptoms.

Results of a study published in 2016 involving 404 people in their late teens and early twenties with first-episode psychosis who received this comprehensive therapy were promising (Kane, Robinson, Schooler et al., 2016). This four-part model may be the most effective way of treating and controlling the progression of all psychiatric disorders, not just schizophrenia. Unlike schizophrenia, where antipsychotic treatment following first-episode psychosis is critical, people with disorders such as anxiety and depression may benefit as much, and in some cases more, from nonpharmacological interventions. This may depend on differences in pathophysiology and symptomatology. In all of these disorders, addressing biological, psychological, and social dimensions could do much to modulate neural and mental functions and improve their quality of life.

Antidepressant therapy in the form of SSRIs or SNRIs has been an improvement over the older-generation tricyclics and monoamine oxidase inhibitors. This is especially the case regarding side effects. Newer-generation antidepressants have side effects, but they tend to be more moderate and thus less likely to result in nonadherence and relapse. Still, some of these drugs may have severe side effects. Some patients taking the SSRI paroxetine have experienced akathisia. This is a psychomotor disturbance characterized by extreme agitation and restlessness. In a case reported in 2017, drug-induced akathisia caused suicidal ideation in a patient with depression who took his own life (Rabin, 2017).

Many studies have shown that a combination of antidepressant therapy and CBT produces better outcomes for patients with depression than drug therapy alone (Cuijpers, Sijbrandijs, Koole et al., 2013; Dubicka, Elvins, Roberts et al.,

2010; Wetherall, Petkus, White et al., 2013). Because psychosocial factors may be as critical as neurobiological factors in the etiology and symptomatology of major depression, CBT and pharmacology are complementary treatments. This technique works by enabling patients to reframe their beliefs, and identify and modify negative thoughts that generate a cycle of fearful thinking or impaired mood. CBT can be especially effective for unipolar depression and GAD, with positive outcomes in some forms of OCD as well. It is a good example of mind–brain interaction, where reframed beliefs can modulate prefrontal cortical function in a top-down manner and improve the impaired cognitive and emotional processing associated with these disorders. The modulating effects of the mind on the brain may also extend to limbic regions to which the PFC projects. One obvious advantage of CBT is that it avoids the adverse effects of antidepressants and anxiolytics. In severe forms of MDD, neural and mental dysfunction may be too extensive to be amenable to psychotherapy alone. Even with current forms of pharmacotherapy, many people with depression remain symptomatic. There is thus a need for newer-generation psychotropic drugs with different mechanisms of action.

Brain-level explanations for psychiatric disorders such as MDD identify dysfunction of neural circuits and neurotransmitters and connections between them. Drugs target neurotransmitter receptors associated with an excess (antagonists) or deficit (agonists) of circulating levels of neurotransmitters. As I mentioned at the beginning of this chapter, one explanation for poor response rates of patients with depression to antidepressant drugs is that they target monoamines, and these may not be the appropriate target. One recent study suggests that these low response rates may be due to poor selectivity of dopamine receptors. This is also a problem in selecting drugs for bipolar affective disorder. The identification of crystal structures in the D4 dopamine receptor and selective dopamine agonists may lead to the development of antidepressant drugs that would result in symptom control with fewer side effects (Wang, Wacker, Levit et al., 2017). This assumes that dopamine is the critical neurotransmitter. Neurotransmitters other than serotonin and dopamine may have a greater role in depression and other disorders. Studies have shown that the glutaminergic NMDAR noncompetitive antagonist ketamine produces rapid and sustained antidepressant effects after a single dose in patients with depression (Zanos, Moaddel, Morris et al., 2016; Zarate, Singh, Carlson et al., 2006). This is in contrast to monoaminergic antidepressants, which can take weeks or even months to produce a response, or no response at all.

These studies are significant because, against the general trend in psychopharmacology research, the pharmaceutical industry is funding them. In a more recent study, intranasal esketamine resulted in rapid improvement of depressive symptoms, including suicidal ideation, when compared with a placebo (Canuso, Singh, Fedgchin et al., 2018). While ketamine is associated with significant side effects, especially toxicity, researchers could regulate the metabolism of the drug to reduce or prevent them without weakening its positive effects. Ketamine "decreases the abnormally high levels of neural excitation and resting-state activity in depression" (Northoff, 2016, p. 95). The drug's "action seems to normalize abnormally high levels of arousal and excitation from which these patients suffer on a mental level" (Northoff, 2016, p. 95).

Despite its therapeutic potential, ketamine may have limitations as an antidepressant. These limitations reflect insufficient knowledge of its safety and efficacy for mood disorders. Treating these disorders with ketamine would be an off-label use of the drug distinct from its primary use as an anesthetic. At least five issues need to be addressed to gain the necessary knowledge and approval for clinical use (Naughton, Clark, O'Leary et al., 2014; Sanacora, Frye, McDonald et al., 2017; Zorumski and Conway, 2017).

First, there must be careful selection of patients. Because the risks and benefits are not known and it would be experimental therapy, ketamine should not be first-line treatment but an option for patients whose depression was treatment refractory. In addition to monoamine-mediated antidepressants, CBT, ECT, and comorbidities such as psychosis and substance abuse would be exclusionary conditions. Second, therapeutic levels of "dose, duration of infusion and route of administration for ketamine" (Zorumski and Conway, 2017, p. 405) are not well understood. Because of differences in patients' brains and variability in their responses to other drugs, there may be one standard protocol for route of administration, but different standards for dosing and duration of ketamine for patients. Dosing is especially important in avoiding toxic levels of the drug in the brain. Third, the "antidepressant effects of ketamine are transient, usually abating in about 1 week" (Zorumski and Conway, 2017, p. 406). Unlike other antidepressants, this is a trade-off from its rapid initial effect. It would require repeated infusions, which could be burdensome for patients having to travel regularly to medical clinics. Fourth, ketamine may have dopaminergic effects that can improve mood but also lead to abuse. Substance abuse and cognitive impairment could result from dosing above an optimal level (Sanacora, Frye, McDonald et al., 2017; Freedman, Brown, Cannon et al., 2018; Kokkinou, Ashok, and Howes 2018). Fifth, ketamine can have psychotomimetic effects. It is not known whether other drugs used to dampen these effects and prevent psychosis would also dampen the antidepressant effects on mood. Presumably, researchers could do this by regulating the metabolism and dosing of ketamine.

More research consisting of placebo- or active controlled clinical trials with a significant number of subjects is necessary to answer questions about the dosing, duration, and frequency of ketamine administration for depression. The research will also have to answer questions about its interactions with other drugs, as well as its effects on bodily systems outside of the CNS. All of these questions require resolution in order to know whether ketamine will become a preferred treatment for depression.

Results from some experiments suggest that the hallucinogen psilocybin could be a treatment for anxiety and depression when combined with psychological support. A study testing this drug on patients with advanced breast, gastrointestinal, and blood cancers resulted in a significant reduction in mental distress (Ross, Bossis, Guss et al., 2016). The drug induces an altered state of consciousness in which there is a substantial change in one's experience of space and time. In addition to peacefulness and an increased feeling of altruism, some people taking psilocybin have reported experiencing a dissociation of the self from the body. Others have reported experiencing a dissolution of the self into the world, leaving no clear boundary between them. The control drug in the study just mentioned was niacin, which has no discernable effect on the content of mental states. This leaves open the possibility of a placebo effect of psilocybin, though it is unlikely that a person would have the same experience from a placebo.

The design of the trial was problematic. Subjects in the experimental group would quickly know that they were in this group from the effects of the drug on them. More importantly, there are significant differences between patients or research subjects with advanced cancer and a limited life expectancy and those with chronic anxiety or depression over many years regarding acceptable risks. Cancer patients experience these symptoms as a secondary response to cancer. The subjects in the psilocybin study experienced psychological distress related to a somatic disease. Depressed patients have these symptoms as a primary response to a psychiatric disorder. It is also significant that hallucinogens can induce psychosis. This may be acceptable as a form of palliative care in the last weeks or months of one's life. But drug-induced psychosis in psychiatric research is not acceptable because of the risk of harm to research subjects and possibly others. Rather than ameliorate symptoms, psilocybin could introduce a second psychopathology in addition to anxiety or depression. The investigators in the psilocybin study noted that schizophrenia would be an exclusionary condition given the risk of psychosis. This exclusion could also be applied to the subtype of depression with a predisposition to psychosis.

The idea of dissolving the self with psilocybin seems to offer a way of resolving the problem of excessive self-focus in depression. Yet if the drug produced the experience of dissociation of the self from the body and the environment, then it could have the opposite effect of increasing self-focus. Dissociation of the self from the body and environment could undermine agency by undermining the embodiment and embeddedness that are necessary for a person to form and execute action plans. By altering consciousness and distorting information from the body and the world, the drug would impair the capacity for goal-directed behavior. Even if psilocybin caused a person to feel more altruistic, the altered cognition from the drug would weaken her capacity to translate this feeling into action. The altered content of the person's mental states would interfere with the capacity for reasoning and decision-making.

Admittedly, these considerations are speculative. A more recent study of psilocybin as a treatment for depression as a primary psychiatric disorder provides a more solid empirical basis for assessing the therapeutic potential of the drug (Carhart-Harris, Roseman, Bolstridge et al., 2017). In the 19 patients participating in the study, there was increased resting-state blood flow and functional connectivity measured by fMRI following administration of the drug. All the patients experienced decreased depressive symptoms 1 week after treatment, and approximately half had symptom improvement at 5 weeks. The study authors point out that "its findings suggest that changes in brain activity observed just one day after a high-dose psychedelic experience are very different to those found during the acute psychedelic state. Specifically, whereas the acute psychedelic state in healthy volunteers is characterized by modular disintegration and global integration, there are trends toward modular (re)integration and minimal effects on global integration/segregation post-psilocybin for depression" (Carhart-Harris, Roseman, Bolstridge et al., 2017, p. 2). The authors acknowledge that the small number of subjects and the absence of a control arm limited the statistical significance of the study's results.

Many randomized, placebo-controlled clinical trials are necessary to determine whether either or both of these rapid-acting drugs would be safe and effective treatment for anxiety and depression. While the research is still at a preliminary stage, ketamine seems more promising than psilocybin as a therapeutic agent for these disorders. As an anesthetic agent, ketamine is delivered intravenously, which requires careful monitoring to reduce the risk of neurological and psychological sequelae from high concentrations that could be toxic to the brain. Multicenter trials are currently being conducted on ketamine. An intranasal version of the drug may be on the market in the next 2 years. If ketamine were proven to be a safe and effective treatment for depression, then it could radically transform the neurophysiological model for understanding and treating this and other psychiatric disorders. Its rapid-acting neuromodulating effects on glutaminergic pathways could overcome the limitations of monoaminergic drugs and be more beneficial for patients. Studies of the psychedelic phenomenology of compounds such as subanesthetic ketamine, psilocybin, and lysergic acid diethylamide may shed light on the complex relations between the level and content of consciousness. They may support the hypothesis that psychiatric disorders are disorders of consciousness (Schartner, Carhart-Harris, Barrett et al., 2017).

Other innovative treatments may develop for anxiety, panic, and PTSD based on the hypothesis that they are disorders of memory content in a dysregulated fear memory system. Pharmacological blockade of memory reconsolidation may become a therapeutic option for these disorders (Pitman, 2015). Memories that have been consolidated need to be reconsolidated, or updated, to remain stored as information in the brain (Nader, Schafe, and LeDoux, 2000; Nader and Einarsson, 2010). This occurs when they are retrieved in conscious or unconscious recall of the original experience. One way of treating PTSD would be to weaken or erase the memory representation or trace in the amygdala by disrupting reconsolidation. This would occur during or immediately after retrieval because memories are labile and susceptible to alteration at this time. Psychiatrist Roger Pitman explains, "For reconsolidation blockade, or updating, to be successful, two steps are required: first, the problematic memory must be destabilized; second, its re-stabilization (reconsolidation) must then be prevented or modified (updated)" (2011, p. 2, 2015).

The technique of extinction training can weaken conditioned fear responses to cues associated with the memory of the original experience (Kindt, Soeter, and Vervliet, 2009). The subject learns to dissociate the memory of the experience from the cues, which weakens the emotional content of the memory and the patient's response to it. Similarly, conditioning can allow fear memories to be updated with nonfearful information provided during reconsolidation (Schiller, Monfils, Raoi et al., 2010). This may eventually allow more recent normal episodic and semantic memories to replace older fear memories in the brain and mind's information store.

Reconsolidation blockade using drugs may have greater therapeutic potential than behavioral interventions for these memories. The beta-adrenergic receptor antagonist propranolol can interfere with noradrenergic mechanisms and weaken the emotionally charged content of the memory while leaving its cognitive content intact (Pitman, Sanders, Zusman et al., 2002; Lonergan, Oliveira-Figueroa, Pitman et al., 2013). Yet the fact that the emotional trace of the memory is weakened but not erased using behavioral techniques and propranolol leaves open the possibility that aversive stimuli could reactivate its emotional representation and reactivate the psychopathology. As Ryan Parsons and Kerry Ressler point out, these stimuli "can sensitize patients with fear-related disorders and lead to worsening of the disorder" (2013, p. 151).

A more effective form of reconsolidation blockade would be one that not just weakened but erased the emotional trace of the memory. Because reconsolidation requires protein synthesis, a drug that blocked protein synthesis could block reconsolidation. Infusion of a protein synthesis inhibitor such as anisomycin into the basolateral amygdala during memory retrieval could prevent reconsolidation and erase any trace of the memory (Agren, Engman, Frick et al., 2012; Parsons and Ressler, 2013; LeDoux, 2015, pp. 281–282, 301–309; Soeter and Kind, 2015). The drug would do this by interfering with long-term potentiation (LTP) and the transcription factor cyclic-AMP response element binding-protein (CREB), both of which regulate protein synthesis and its effects on mechanisms regulating long-term memory. The drug would erase the memory, not by ablating it, but by selectively weakening or inactivating neurons and synaptic connectivity within the memory trace. These neurons would be localized within a discrete region of the amygdala. Functional imaging during retrieval of the fear memory could identify these neurons and confirm their inactivation after infusing the drug. This could eliminate the possibility of reactivation of a heightened emotional response to stimuli associated with the memory if there were no trace to be reactivated. Erasing pathological fear memories through pharmacological blockade of reconsolidation has been attempted only in animal models. As it is still a hypothetical intervention in humans, any claims about erasing these memories as therapy for anxiety, phobia, panic, depression, and PTSD must be made tentatively.

There are a number of challenges in using this intervention as therapy for these psychiatric disorders. One challenge is that the longer a memory has been stored in the brain, the more difficult it is to destabilize and alter it. Parsons and Ressler note that "older and stronger memories are less susceptible to disruption after retrieval" and that "it may prove difficult to disrupt traumatic memories after retrieval because these memories are most certainly strong and in many cases have persisted for some time" (2013, p. 151). Older memories may be less susceptible to disruption after retrieval due to strengthened synaptic connectivity from the effects of LTP, cyclic-AMP response element binding-protein CREB, and protein synthesis. To be effective, reconsolidation blockade would have to occur not long after the memory had been encoded and consolidated in the hippocampus and amygdala.

Another challenge is selectivity. Even if the targeted neurons constituting the memory trace were localized in a discrete region of the basolateral amygdala, it is not clear that these neurons could be inactivated while leaving other neurons associated with other normal memories intact. It is not known whether the drug would have expanding effects in normal functioning adjacent nuclei. Not all memories of fearful events are maladaptive or pathological. Many are adaptive and necessary for survival by enabling us to recognize and respond appropriately to external threats. Weakening or erasing these memories could make us vulnerable to these threats or produce a new psychopathology. Nor is it known whether a protein synthesis inhibitor or other means of erasing fear memories would affect normal emotional memories mediated by other regions of the limbic system and prefrontal regions to which it projects. As with the other novel interventions I have considered, these questions can be answered only after a sufficient number of clinical trials on memory modification involving a sufficient number of human subjects have been conducted.

A novel treatment for PTSD is already in an advanced experimental phase for humans. In May 2017, the US Food and Drug Administration (FDA) approved phase III clinical trials to test the drug MDMA as therapy for the disorder (Maxmen, 2017). Preliminary results of studies have shown that the drug reduced anxiety and nightmares and improved information processing in some subjects. These effects are associated with the drug's ability to decrease activity in the amygdala and increase activity in the PFC. It does this by increasing circulating levels of serotonin in the brain. This drug and psilocybin are similar in that both have a psychedelic compound that alters cognitive and emotional processing. MDMA would be used therapeutically in combination with psychotherapy in controlled settings of psychiatric research and practice.

Uncontrolled use of MDMA could result in toxicity and lethal overdosing, as has occurred among some people using it as a recreational drug. One neurophysiological risk of chronic use of the drug at higher doses is the serotonin syndrome. This syndrome occurs in approximately 14–16% of persons who overdose on SSRIs. Symptoms may include euphoria, drowsiness, hyperactive reflexes, rapid muscle contractions, hyperthermia, confusion, hypomania, and, in severe cases, coma and death (Boyer and Shannon, 2005). This risk is greater than the risk of using SSRIs for depression or anxiety. While SSRIs prevent reuptake of serotonin in the synaptic cleft in these disorders, MDMA could increase circulating levels of serotonin in brains where they may be normal. Even if the risks associated with chronic use of MDMA were minimal, the drug would not weaken or erase the memory of the experience that triggers PTSD. Combined with psychotherapy, the drug could ameliorate some of the symptoms of PTSD by modulating the neural dysfunction underlying them. Still, it is questionable whether MDMA's mechanism of action would allow it to target the neural source of the disorder precisely enough to eradicate it.

A major problem in identifying safe and effective pharmacological treatments for psychiatric disorders is the heterogeneity of their pathophysiology and symptoms. This can result in variable responses to them among patients. Genetic, epigenetic, neurobiological, neuroimmune, neuroendocrine, psychosocial, and environmental factors have been implicated in these disorders. It is difficult to identify which of these factors have a greater role in the development of different types and subtypes of these disorders. It is also difficult to explain why some conditions respond to drug therapy while others remain treatment-resistant. This complicates efforts to arrive at an overarching hypothesis for their underlying neurobiology. Indeed, the idea that there could be such a hypothesis may be misguided.

Paul Holtzheimer and Helen Mayberg state that "the current construct of depression, as defined for the purposes of clinical and basic research, has lost its utility" (2011, p. 2). They point to the "inadequacy of available antidepressant treatments" and conclude that, "a shift is needed in the definition of depression and the research agenda going forward" (2011, p. 2). One way of making progress is to shift away from the monoamine hypothesis as the basis for understanding and treating psychiatric disorders. Instead of focusing mainly on serotonin in depression, psychopharmacology could be designed to modulate transmission in glutaminergic pathways and their interactions with neural circuitry. Similarly, instead of focusing mainly on dopamine in schizophrenia, psychopharmacology could aim at modulating interaction between gamma-aminobutyric acid (GABA) and glutamate. This is supported by comments in an editorial by Anissa Abi-Dargham: "A core pathology in schizophrenia is the imbalance in inhibition and excitation in cortical circuits related to alterations in the inhibitory neurotransmitter gamma-aminobutyric acid (GABA) and the excitatory neurotransmitter glutamate, resulting in suboptimal synchronization of neural circuits needed for cognitive function" (2015, p. 1062). Dysfunction in the NMDAR may be the key neurotransmission abnormality in both major depression and schizophrenia. This is one reason why ketamine has considerable therapeutic potential. It is also possible that future psychotropic drug therapies will be based on neural mechanisms that have not yet been discovered.

One way of improving response rates to drug therapy is to adopt a symptom clustering approach (Chekroud, Gueorguieva Krumholz et al., 2017). In depression, for example, identifying clusters of symptoms may be one way of measuring severity and lead to more accurate prediction of responsiveness to antidepressant medications. While in general there are differences in symptoms across psychiatric disorders, there is overlap in symptoms between particular disorders. For example, people with a subtype of MDD and GAD associated with a hyperactive fear memory system have similar symptoms. There are also similarities in symptoms of people with a different subtype of depression and the negative subtype of schizophrenia, where flat affect, anhedonia, and avolition are associated with a dysfunctional reward system. Selecting a drug that could treat symptoms in a cluster could produce greater benefit than one targeting isolated symptoms. Clustering may have limited therapeutic value, however, in diseases with mixed states, as in BD, or in diseases with very different symptom subtypes, such as schizophrenia. Even where there are commonalities and overlap between mental diseases, treating symptom clusters with a drug would not automatically result in symptom relief for everyone who took it. As noted by Insel in a passage cited in Chapter 1, treatment responses depend not just on symptoms but also on biological factors that underlie symptoms.

Clustering has to include a larger set of data from genetics, neuroimaging, electrophysiological recording, and cognitive and emotional processing. Nevertheless, symptom clustering could lead to more targeted drug therapy for overlapping disorders. With close monitoring of symptoms over time rather than at one time, clustering motor and mental symptoms could result in more effective treatment than disorder- and symptom-specific approaches. This could limit the nondiscriminating effects of drugs, reduce side effects, and benefit a significant number of patients.

A more promising approach to treatment may be to combine psychiatric genetics with structural and functional imaging to identify biomarkers for abnormalities in brain regions mediating cognition, mood, and motivation. Psychiatric genetics would involve investigating how genes regulate synaptic connectivity in dopaminergic, serotonergic, glutaminergic, and GABAergic systems, as well as how genes encode receptors and signaling proteins for neurotransmission. Identifying dysfunction in brain regions with neuroimaging could help to clarify differences between unipolar and bipolar depression, for example, and result in more accurate diagnosis of these disorders. More careful drug selection based on these biomarkers could help to prevent or control manic and depressive episodes. It could help to avoid situations in which controlling one set of symptoms resulted in exacerbating others. Currently, the most promising area of biomarker research in psychiatry is predicting responses to different treatments.

In a study involving patients with MDD, hypometabolism in the insula displayed by functional neuroimaging (PET) was associated with a positive response to CBT in symptom reduction but a poor response to the SSRI escitalopram. In contrast, hypermetabolism in the insula was associated with a positive response to the drug and a poor response to CBT. The study showed that a treatment-specific biomarker could guide treatment selection for patients with MDD (McGrath, Kelley, Holtzheimer et al., 2013). Another imaging study of schizophrenia patients with first-episode schizophrenia showed cortical–striatal dysconnectivity. The researchers hypothesized that increased functional connectivity of the striatum with prefrontal and limbic regions may be a biomarker for improvement of symptoms from antipsychotic medication (Sarpal,

Robinson, and Lencz et al., 2015). A third study using voxel-based morphometry showed greater reductions in gray matter volume in the hippocampal formation and amygdala among individuals with bipolar depression compared with individuals with unipolar depression. This finding can help to clarify diagnosis and improve treatment for patients at different points along the depression spectrum (Redlich, Almeida, Grotegerd et al., 2014). Using imaging to confirm differences between unipolar and bipolar depression could overcome the challenges of treating mixed manic and depressive states and avoid antidepressants that could trigger mania. Imaging identifying critical biomarkers could optimize treatment for BD.

By identifying specific signatures of dysfunctional neural connectivity and neurotransmission and combining it with genetic and environmental analysis, biomarker research could promote precision medicine in psychiatry (Jameson and Longo, 2015). It could promote more accurate prediction and confirmation of how and why individuals respond, or fail to respond, to different treatments. Still, genetics and imaging biomarkers alone will not enable psychiatrists to predict whether a patient will respond to pharmacotherapy or the extent to which she will respond. Again, this is because of the heterogeneity of pathophysiology and variability of symptoms among patients. It is unlikely that identifying particular brain biomarkers, such as the one reported by McGrath and coauthors, will have a significant impact on treating psychiatric disorders in general. Although the identification of more neuroanatomical and neurophysiological signatures through genetic analysis and neuroimaging will contribute to a better understanding of psychiatric disorders, it will not provide a complete explanation of different response rates to psychotropic drugs. This depends on other factors in the body, brain, and mind in addition to gene expression, neuroanatomy, and neurophysiology.

There is also the risk of psychological harm to patients if they have unreasonable expectations about benefit based on an overly optimistic interpretation of brain biomarkers and fail to respond to treatment. More tailored therapies based on advances in neuroscience will not always result in a positive response to these therapies. "Precision" medicine thus will always involve some degree of uncertainty in psychiatry. This has to be included in the informed consent process in research and clinical settings to reduce the risk of harm to research subjects and patients.

The future development of potentially safer and more effective therapeutic drugs for psychiatric disorders remains unclear. In 2013, Steven Hyman spelled out a major problem that may preclude the realization of this potential. "During the past three years, the global pharmaceutical industry has significantly decreased its investment in new treatments for depression, BD, schizophrenia and other psychiatric disorders. Some companies have closed their psychiatric laboratories entirely . . . This retreat has occurred despite the fact that mental disorders are not only common worldwide but . . . there is, moreover, vast unmet medical need. . . . This withdrawal reflects a widely shared view that the underlying science remains immature and that therapeutic development in psychiatry is simply too difficult and too risky" (Hyman, 2013, p. 2). What is risky here is not the possible physiological effects on patients but the financial effects on the pharmaceutical industry. The estimated profit from marketing drugs might not outweigh the cost of developing and testing them. There may not be enough of a return on their investment to justify funding studies of psychotropic drugs to determine their safety and efficacy. The fact that all major pharmaceutical companies have stopped or markedly decreased their investment in psychopharmacology has created a therapeutic vacuum in psychiatry.

This raises a social justice issue. In principle, patients with medical needs in general and psychiatric needs in particular have a right to receive therapy that will ameliorate their symptoms. Insofar as they do not benefit from psychotherapy and can benefit from pharmacotherapy as first-line treatment, presumably they would have a right to access psychotropic drugs. As a matter of economics and financial survival, though, pharmaceutical companies are not obligated and cannot be expected to develop and test new drugs without considering cost and profit. Data indicating that a significant number of patients with depression, for example, do not benefit from psychotropic drugs is another disincentive to continue drug development. This problem is similar in some respects to social justice issues regarding the role of device manufacturers in enabling people to participate in clinical trials testing the safety and efficacy of DBS, which I discuss in Chapter 4.

Magnitude of the problem is greater with psychotropic drugs because they are the first-line treatment for psychiatric disorders and are taken by a much larger number of patients. Many could benefit from novel therapeutic agents. This is an issue requiring coordinated work by medical professionals, health policy analysts, political representatives, and patient advocates to promote rather than thwart the development of next-generation, rapid-acting, and safe antidepressant, antipsychotic, and other psychotropic drugs. In schizophrenia, drugs modulating glutaminergic transmission in the brain might not just reduce psychotic symptoms but also the metabolic and cardiovascular side effects of typical and atypical antipsychotics. These are more debilitating than the side effects of antidepressants. This could reduce the incidence of nonadherence among patients with schizophrenia. Despite current knowledge of the abnormal neural circuitry and neural transmission associated with psychiatric disorders, a better understanding of the underlying science of the brain and mind is necessary for the development of new psychotropic drugs that will maximize benefit and minimize harm for the millions of people who suffer from these disorders. Many people with severe psychiatric disorders do not respond to current pharmacotherapy and will not respond to novel psychotropic drugs in the future. They must turn to alternative forms of neuromodulation.

Much of the neuroethics literature has been devoted to discussion of reasons for and against cognitive and moral enhancement using psychotropic drugs. The idea is that these drugs could enable people to perform better on cognitive tasks or become more responsive to moral reasons for not harming others. In the 1990s and early 2000s, there were anecdotal reports of people "enhancing" normal levels of mood by taking SSRIs (Kramer, 1993, 2005, 2016). Research showing that antidepressants for mild to moderate depression were no better than placebos cast suspicion on these reports (Kirsch, Deacon, Huedo-Medina et al. 2008; Fournier, DeRubeis, Hollon et al., 2010). There have been recent reports that the wakefulness-promoting drug modafinil can enhance episodic and working memory in some patients whose depression is in remission (Lyon, 2017). Yet if these cognitive functions are impaired to begin with, then it is inaccurate to describe modafinil as an enhancer for these patients. There are also risks. Sleep disturbances are a common symptom of depression. Altering normal sleep–wake cycles and circadian rhythms could disrupt homeostasis and cause a relapse of the disorder. The ability to move between sleep and attention states is an adaptation to the environment. If the brain is in a constant state of attention, then some regions mediating cognition could become overloaded with information. This could impair reasoning and other cognitive functions (Zhang, Zhu, Zhan et al., 2014). In this regard, unnecessary wakefulness can be more problematic than unnecessary sleep.

Conducting the research necessary to determine whether these drugs had these effects and that they were not just a placebo response would be conceptually and ethically problematic. It is doubtful that tinkering with neurotransmitters alone will improve a person's academic or athletic performance. Nor will a psychotropic drug by itself make a person more cooperative or altruistic. More importantly, the research would expose healthy subjects to potentially toxic levels of biochemically active substances. Hyman points out that testing toxic chemicals in people "who have no clear illness is hugely unlikely to get the go-ahead in our current climate" (2013, p. 20). Researchers intending to conduct clinical trials testing the presumed enhancing effects of the drugs on cognition or moral sensitivity could have difficulty receiving ethics approval to conduct them. The risks entailed by exposing normal brains to potentially toxic levels of drugs, and lack of criteria for measuring long-term outcomes of enhancement, would make pharmaceutical companies reluctant to fund trials testing cognition-enhancing effects of drugs. They would likely be even more reluctant to fund enhancement studies than studies aimed at developing theories for psychiatric disorders.

Not all studies of cognitive enhancement involve toxic levels of drugs. A recent placebo-controlled experiment showed that methylphenidate and modafinil enhanced chess performance when players were not under time pressure (Franke, Gransmark, Agricola et al., 2017). The investigators concluded that the drugs may have had this effect by enhancing reflective decision-making processes. Still, the study tested the drugs' effect on a specific cognitive task rather than on cognitive functions in general. It also showed that, "under time constraints, more reflective decision-making may not improve or even have detrimental effects on complex task performance" (Franke, Gransmark, Agricola et al., 2017, p. 248). Insofar as these detrimental effects are associated with the stimulants, they may be an example of trade-offs in cognitive enhancement. Enhancing some cognitive functions may come at the cost of impairing others.

Some proponents of enhancement argue that there is no clear demarcation between therapy and enhancement (Harris, 2007). There is no significant difference between improving neural and mental functions to normal levels and raising them above these levels. Depending on what these effects are and where they fall along a functional continuum, some interventions described as therapies could also be described as enhancements. Nevertheless, in severe psychiatric disorders, the distinction between therapy and enhancement should be upheld. Psychopharmacology for these disorders is correctly described as therapy because it aims to restore dysfunctional neural and mental functions to normal levels. "Normal" is consistent with any process that restores or maintains homeostasis in the brain and body of the organism and enables a person to perform a range of motor and mental tasks. The very idea of enhancement for these disorders should be questioned. Healthy brains and minds require optimal levels of neurotransmitters and connectivity between neural circuits. This ensures a balance between excitatory and inhibitory mechanisms in the brain. Raising these mechanisms above optimal levels could result in manic or compulsive behavior that could harm the patient and others. Based on studies of the potential benefits and side effects of cognition-enhancing drugs in adults and especially the elderly, Sharon Straus states that "there is no high-quality evidence to support the use of cognitive enhancers in healthy people" (cited by Lyon, 2017, p. 4).

Many severe psychiatric disorders fail to respond to drug therapy, and the disorders remain treatment-resistant. Among people with MDD, as many as 30% may remain symptomatic following first-line treatment (Holtzheimer and Mayberg, 2010, p. 1437). It is possible that further development of designer receptors exclusively activated by designer drugs (DREADDS) would lead to more effective psychopharmacology for these disorders. DREADDS are chemogenetically engineered proteins that can regulate presynaptic release of glutamate and other neurotransmitters as well as synaptic transmission in neural circuits (Roth, 2016). The chemogenetic properties of these drugs may allow for a degree of specificity regarding dysfunctional neural targets that is lacking in existing psychotropic drugs. Like other novel drugs, a significant number of human clinical trials would have to be conducted to achieve a better understanding of their mechanisms of action, dose toxicity, and potentially adverse effects.

Nonpharmacological interventions have been effective in treating some of these disorders. These interventions involve different types of neuromodulation. They also involve different models for weighing potential and actual benefit against potential and actual harm. I discuss them in the remainder of this chapter and in Chapter 4.

## Invasive versus noninvasive treatments: a misleading distinction

Ethical questions about treatments for psychiatric disorders often revolve around invasiveness. This falls along a medical and ethical continuum. Generally, more invasive treatments entail greater risks than less invasive treatments. It is more difficult to ethically justify the first type than the second type. But more invasive treatments may offer greater benefits, despite their risks. Two types of risk need to be considered: the risk associated with the neurointervention; and the risk associated with not treating a chronic psychiatric disorder. The potential benefit of more or less invasive treatments need to be assessed against both types of risk. The fact that DBS involves intracranial neurosurgery and activation of circuits in the brain does entail certain risks. Yet the nondiscriminating effects of psychotropic drugs in the brain involve their own set of risks, despite being less invasive. Indeed, the very concept of invasiveness needs critical examination in order to determine its significance in the ethical justification of intervening in the brain. It is important to examine this general concept and some of its ethical implications before discussing specific ethical questions raised by specific nonpharmacological interventions.

A typical definition of an invasive technique in clinical neuroscience is one that penetrates the skull and involves direct contact of a probe or other instrument with neural tissue. The *Oxford English Dictionary* (*OED*) defines a noninvasive medical treatment as "a diagnostic or therapeutic procedure that does not require the insertion of instruments . . . through the skin or into a body cavity." A second medical definition of "noninvasive" says that it involves "not spreading into adjacent tissue from an initial site of development or colonization" (*OED*, 2003, p. 1057). The implantation of electrodes in the brain in DBS and neural ablation are examples of invasive techniques in psychiatric treatment. "Noninvasive" suggests a procedure in which the skull is intact and no device is implanted in the brain. Yet the distributed effects of ECT and the potential of the effects of TMS and tCS to spread beyond targeted regions in the brain suggest that these techniques should also be described as invasive. Another invasive technique not involving intracranial surgery is Gamma Knife˚ radiosurgery (GKR). The procedure consists in directing a focused beam of gamma radiation to a particular site in the brain. It has been used to resect tumors and malformations in the brain, as well as a form of neural ablation for dystonia and OCD. Despite the focused beam and the absence of intracranial surgery, the effects of the Gamma Knife˚ can spread beyond the targeted area to adjacent healthy tissue. This may result in neurological and psychiatric sequelae even though there is no cutting through the skull.

Nick Davis and Martijn van Koningsbruggen point out that the potential for expanding effects on neural circuits and tissue not targeted by nonsurgical techniques "is in itself contrary to the definition of 'noninvasiveness'" (2013, p. 1). Focusing on TMS and tCS, the authors argue that these techniques are invasive insofar as "induced currents spread from the point of delivery through the brain (and nearby tissues) to adjacent regions. This spread is large in the case of tCS compared to the relatively focal sphere of stimulation in the clearly invasive procedure of DBS" (2013, p. 2). Davis and van Koningsbruggen further argue that the different neuromodulation technique of optogenetics should also be classified as invasive, "since the stimulation (light) must pass through multiple layers of tissue, and possibly beyond, to activate the target cells . . ." (2013, p. 1). These authors are referring to the nonimplantable form of optogenetics, and this underscores their point about invasiveness. They recommend that TMS and tCS "be referred to simply as 'brain stimulation,' without the potentially misleading qualifier of 'noninvasive'" (2013, p. 2).

Similar remarks apply to ECT for unipolar and bipolar depression. Seizure induction in this technique is another form of stimulation with effects that may expand beyond the brain region identified as the source of dysregulation. Not all effects of neurostimulation would necessarily be harmful. Apart from whether they are positive or negative, a focal sphere of stimulation does not preclude the possibility of expanding effects beyond the targeted area. They may occur from procedures that penetrate the skull and from procedures that do not. "Noninvasive" may create the illusion of safety or minimal risk. Intracranial surgery and implantation of a device in the brain entail risks of infection, edema, and hemorrhage that nonsurgical procedures avoid. Nevertheless, the fact that ECT, TMS, tCS, and other procedures can alter brain function, and that this alteration may be distributed across regions of the brain, indicates that a patient or research subject can be exposed to risk even when the skull is not cut open and no device is implanted in the brain.

All forms of electrical brain stimulation can alter neural circuits and tissue with intended and unintended consequences. Any technique that has these effects in the brain is invasive in the broad sense of the term and entails some risk. Whether a procedure is invasive or noninvasive is more than a function of whether it involves intracranial surgery. Accordingly, the distinction between invasive and noninvasive techniques that apply electrical stimulation to the brain should be replaced by the distinction between more and less invasive techniques. To fully inform patients and research subjects of the risks in undergoing these procedures and prevent misunderstanding and potential psychological harm from unexpected outcomes, researchers and practitioners should adopt the second *OED* definition of "invasive." They should include information about altering circuits or tissue at a targeted site, as well as the possibility of altering nontargeted circuits or tissue, in explaining the nature, purpose, and potential effects of neurostimulation techniques for psychiatric disorders. They would be obligated to do this because of their duty of nonmaleficence in preventing harm to patients and research subjects.

Replacing the binary invasive versus noninvasive distinction with the distinction between more and less invasive neuromodulating techniques suggests that the mechanisms and effects of these interventions in the brain and mind fall along a continuum. They involve differences of degree rather than kind. More importantly, what matters is not just whether an intervention is more or less invasive, but what the potential benefits are and how these weigh against the risks. Intuitively, the more invasive a procedure is, the more risk it entails and the less likely it is to benefit patients. But more invasive procedures may have a more favorable benefit–risk ratio. This is especially the case when a disorder has not responded to less invasive treatments and the risk of harm from a treatment-resistant disorder is significant.

## Electroconvulsive therapy

Developed in the late 1930s, ECT for the treatment of unipolar and bipolar depression consists in applying electrical current to the scalp to induce seizures in regions of the brain implicated in these disorders. Patients are anesthetized during the procedure. Although psychiatrists do not completely understand the mechanisms behind the effects of ECT, the seizures can have a modulating effect on dysfunctional circuits and relieve depressive symptoms for some patients (Lisanby, 2007). Its most important property is its rapid onset of action, which can prevent suicide in patients with acute depressive episodes. Antidepressant therapy typically precedes and follows a number of applications of the technique. "A course of ECT is typically 6 to 12 treatments, administered three times weekly (in the United States) or twice weekly (in Britain) . . . It is widely used in geriatric depression" (Goodman, 2011, p. 1785). The technique has also been used for bipolar mania and catatonia in schizophrenia (Goodman, 2011, p. 1785). It may seem paradoxical that inducing seizures could have a therapeutic effect, but the seizures can increase concentrations of serotonin and the major inhibitory neurotransmitter GABA in the cerebral cortex. Since these neurotransmitters are involved in mood regulation, the therapeutic effects of ECT can restore normal levels of mood in some depressed patients (Sanacora, Mason, Rothman et al., 2003; Husain, Rush, Fink et al., 2004). ECT may also modulate activity in the HPA axis, dysregulation of which has been associated with anxiety and some forms of depression. In addition, results of a recent study of ECT suggest that the brain activity it induces could promote neuroplasticity and neurogenesis (Dukart, Regen, Kherif et al., 2014).

Ken Kesey's 1962 novel, *One Flew Over the Cuckoo's Nest*, and especially the 1975 film version with Jack Nicolson, misleadingly depicted ECT as a barbaric procedure (Kesey, 1962). The book and film generated a critical reaction to and mistrust of psychiatry. They contributed to the antipsychiatry movement led by Szasz in the 1960s and 1970s and the stigma associated with mental illness in general. Arguably, this novel and film have generated more misunderstanding of mental illness and have done more to damage the reputation of psychiatry than any other media form. A fair and accurate description of research on ECT and its effects on brain and mental function can help to disabuse the public of a negative perception of the technique. This can shift the focus from the observable behavior of those undergoing the procedure to its therapeutic potential while acknowledging its risks.

Studies indicate that ECT can be especially effective in treating unipolar depression in older adults by modulating dysfunctional frontal–striatal–limbic pathways. Response rates have been higher in older patients with the psychotic subtype of depression in this cohort. The rapid onset of psychosis among many patients in this group underscores the importance of ECT's rapid onset of action. Still, as Sarah Lisanby points out, "although ECT is more effective than antidepressant medication in this group, it is typically reserved for use after several medication trials because of it relatively higher risk of side effects" (2007, p. 1941). In addition to the risk of general anesthesia, the most problematic of these effects is the retrograde amnesia that a significant number of patients experience after undergoing the technique. A recent controlled study showed that there was no significant association between ECT and the risk of dementia over a median follow-up period of five years (Olson, Rozing, Christensen et al., 2018).

Combined with potential cognitive impairment and comorbidities in elderly patients with depression, the higher risk of side effects from ECT compared with pharmacology may make these patients a vulnerable group in need of protection. In particular, there may be questions about whether these patients have the cognitive and affective capacity to give informed consent to undergo the procedure. Discussion between the patient and the practitioner, as well as family, is necessary to determine whether they have sufficient mental capacity to consent. As a matter of fairness, elderly patients with depression who have not responded to CBT and drug therapy should have the same opportunity to benefit from ECT as younger patients with depression who have benefited from it. Nevertheless, the greater likelihood of cognitive impairment among the elderly highlights the need for caution among practitioners in explaining the potential benefits and risks of the procedure and obtaining informed consent from patients. This is particularly the case in patients with what Lisanby describes as "depression-executive dysfunction syndrome" associated with vascular neurodegenerative factors (2007, p. 1940).

Lisanby further states that "the decision to use ECT depends on several factors, including the severity and chronicity of the patient's depression, the likelihood that alternative treatments would be effective, the patient's preference, and the weighing of risks and benefits" (2007, p. 1941). Severity and chronicity and a poor response to antidepressant therapy would justify offering ECT as an alternative treatment. Yet this would depend on the patient's understanding of the known and potential side effects of ECT and the ability to process this information in deciding to undergo the procedure. As part of this process, the practitioner would be obligated to inform the patient that maintenance ECT may be necessary even if the depression goes into remission after one or several sessions.

One of the problems with this technique is that its effects can be nonspecific, spatially unfocused, and distributed over different brain regions. Some of these regions may not have any of the dysfunction in regions associated with unipolar or bipolar depression. Although ECT is typically described as a noninvasive procedure, these effects could make it invasive on the broader interpretation of the concept. Studies have demonstrated that more precise placement of electrodes on the right side of the head and unilateral activation of the right hemisphere relieved symptoms and had fewer side effects in two groups of patients with unipolar and bipolar depression (Goodman 2011; Dukart, Regen, Kherif et al., 2014). Another challenge in using ECT is that patients within these two groups may respond differently to it because of differences in the underlying pathophysiology. Still, inducing more specific seizure activity can improve mood in both groups and reduce the risk of triggering mania in those with bipolar depression. More speculatively, the potential neuroplastic and neurogenerative effects of ECT may go some way toward explaining its efficacy in older adults with depression. Many of these patients have age-related neurodegeneration associated with impaired cognition and mood. These effects could help to control the disease and its symptoms. This is an example of how one form of depression may be more of a neurodegenerative than a neurodevelopmental disorder.

Cognitive impairment and retrograde amnesia are the most common adverse effects of ECT. The induced seizures seem to disrupt memory consolidation in the hippocampus and long-term memory storage in the neocortex. More focal seizure induction that avoids the hippocampus and memory storage sites in the neocortex might be one way of reducing the incidence of memory loss (Lisanby, Maddox, Prudic et al., 2000). For many patients undergoing ECT, any retrograde amnesia is temporary and resolves after a relatively short time. For others, however, it does not resolve and can be severely debilitating. Patients who experience only short-term amnesia may find the trade-off between even temporary relief and memory loss to be acceptable. In contrast, those who experience permanent loss of episodic memories extending back 10, 15 years or more, will likely find the trade-off between even sustained relief and amnesia to be unacceptable. There is variability in the incidence, degree, and duration of memory loss and recovery among patients. Consistent with the pattern of responses to other treatments for psychiatric disorders in general and depression in particular, each patient's experience with ECT will be unique.

Nevertheless, as Wayne Goodman points out, "reports of permanent erasure of some personal memories after ECT cannot be ignored" (2011, p. 787). Goodman explains the idea of trade-offs as follows: "The uncertain risk of memory loss must be considered in the context of the gravity of the underlying illness. Many patients undergo ECT only after other treatment options have been exhausted. Decisions about ECT require full participation of the patient in a robust informed consent process that acknowledges gaps in our knowledge about the extent of personal memory loss" (2011, p. 1787). The information from which patients make these decisions will always involve some degree of uncertainty. Depending on their experience with depression and attitudes about short- and long-term amnesia, different patients may interpret this uncertainty differently in weighing the potential benefit and risk of undergoing or continuing to undergo ECT.

I have noted the incomplete knowledge of the mechanisms of ECT. But the side effect of amnesia may provide a clue to a better understanding of it. In a recent study, a single ECT session for patients with unipolar depression disrupted reconsolidation of emotional episodic memories (Kroes, Tendolkar, van Wingen et al., 2014). Episodic memories must be retrieved to be reconsolidated, and the study showed that administering ECT interfered with memory retrieval. I described PTSD, panic disorders, and anxiety disorders as disorders of memory content involving the fear memory system. The persistence of emotionally charged memories of traumatic or disturbing experiences might also have a causal role in the pathophysiology of some forms of depression. These memories can have a deleterious influence on sensory and emotional processing and result in impaired cognition, mood, and volition.

The disruption of reconsolidation of these memories by ECT could provide a therapeutic explanation for the retrograde amnesia caused by ECT. Losing some memories may not be an adverse effect but a serendipitous benefit of the technique. Limited retrograde amnesia resulting from ECT may rid some patients of these memories and restore some degree of cognitive and emotional function. It may be particularly beneficial for elderly patients with depression who are not candidates for CBT because of cognitive impairment. Amnestic mechanisms beyond the patient's conscious control might not be a memory disorder but the brain's way—with the help of ECT—of modulating a dysregulated fear memory system. Of course, this is not the case where ECT results in significant, permanent retrograde amnesia of pleasant episodic memories as well as disturbing fear memories. There is no identifiable selectivity mechanism to explain why some memories are lost and others retained following ECT. Accordingly, one must be circumspect in making claims about salutary amnestic effects of this technique. Any explanation for such a mechanism would be different from an explanation of pharmacologically induced amnesia for disorders of memory content.

Researchers have found that DBS may promote neurogenesis in the hippocampal–entorhinal circuit and enable the encoding of new memories (Laxton, Tang-Wai, McAndrews, et al., 2010). In a very different study outcome, stimulation of the medial temporal lobe during the delay between memory encoding and recall selectively enhanced forgetting in a small group of human subjects (Merkow, Burke, Ramayya et al., 2017). If there are at least some similarities between the effects of DBS and ECT in disrupting reconsolidation of disturbing memories, and if these memories have a role in the pathogenesis of depression, then this finding further supports the idea that some of the amnestic effects of ECT might be therapeutic. The extinction of these memories may serve an adaptive purpose.

Admittedly, this hypothesis is speculative and raises open questions for research. Clinical trials would be necessary to test the idea that some degree of amnesia from the technique might be beneficial. The possible salutary effects of some memory loss would have to be weighed against what can be severe retrograde amnesia for some patients. Still, it may offer an alternative explanation of what has been the most serious side effect of ECT. The plausibility of this hypothesis would depend on which memories were affected by ECT's disruption of memory reconsolidation. Research clearly demonstrating positive effects of ECT on emotionally charged fear memories would be necessary for investigators and practitioners to explain the possible benefit of a limited degree of retrograde amnesia to patients and research subjects before they consent to undergo the procedure.

## Transcranial magnetic stimulation and transcranial current stimulation

In TMS, an electrical current passing through a coiled wire placed on the head creates a magnetic field that can penetrate the skull (Valero-Cabre, Amengual, Stengel et al., 2017). Magnetic pulses generate electrical potentials in the brain. These depolarize neurons and trigger action potentials in brain regions underlying the coils. The effects of a single pulse of TMS may last only a few milliseconds. Repeated pulses in repetitive transcranial magnetic stimulation (rTMS) may have more sustained effects. The pulses may induce long-term potentiation in the target cells and promote neuroplasticity (Nitsche, Boggio, Fregni et al., 2009). The general term "tCS" refers to procedures generating direct (tDCS) or alternating current (tACS) stimulation. In these techniques, the experimenter or practitioner typically delivers pulses of low-frequency electrical current for 10–20 minutes (Davis and van Koningsbruggen, 2013, p. 1). TMS and tCS involve different ways of inducing electrical activity in the brain. The effects of this activity depend on such factors as the amplitude and duration of the current, the region to which it is applied, and each person's unique neural circuitry.

TMS and tCS have been used experimentally for AN (Coman, Skarderud, Reas et al., 2014) and schizophrenia (Dougall, Maayan, Soares-Weiser et al., 2015). They have been used most frequently for depression (Nitsche, Boggio, Fregni et al., 2009; Slotema, Blom, Hoek et al., 2010; Palm, Schiller, Fintescu et al., 2012; Brunoni, Boggio, Ferrucci et al., 2013). Repeated stimulation in rTMS appears to have neuromodulating effects that can improve cognition and mood. Unlike DBS, these techniques do not require implanting devices in the brain and thus avoid the risk of infection, edema, and other sequelae associated with neurosurgery. They are less expensive than DBS, can be administered in outpatient clinics and the machinery can easily be removed from the head.

Even if TMS and tCS are invasive procedures in the broad sense of the term, they are less invasive than procedures involving intracranial surgery and thus entail fewer risks. For this reason, the capacity threshold necessary for consent to TMS may be lower than it is for DBS.

The neuromodulating effects of these techniques may be limited, however. Cognitive and mood disturbances involved in MDD, schizophrenia, and AN involve dysfunction in cortical, limbic, and subcortical regions. TMS can only activate the first 1 centimeter of cortex (Deng, Lisanby, and Peterchev, 2013; Widge and Moritz, 2015, p. 236). It may positively influence how the PFC projects to the amygdala and ventral striatum and have indirect salutary effects in these regions. But these effects may be too weak for significant improvement in symptoms. Another limitation of TMS is that its effects are transient and in this respect analogous to the effects of psychopharmacology. The effects of rTMS might not be sustained for long periods. Pulses of stimulation in advanced versions of TMS and tCS may be able to penetrate more deeply in the brain, though it is not known whether these effects would be weaker in subcortical regions. There is also the possibility that the pulse delivered to the cortex would be deflected by the cranium, further limiting its effect in the brain. This may depend on the thickness of the cranium.

In a recent, randomized, double-blind, placebo-controlled study comparing tDCS with the SSRI escitalopram, the results showed that the technique was not as effective as the medication in relieving depressive symptoms over a 10-week period (Brunoni, Moffa, Sampaio-Junior et al., 2017). The technique also produced more adverse events than the drug. One reason for caution in interpreting these results is that many studies testing TMS and tDCS have had flaws in trial design. In the study just mentioned, patients in the medication group became aware that they were receiving the drug when they experienced side effects. This interfered with the attempt to do a double comparison between the drug and a placebo, on the one hand, and tDCS and sham tDCS, on the other. In addition, it was not clear what the optimal level of electrical current delivered to the targeted region should be or what the expected effect was on the targeted circuit (Lisanby, 2017). Improved trial design may clarify the neurophysiological mechanisms of TMS and tDCS and establish whether they can be as effective as other interventions in treating depression or other psychiatric disorders.

The ethical questions generated by TMS and tDCS are less about their efficacy and more about their safety (Horvath, Perez, Forrow et al., 2013). In light of the problems with trial design just mentioned, appropriately designed placebo-controlled studies are necessary to gain a better understanding of their positive and negative effects in the brain. There is also a need for adequate regulation of the technique. Like other interventions for psychiatric disorders, differences in people's brains will result in variable effects among those who undergo these techniques. Repeated pulses of current to cortical regions could improve cognition and mood by modulating hyperactive or hypoactive frontal–limbic circuits. Nevertheless, electrical stimulation of the brain beyond optimal levels may cause more adverse effects than the headaches reported anecdotally by some who have used these techniques. Repeated pulses in rTMS could cause unintended seizures from excessive excitatory activity in the cortex. While ECT also induces seizures, these are part of the intended mechanism to relieve depressive symptoms. One cannot assume that seizure-related effects of TMS or tCS would also be therapeutic.

Of particular concern is how repeated electrical stimulation might affect the brains of children and adolescents (Davis, 2014). As their brains are still developing, it is unclear whether or how electrical stimulation of neural circuits might affect the balance between inhibitory and excitatory mechanisms in cortical networks or their projections to limbic and subcortical networks. In particular, it is unclear whether or how electrical stimulation would affect synaptic pruning, the natural process of eliminating redundant synapses overproduced in the early years of life. Dysregulated synaptic pruning may be the cause of abnormalities in the volume and thickness of cortical gray matter displayed by imaging of adolescents and young adults with schizophrenia. Its effects may also appear later in life in older adults with bipolar depression and other disorders (Paus, Keshavan, and Giedd, 2008; Boksa, 2012). This uncertainty provides reasons for caution in stimulating the brains of people in these cohorts.

Another difference between these electrical stimulation techniques and ECT and DBS is that the latter two procedures typically occur in a controlled clinical or research setting. In addition, pulses of electrical current from TMS and tDCS are not as focused as the electrical stimulation in DBS. Because these less invasive techniques do not allow the practitioner to probe neural circuits and directly observe the effects of stimulation as in the more invasive technique, it may be more difficult to control any expanding effects on healthy neural tissue and circuits. Neurological and psychological changes from transcranial stimulation may persist for weeks after the end of a session. These changes may not always be salutary or benign (Davis and Koningsbruggen, 2013). They are difficult to predict because of the technique's imprecise and only partly understood mechanisms of action. All of these considerations underscore the need for constant monitoring of patients and research subjects during and between stimulation sessions. This can be challenging. Therapeutic benefit from TMS requires daily outpatient visits for several weeks (Lozano, 2017, p. 1097). A person with a psychiatric disorder may feel better after one or several applications, or may feel burdened by having to travel daily to the treatment site, and not follow up with additional treatments. Nonadherence could compromise the intended therapeutic purpose of the technique. A patient may be unaware, or not sufficiently aware, of the potential for delayed adverse effects and the possibility of relapse in cases where the technique temporarily has relieved symptoms. The importance of monitoring and completing a course of TMS or tCS therapy must be included in the informed consent process. Continuity of care is crucial.

The portability, relatively low cost, and irresponsible media accounts of the efficacy of these stimulating devices may lead some patients with psychiatric disorders to use them for self-treatment (Lott-Schwartz, 2012). The perception of TMS and tCS as safe for this use may reflect the view that they are noninvasive and as such without much, if any, risk (Cohen Kadosh, Levy, O'Shea et al., 2012; Davis and Koningsbriggen, 2013; Dubljevic, Saigle, and Racine, 2014). Patients may have an oversimplified view of the device's mechanisms of action and apply it at home in an untrained and unsupervised setting. They may mistakenly believe that they can operate it on their own without only positive and no negative effects. It would only enhance their experience of TMS or tCS under medical supervision. This entails a risk of operating the device incorrectly and overstimulating the brain with too much current. For those on antidepressant or other psychotropic or nonpsychotropic medications, there would be the additional risk of adverse interactions with these other treatments. The limited knowledge of the effects of TMS and tCS for psychiatric disorders is from applications in controlled experimental settings. Without psychiatric supervision, the use of these techniques on one's own could exacerbate depression or other disorders and result in self-harm.

In fact, the risk goes beyond a potential worsening of depressive or other psychiatric symptoms. One case of self-administered tCS resulted in temporary respiratory paralysis (Dubljevic, Saigle, and Racine, 2014). While this is a rare adverse event, it illustrates that there are significant risks to unsupervised use of these techniques, despite being "noninvasive" in the narrow sense of the term. Uncertainty about short- and long-term effects of electrical brain stimulation and the potential harm to its recipients warrant restricting its use to settings with constant medical supervision.

In the United States, TMS and tCS are largely unregulated. Government agencies such as the FDA, the National Institute of Mental Health, and professional psychiatric and neurological organizations need to formulate, implement and enforce regulations for appropriate use of these techniques. The European Commission went some way in this direction with the publication of *Medical Devices: Guidelines Document—Classification of Medical Devices* (2014). This followed a policy paper from the Institute of Science and Ethics at Oxford University (Maslen, Douglas, Cohen Kadosh et al., 2012) and a paper by

Roi Cohen Kadosh and coauthors on the neuroethics of noninvasive brain stimulation (Cohen Kadosh, Levy, O'Shea et al., 2012). The guidelines should be based on a meta-analysis of clinical trials testing the safely and efficacy of the techniques and peer review of these results. Manufacturers of these devices also have an ethical obligation to inform psychiatrists, government agencies, professional organizations, and the media of the mechanisms of action of TMS and tCS, as well as what research and development has revealed about their effects in the brain.

All of these groups have a collective obligation to inform users of these techniques of their therapeutic potential and limitations. This includes an obligation to emphasize the uncertainty about short- and especially long-term neural effects of single and repeated pulses of electrical current. This information should lead to appropriate regulation and selection criteria for patients with depression, AN, schizophrenia, or other disorders receiving TMS or tCS for investigational or therapeutic purposes. Expanding insurance coverage for TMS and acquisition of the device by private practitioners in the United States is increasing accessibility for patients. Thus underscores the importance of having universal quality control and ethics standards to protect patients from harm.

Transcranial stimulation has also been used to enhance normal cognitive capacities in healthy subjects. There have been experiments testing its potential to improve moral decision-making as well (Young, Camprodon, Hauser et al., 2010). In an experiment using this technique to test the learning and application of mathematical information, researchers found that stimulating an area of the subjects' parietal cortex enhanced the ability to learn new mathematical information but impaired the ability to apply this information. Stimulating an area of the PFC had the opposite effect of enhancing the ability to apply existing information but impairing the ability to learn new information (Iuculano and Cohen-Kadosh, 2013). The results of this study suggest that there are optimal levels of interconnected cognitive functions mediated by optimal levels of interconnected neurotransmitter and neural circuit activity. It shows that techniques that improve some cognitive functions may interfere with others. In this respect, the outcome of the transcranial stimulation experiment is similar to the outcome of the study demonstrating that psychostimulants could enhance chess performance but also have detrimental effects on complex task performance.

In a meta-analysis of studies on the enhancing effects of tDCS, Jared Horvath and coauthors concluded that the technique did not have a significant positive outcome in a number of cognitive and motor tasks when compared with sham control groups (Horvath, Forte and Carter, 2015). The results of the study offer further support for the claim that justification for intervening in the brain with TMS, tDCS, or any other technique to raise cognitive and emotional functions to normal levels is stronger than any justification for trying to raise them above these levels. As a case I present in Chapter 5 illustrates, trying to raise these functions above optimal levels may result in psychopathology. The most defensible purpose of intervening in the brains of people with major psychiatric disorders is to restore normal neural and mental functions. When the disorders are severe, there are good reasons for skepticism about the very idea of enhancing cognitive and emotional capacities.

## Temporal interference

A novel form of neuromodulation that may have greater therapeutic potential and a superior benefit–risk ratio than other techniques is TI. Unlike TMS and tCD, where the electrical current weakens as it passes through the cortex, electrical current in TI can penetrate and modulate activity in subcortical regions of the brain. This is significant because many of the dysfunctional neural circuits implicated in psychiatric disorders are in these regions. TI can have this effect without disturbing cortical neurons. This gives it a higher level of specificity than the other two techniques and thus reduces the probability of expanding effects on nontargeted normally functioning circuits. TI uses two intersecting, high-frequency, oscillating electromagnetic fields to create a low-frequency envelope that can increase neural activity at deeper levels. Because a source outside of the brain generates the electrical fields and interference, it could obviate the need for intracranial surgery. This would make it a viable alternative to DBS because it would avoid the risk of infection, bleeding, and seizures from cutting through the skull and implanting and activating electrodes in the brain. It might also be preferable to DBS if it had the same neuromodulating effects as this more invasive technique.

Strictly speaking, TI is a form of noninvasive brain stimulation. In the broad sense I have described, though, it is invasive because it can cause changes in the brain by activating neurons in specific regions. An experiment using animal models led by Nir Grossman has shown that the high-frequency fields in TI do not increase the temperature of brain tissue beyond a normal level. In this way, it can modulate neural circuits and avoid unintended thermal ablation of neural tissue (Grossman, Bono, Dedic et al., 2017). Researchers have been able to activate neurons deep in the hippocampus without affecting neurons in the cortex between the extracranial source of the interference and the subcortical target. A number of trials will be necessary to determine whether researchers will be able to convert high-frequency fields into a low frequency envelope in the human brain. This is the crux of its neuromodulating potential.

Just because TI is not as invasive as DBS does not mean that it would be safer or more effective than this technique in all respects While the mice in the study by Grossman and coinvestigators did not experience seizures, it cannot be assumed that a high-frequency electrical current would not induce them in the human cortex. This is one of a number of questions about safety in this example of translational neuroscience. Moreover, recording and monitoring neural activity and cognitive and emotional processing in TI may not be as accurate as it is in DBS. The first technique would not have the same probing ability or facility of parameter adjustment as the second. There are questions about its potential efficacy as well. Like TMS, rTMS and tCS, one of the limitations of TI is that the cranium may deflect the electrical current and interfere with its activation of subcortical neurons.

Even if the electrical current from TI penetrated deeper in the brain than the current from these other techniques, the cranium could deflect current from the source and prevent it from reaching its target. Cranial thickness can vary among patients and can affect how deeply and accurately pulses from a device can penetrate the brain. In addition, "brain stimulation with interfering electrical fields would require ongoing access to specialized equipment and personnel. The application of continuous ongoing stimulation—as is required for some conditions, such as Parkinson's disease—is often challenging, Patients with implanted stimulating electrodes and a pulse generator [as in DBS] do not have these constraints, can receive stimulation 24 hours a day, and are not required to adhere to a demanding regimen of visits" (Lozano, 2017, p. 1097). This raises the possibility of nonadherence and underscores how tolerability of TI will be necessary to establish its efficacy. Nevertheless, preliminary results of studies of TI in animal models suggest that it could provide a more effective form of neuromodulation than many or most techniques currently in use in clinical and experimental settings.

## Placebos in the clinical psychiatric setting

Ted Kaptchuk and Franklin Miller point out that "In a broad sense, placebo effects are improvements in patients' symptoms that are attributable to their participation in the therapeutic encounter, with its rituals, symbols and interactions" (2015, p. 8). What induces these effects is not whether the patient receives a biochemically inert or active pill or infusion, but the context in which he receives it. This includes the condition being treated, the patient's beliefs about his condition, the expectation that his condition will improve with the treatment, and the experience the patient has had with medical interventions in general. Kaptchuk and Miller note that "placebo effects do not alter the pathophysiology of diseases beyond their symptomatic manifestations; they primarily address subjective and self-appraised symptoms" (2015, p. 8). Fabrizio Benedetti explains that the placebo effect is "a psychobiological phenomenon" that is "triggered by the psychosocial context around the patient and the therapy" (2009, p. 19). Expectation and learning play critical roles, and "conditioned placebo responses are consciously mediated by complex cognitive factors" (2009, p. 19). These responses "may have emerged during evolution as a defense mechanism of the body" (2009, p. 19). Placebo responses may be one mechanism of a human organism's natural adaptive capacity.

As the subjective quality of experience may have a causal role in some psychiatric disorders, the psychology of placebo responses from some patients with these disorders can be effective in controlling symptoms. There is some overlap between CBT and placebo responses in that symptom relief depends on the patient's psychology. Unlike CBT, though, where the aim is to help the patient to reframe her conscious beliefs about herself and her relation to her environment, placebo responses rely on unconscious conditioning and suggestion as well as conscious expectation of symptom relief. The original meaning of "placebo"— "I shall please"—captures the idea of an expectation to improve.

There is considerable variation in placebo responses among patients with different psychiatric disorders. Placebos tend to be more effective in patients with panic disorder, mild to moderate depression, and GAD (Brown, 2012, p. 7). Interestingly, these are among the conditions that respond to CBT. This may be explained by a greater degree of mind–brain interaction in these disorders than in others. Many patients with these conditions get "almost as much relief with placebo as they do with conventional treatment" (Brown, 2012, p. 23). Some studies have indicated that, among patients with mild to moderate depression, SSRIs are no more effective than placebos. Any positive response to a SSRI may be nothing more than a placebo response (Kirsch, Deacon, Huedo-Medina, et al., 2008; Fournier, De Rubeis, Hollon et al., 2010). These responses are much lower among persons with severe depression and OCD. Placebo "benefits only 20% to 30% of those with severe depressive illness, but it brings relief to a greater proportion (50% to 70%) of patients with less severe depression" (Brown, 2012, p. 28). Those who have been depressed for an extended period (6 months or longer) do less well than those whose depression has been of shorter duration. Fewer than 20% of those with OCD improve with placebo.

One possible explanation of why antidepressants are not very effective in patients with mild to moderate depression is that the brain is able to restore or maintain homeostasis by counteracting internal stressors from the body and external stressors from the environment. Antidepressants may be redundant in these cases. If these drugs have no positive but only negative effects, then there are good reasons for questioning their use in mild to moderate depression. Placebos and CBT may be beneficial because of their ability to regulate mind–brain interaction in these types of depression and other disorders. It should be emphasized that meta-analyses consistently show that antidepressants are more effective than placebos in major (moderately severe to severe) depressive disorder (Cipriani, Furukawa, Salanti et al., 2018).

Cognitive impairment in the form of hallucinations and delusions in the positive subtype of schizophrenia appears to preclude insight into the disorder and the motivation necessary to drive a patient's expectation for improvement. A certain degree of intact cognitive function associated with belief and expectation is necessary for a placebo response. This is one reason why these responses do not occur among people with the severe cognitive impairment of Alzheimer's disease (Benedetti, 2009, pp. 131–135). In moderate and especially advanced Alzheimer's, the lack of incongruence between the patient's actual pathological mental states and the normal mental states she ordinarily would want is a further impediment to a placebo response. In neurological and psychiatric disorders with less cognitive impairment, the patient's belief that she has a disorder and that she will improve could promote such a response. Lack of insight into a disorder and lack of a desire to improve could preclude an expectation to improve.

In less severe forms of schizophrenia, some patients may have enough cognitive capacity and expectation of improvement to enable a placebo response. In the negative subtype of the disorder, this would depend on the extent of avolition and anhedonia, both of which would seem to preclude a motivation to improve. In the positive subtype, it would depend on whether the patient was in a remitting or relapsing phase with psychosis. Intuitively, these symptoms would make it difficult to induce a placebo response in either group of patients. But there has been a reported increase in the incidence and degree of these responses in schizophrenia clinical trials (Kinon, Potts, and Watson, 2011; Alphs, Benedetti, Fleischhacker et al., 2012). Data from these trials suggest that patients with less severe forms of this disorder may have the cognitive and emotional capacity for these responses. They may have these responses not just from their interactions with clinicians, but also from their interactions with researchers.

Although placebo responses in research are different from placebo responses in the doctor–patient relationship, the beliefs and expectations of controls in a schizophrenia clinical trial may enable these responses. They could confound questions about the efficacy of experimental antipsychotic drugs. This situation would be similar to the effect of placebo responses from controls in a depression trial confounding questions about the efficacy of antidepressant drugs. It may be difficult to completely separate placebo responses in psychiatric practice from those in psychiatric research if a patient or research subject has the same motivational states in the two settings.

Genetics may explain why some psychiatric patients respond or fail to respond to placebos. Genes regulating dopaminergic pathways can influence how the brain and mind respond to sensations and symptoms (Hall, Loscalzo, and Kaptchuk, 2015). Suggestion and other psychological techniques used to induce placebo responses may allow some patients to control their symptoms and experience relief from them. There is variation in how genes code for dopamine in people's brains, and this can result in variable placebo responses—or no response—in patients. In addition to neuroimaging biomarkers, genetic information about which patients would be more likely to respond to placebos could be another component of precision medicine and personalized treatment in psychiatry. It could clarify critical aspects of the brain–mind relation in different patients and its role in symptom relief. In light of research showing that patients respond to placebos even when they know that they are receiving them, ethical concerns about deception would not arise (Kaptchuk, Friedlander, Kelley et al., 2010).

Based on the relevant genetic information, a psychiatrist could explain the placebo response to a patient and recommend that placebo be part of their therapy. Still, there would be ethical concerns about how to obtain the relevant genetic information. Patients would have to consent to undergo testing to reveal information not only about their genes but also about the role of gene expression in their brains. This would be justified when the psychiatrist explained that it would be part of their treatment plan. However, this information would be confidential between the psychiatrist and patients and would have to be protected from unauthorized access by third parties. In addition, genetic variation influencing responses to placebos may also influence responses to psychotropic drugs. This could complicate knowing the efficacy of the drug because it would be difficult to separate the placebo effect from the drug effect.

Genetics could also exclude patients more likely to have placebo responses from participating in clinical drug trials with a placebo control group. This would be unfair to those who want to contribute to and may subsequently benefit from research because the interaction between genetic and neurobiological factors causing these responses would be beyond their control. It would be a natural form of unfairness without any viable resolution. On the other hand, patients with genes more likely to induce a placebo response could be given a placebo to enhance the effects of a psychotropic drug. Placebo would not be contraindicated because it would not interfere with the drug's biochemical mechanism. A placebo would not replace the drug but would be used in addition to it in combination therapy. Again, though, these effects would be more likely to occur in patients with less severe forms of psychiatric disorders and certain levels of intact cognitive and emotional functions. Placebo responses depend on a patient's capacity for belief in and expectation about a therapeutic outcome.

Similarities between neurological and psychiatric disorders can shed light on interacting neurobiological and psychological processes in placebo responses. In Chapter 1, I described how symptoms of neurological and psychiatric disorders overlap, and that this supports relaxing the categorical distinction between them. Studies using PET imaging of subjects with PD have confirmed the release of endogenous dopamine in the striatum in response to placebos (de la Fuente Fernandez and Stoessl, 2002; Benedetti, 2009, pp. 104–106). Presumably, psychogenic factors should not induce such a neurophysiological response in a movement disorder. Yet these studies show that some patients with this type of disorder may respond to these factors in this way.

PMDs may be the best example of this phenomenon because their etiology and psychomotor and psychological symptoms are similar to some of the symptoms in anxiety and depression. Like the behavioral changes in GAD and MDD, PMDs involve abnormal movements that arise as unconscious and conscious manifestations of psychosocial stress (Shamy, 2010). Like depression and anxiety, PMDs correlate with dysfunctional connectivity between prefrontal and limbic regions. There is also dysfunctional connectivity between motor cortices and limbic areas (Benedetti, Carlino, and Pollo, 2011; Rommelfanger, 2013). These findings are consistent with the view that PMDs are associated with dysfunction in motor and limbic circuits of the basal ganglia. As these circuits are in close proximity to each other, abnormalities in one circuit could affect the others and account for the characteristic psychomotor symptoms in PMDs. Karen Rommelfanger claims that "the prognosis and successful treatment of PMDs are highly dependent on the patient's belief that they have a PMD and that they will get better. Because of the powerful role of belief in PMD . . . and the poor prognosis for patients with currently available treatment options, some neurologists advocate placebo therapy for PMDs" (2013, p. 352). Another reason why placebos might be effective in relieving symptoms of PMDs and some psychiatric disorders is that psychosocial stressors are a key factor in their etiology. Placebos could positively influence a patient's perception of these stressors and downregulate his response to them. One difference between PMDs and MDD is that a number of pharmacological and psychological treatments other than placebos are available for the latter. PMDs may be more difficult to treat with placebos or other forms of suggestion when these psychological techniques cannot be combined with other therapies and are offered as the only treatment.

Rommelfanger's comments suggest that patients with PMDs who are more likely to respond to placebos are those with insight into their disorder and who experience it as ego-dystonic. The patient believes or knows that she has the disorder, and feels distress from the incongruity of the psychomotor symptoms she has and the psychomotor capacities she wants to restore. Her desire to rid herself of the symptoms motivates her to seek treatment. These attitudes can generate an expectation to improve that can result in actual improvement. The treating neurologist or psychiatrist can use these attitudes to elicit a placebo response that might relieve motor and nonmotor symptoms. A psychiatrist can use these same attitudes to elicit a placebo response in patients with moderate MDD or GAD. The patient's belief and expectation about improvement may have a top-down effect on cognitive and emotional functions that could modulate activity in prefrontal–limbic–striatal pathways involved in expectation and reward processing (Rommelfanger, 2013, p. 353). The comparison between depression, anxiety, and psychogenic movement disorders is also appropriate because they all involve a similar phenomenology of impaired agency and behavior control. They all involve some form of avolition, with difficulty forming and executing action plans. In all of these disorders, unconsciousness conditioning, conscious expectation, and trust between the patient and physician are critical in generating and possibly sustaining a placebo response.

A weak or no response to a placebo by a patient with a neuropsychiatric disorder may reflect extensive dysregulation in distributed neural networks. This could make the disorder refractory to psychological techniques designed to reframe beliefs or other mental states. Significant anatomical and functional changes in neural circuits in diseases with lower response rates to placebos may be the result of their chronicity (Mayberg, Silva, Brannen et al., 2002). The longer one has had a severe mental illness and the more extensive neural dysfunction there is, the less likely will techniques involving psychological processes be able to modulate this dysfunction and its manifestations at the mental level.

One question that arises is whether there would be a stronger ethical justification for providing placebos for conditions in which there are more positive placebo responses to them. If a placebo can relieve symptoms of some psychiatric disorders without causing any adverse effects, then there would seem to be a compelling ethical reason to prescribe it to patients with these disorders. Yet this raises the related ethical question of how a physician who believes that he would be discharging his obligations to benefit and not harm a patient would weight these against his obligation to respect the patient's autonomy and provide him with all relevant information about the proposed intervention (Beauchamp and Childress, 2012, Chapters 4–6). This hinges on the issue of deception in the doctor–patient relationship.

Most discussions of the ethics of placebos in psychiatric and other clinical settings focus on whether their use is deceptive or nondeceptive (Brody, 1982). Deceptive use consists in deliberately misinforming or not informing the patient of the actual biochemical properties of the pill or infusion they are providing to him. The physician misleads the patient into believing that the intervention has a psychoactive mechanism of action that it lacks, or a mechanism not indicated for the condition for which it is prescribed. This appears to violate the psychiatrist's obligation to respect the patient's autonomy in providing all relevant medical information. This is necessary for the patient to understand the nature and purpose of the proposed treatment and voluntarily accept or refuse it based on this information. In addition to violating patient autonomy, deceptive use of placebos may threaten trust between the physician and patient and have a negative impact on the patient's perception of the caring relationship.

In its 2007 ethical guidelines for the use of placebos, the American Medical Association (AMA) stated that, in the few circumstances in which placebo treatment could be justified, physicians should offer it without deception and accordingly should tell the patient that it is a placebo. The AMA claims that physicians are prohibited from providing "a substance . . . that the physician believes has no specific pharmacological effect upon the condition being treated" (Bostick, Sade, Levine et al., 2008, p. 60). As the American Medical Association suggests, patients can sign a waiver requesting that they not be told whether or not placebo treatment is used. This is consistent with respect for patient autonomy.

Some might claim that nondeceptive use of placebos would undermine its efficacy by undermining the patient's belief that it will be effective. Yet, as noted, contrary to the view that placebo effects require deception, some studies suggest that these effects can be generated and sustained even when patients are told that they are receiving a placebo (Kaptchuk, Friedlander, Kelley et al., 2010). The desire and expectation that one's symptoms will improve seem to override information about the lack of pharmacological properties in the proposed treatment. There seems to be cognitive dissonance between the information the patient receives about the placebo and his belief in its efficacy. Unconscious conditioning based on previous use of prescribed drugs may influence the conscious expectation of benefit. Yet if a therapeutic effect can result from nondeceptive provision of a placebo, then deception will not be necessary to produce this effect. In that case, the issue of deceptive use would not arise.

Still, some authors argue that deceptive use of placebos can be ethically justified (Gold and Lichtenberg, 2014). Thus depends on what counts as "essential" information that a psychiatrist is obligated to disclose to a patient. Placebos are unique among medical interventions in applying the bioethical principles of respect for patient autonomy, nonmaleficence, and beneficence. Unlike typical discussions of these principles, the core issue is not side effects of the treatment but its mechanism of action. Most patients suffering from depression or anxiety are not interested in the theoretical question about the pharmacological properties of the intervention but the practical question of whether it will relieve their symptoms. A patient may not need disclosure of all medical facts about a proposed treatment to make a sufficiently informed decision to accept or refuse it. If only some of these facts are necessary for this decision, then the psychiatrist may not be obligated to disclose all information about a treatment and could permissibly withhold some of it.

Not all patients are interested in knowing all the properties of a treatment. Most only want to know its probable positive or negative effects on them. Some might claim that it would be paternalistic and as such a failure to respect patient autonomy to withhold any of this information. But disclosing information that may not be relevant to the patient's condition and which he does not want may also be paternalistic and a violation of patient autonomy (Gold and Lichtenberg, 2014, p. 222). Azgad Gold and Pesach Lichtenberg claim that "unless the physician knows, or reasonably assumes, based on personal acquaintance, that her patient is interested in being informed about the mechanism of action of the proposed intervention, she is not obligated to disclose this sort of information. When the preferences of the individual patient for the extent of disclosure are unknown, disclosing potentially unneeded information may be as paternalistic as concealing such information" (2014, p. 222).

Some depressed or anxious patients' cognitive and emotional capacities may be impaired to the point where they can only process a limited amount of information. They may feel overloaded by information about the properties of the intervention, including possible side effects. This could impair their ability to decide whether to have it. But difficulty in processing information and making decisions is less likely in mild to moderate depression, where the incidence of placebo responses tends to be higher. In these cases, the issue is not whether they can or cannot process information about pharmacology. Rather, the issue is that they may need only a minimum of pharmacological information to consent to placebo treatment.

In MDD, variability in responses to different antidepressants supports the view that the efficacy of these drugs is not solely a function of their biochemical properties. Differences in how patients' brains are wired, genetic and epigenetic factors in neural function, the role of their mental states in the etiology of the disorder, and their attitudes toward the treating psychiatrist can influence these responses. The lack of a satisfactory explanation of variability in patient responses to antidepressants indicates that the mechanism of action of these drugs is not well understood. This has important ethical implications for disclosing information about these drugs. Telling a patient that a drug such as paroxetine inhibits the reuptake of the neurotransmitter serotonin and increases its availability in the synaptic cleft will not matter to her if it does not relieve her symptoms or is not part of an explanation for its failure to do so. Nor will it matter to a patient taking venlafaxine whether the psychiatrist explains that the drug inhibits the reuptake of serotonin and triggers the release of nor-epinephrine at higher doses. It seems misguided to charge that a psychiatrist fails to respect patient autonomy in not informing her that a placebo has no pharmacological mechanism of action when the mechanism of the antidepressant is not well understood by the psychiatrist. It does not serve any informative or therapeutic purpose to tell a patient that a placebo is biochemically inert. This would be included in what Gold and Lichtenberg describe as "unneeded" and unhelpful information.

These same authors appeal to the uncertainty of pharmacological effects of drugs in assessing the ethical permissibility of prescribing placebos. They state: "The criteria for evaluating the moral status of an intervention should focus on the reason of whether the *physician* believes—based on empirical data—the intervention will be effective; the effectiveness should not be limited to its 'specific pharmacological effect'. The everyday medical practice is abundant in situations in which physicians provide interventions whose specific pharmacological effect is unknown" (Gold and Lichtenberg, 2014, p. 221). This point applies not only to placebos but also to off-label uses of drugs for depression, anxiety, and other psychiatric disorders. Gabapentin is one example of a drug used to relieve somatic symptoms of depression and anxiety despite its primary use as an anticonvulsive agent. These considerations may support the view that something less than full disclosure about the nature of a prescribed placebo may be ethically justified. There is a gray area between partial and full disclosure. Even if full disclosure about all of the properties of a proposed treatment is not obligatory for the psychiatrist, a certain amount of information is necessary for a patient to decide to accept or refuse it. But there is no definitive answer to the question of *how much* information about placebos compared with biochemically active agents should be disclosed, or *how* it should be disclosed.

To a certain extent, how much information should be disclosed can be left to the discretion of the treating psychiatrist. Some may be more inclined to disclose or withhold more information about placebos than others. It will depend on the psychiatrist's assessment of the patient's condition and personality and how much information the patient needs and wants to process in making a decision about this, or any, treatment. Some of these assessments may be more paternalistic, while others may show more respect for patient autonomy. Even if they are paternalistic, they would not necessarily be unethical if the patient is not interested in knowing the biochemical properties of the proposed treatment—or lack thereof—and defers to the psychiatrist's judgment in prescribing what will benefit him. These same considerations apply to the question of how much information about a technique used to induce a placebo response in a PMD should be disclosed to a patient with this disorder.

This does not explain away concern about the patient who considers the withholding of information about a placebo a violation of trust. Some patients do not want to know anything more than the fact that the psychiatrist is offering a treatment that could benefit them. Others want to know every detail about the treatment. Misleading them can have a devastating effect on the doctor–patient relationship by eroding the trust that is at the core of this relationship. Gold and Lichtenberg suggest that a nondeceptive and ethically justifiable way of prescribing a placebo would be the following: "I am prescribing a pill which research suggests can be of benefit to you. In your circumstances, I have reason to believe that it will work, with a minimum of side effects" (2014, p. 221). Walter Brown proposes a similar nondeceptive approach to prescribing placebos as an alternative to pharmacotherapy and psychotherapy for depression:

> There is a third kind of treatment, less expensive for you and less likely to cause side effects, which also helps many people with your condition. The treatment involves taking one of these pills twice a day and coming to our office every two weeks to let us know how you are doing. These pills do not contain any drug. We don't know exactly how they work; they may trigger or stimulate the body's healing process. We do know that your chances of improving with this treatment are quite good. If, after six weeks of this treatment you are not feeling better we can try one of the other treatments. (Brown, 1994, p. 266)

Although neither Gold and Lichtenberg nor Brown mention genetics, knowing that a patient had a genetic predisposition to placebo responses would support a reason to believe that her symptoms would improve from receiving a placebo. This genetic information about the particular patient can make a claim about chances of improvement sincere, empirically based, and more than just speculation. With this information, a psychiatrist would be able to provide a more accurate assessment of whether a placebo would be appropriate for the patient.

Based on Brown's empirical data cited earlier, the type of patient to whom these vignettes apply and for whom placebo therapy would be beneficial would be one with mild to moderate depression. It would be justified in cases where the psychiatrist has known the patient for some time and knows that the patient has the cognitive and emotional capacity to respond to a placebo. However, it is

doubtful that a placebo would be of any benefit to a patient with moderately severe to severe depression. The cognitive, emotional, and volitional impairment
would probably preclude the capacity to expect improvement and respond to
the placebo based on this expectation.

Given that many factors influence placebo responses, focusing on the absence of a biochemical mechanism of action of the placebo may reflect a neurobiological reductionist account of treatment that ignores the psychosocial
context in which it is prescribed and received (Gold and Lichtenberg, 2014).
Ethical questions such as how much information about a placebo should be
disclosed to the patient must be framed by whether the physician believes that
a placebo would relieve a patient's symptoms. The beliefs of both the patient
and the physician are critical for generating this effect. The psychiatrist's belief
is based on the patient's behavior in the clinical encounter as a manifestation
of neural and mental processes and the psychosocial factors that shape them.
Benedetti underscores the importance of these factors in the clinical use of
placebos: "Understanding the biological mechanism of placebo effects means
to understand how the psychosocial context affects the patient's brain" (2011,
p. 181). Whether it is ethically justifiable for a psychiatrist to prescribe a placebo
to a patient can only be adequately addressed by understanding how biological,
psychological, and social factors interact in the patient's disorder. Framing this
question within a narrow cognitive model of consent requiring full disclosure
of information ignores the more holistic biopsychosocial framework in which
psychiatric disorders develop and can be mitigated or resolved.

## Neurofeedback

NFB uses EEG or fMRI to enable patients with neurological and psychiatric
disorders to visualize and modulate brain activity and control symptoms in real
time. With fMRI, the technique relies on the patient's own cognitive and emotional responses as she interacts with imaging displaying regional blood flow in
her brain. When they successfully use NFB to modulate neural hyperactivity or
hypoactivity associated with chronic pain, depression, anxiety, or attention deficit hyperactivity disorder, patients exercise more autonomy and control over
their brains and minds than they do when they are passive recipients of brain
stimulation or psychotropic medication (Schermer, 2015). NFB is a form of
self-regulation in the sense that the subject learns to regulate her own brain-
wave patterns and ameliorate symptoms. NFB is appropriately described as a
noninvasive form of neuromodulation because it involves no electrical stimulation from sources inside or outside of the brain. It is also distinctive as a therapy
for neuropsychiatric disorders because it combines biological psychiatry in the

form of functional brain imaging or electrophysiological recording with self-directed psychotherapy as complementary components of treatment.

In one NFB study involving subjects with chronic intractable pain, some were able to regulate activity in the rostral anterior cingulate cortex, which is associated with pain perception. Some of the subjects experienced pain relief by downregulating hyperactivity in this region (de Charms, Maeda, Glover et al., 2005). In a controlled proof-of-concept study using fMRI-based NFB, patients with depression who had not responded to pharmacological or psychological therapies were successfully trained in four NFB sessions to upregulate neural circuits involved in the generation of positive emotions. These included the ventrolateral PFC and insula. This resulted in significantly improved mood among subjects in the active intervention group that was not experienced by controls receiving cognitive techniques other than NFB (Linden, Habes, Johnston et al., 2012).

Successful use of this technique may enable patients with anhedonia to regulate metabolic activity in the ventral striatum of the reward system and experience improved motivation. It may enable other patients to downregulate hyperactivity in the subgenual cingulate region associated with cognitive and emotional disturbances and improve reasoning and mood. Another study testing this same technique trained people with high levels of contamination anxiety to modulate hyperactivity in the orbitofrontal cortex and reduce anxious responses to stimuli (Scheinost, Stoica, Saksa et al., 2013). Other studies investigating the effect of NFB on neural circuits mediating cognitive inhibitory mechanisms in childhood and adolescent attention deficit hyperactivity disorder have had positive results as well (Bakhshayesh, Hansch, Wynchkon et al., 2011).

Perceived loss of control of one's cognitive, emotional, and motivational states and one's environment can be a secondary symptom of MDD, GAD, and panic disorder. By modulating brain activity in response to viewing images or recordings of it on fMRI or EEF, a patient can recover some degree of behavior control impaired by psychiatric disorders. The subject herself is causing salutary changes in her mental states through her cognitive and affective responses to her brain activity. As a form of psychotherapy, it is questionable how effective NFB could be in treating moderately severe to severe psychiatric disorders. Yet it is much safer than DBS, TMS, or tCS because it does not entail any risk of bleeding or other adverse events in brain tissue or circuits beyond the regions the technique modulates. It also avoids the potential side effects caused by interactions between different drugs in the body and brain at the same time, or potentially adverse interactions between psychotropic drugs and electrical brain stimulation. It could be used adjunctively with medication and/

or psychotherapy to improve symptoms. The knowledge that the patient's own cognitive and emotional response to the visual feedback from EEG or fMRI and symptom relief can generate a feeling of control of her condition allows the patient to transform a perceived loss of control from a disease of the brain and mind into an experience of restored control.

There is potential harm from NFB. The belief that the technique provides a person with more control of her neural and mental states than other treatments for depression or anxiety may generate unreasonable expectations about the extent to which she can control them. Failure to successfully manipulate the NFB technique and meet the expectation of symptom relief may harm the patient by thwarting the realization of this goal. This could exacerbate the feeling of loss of control of her brain, mind, and environment. NFB utilizes a combination of unconscious operant conditioning and conscious expectation. While this may appear similar to the placebo response, NFB is different because of the role of real-time visual feedback in these conscious and unconscious processes. Both processes are involved in a patient's use of the technique, and this depends critically on how effectively the practitioner trains the patient to operate it. This underscores the importance of the availability of competently trained clinicians and researchers to provide and monitor the technique, despite the fact that the patient uses it. Effective use of NFB requires a certain level of cognitive, emotional, and motivational capacity, as well as sustained attention and patience. Not all patients with psychiatric disorders have the necessary level of these capacities to engage in NFB. Even those with mild to moderate depression or anxiety may not be able to do this. To prevent or minimize the probability of psychological harm, psychiatrists could identify and recommend certain patients who would be more likely to use the technique successfully.

This may seem unfair to those with more severe depression who lack the mental capacity to use it. It would deny them the opportunity to benefit from a technique that is safer than electrical brain stimulation or psychoactive drugs. Nevertheless, if the patient's behavior indicates that he lacks the mental capacity to effectively engage in NFB, then a psychiatrist may reasonably and fairly conclude that the patient would not be a candidate for it. It is also possible that changes in the brain associated with a less severe disorder would not be amenable to this technique. Excluding patients from research into or clinical applications of NFB would be a way of preventing harm to them. It would thus be ethically justified to discriminate among psychiatric patients on these grounds.

Still, any psychological harm from failing to meet an expectation to use NFB would not be as serious as the harm from adverse drug- or stimulation-induced physiological changes in the patient's brain. Also, insofar as NFB was used as an adjunct to an antidepressant and/or CBT, any risk of harm resulting from unrealized expectations would be mitigated by the fact that it was not the only treatment for the patient. Typically, NFB would be integrated into a broad treatment regimen that included CBT and medication. As it supplements rather than supplants these other therapies and is clearly noninvasive, the potential benefit of NFB outweighs any risk of harm to patients with the cognitive and emotional capacities necessary to use it.

NFB raises social justice issues. Assuming that it was effective, using NFB as an alternative to first-line drug therapy would be expensive and not covered by private insurance in the United States or Medicare in Canada. This would make it available only to the financially better off. It would create a situation in which some patients had access to a treatment and others were excluded from it. Unequal access would be unfair because both the better off and worse off would have a psychiatric disorder through no fault of their own. Access to NFB or a similar nonpharmacological therapy would depend on the ability to pay, which would be unfair when income inequality does not result solely from affected people's actions. This situation conflicts with the theory of luck egalitarianism, whereby the principle of distributive justice requires correcting disadvantages for which individuals are not responsible. It seeks to compensate for the effects of bad luck on their lives (Rawls, 1971, pp. 60 ff.; Segall, 2010, Chapter 7). Insofar as psychiatric disorders befall people through bad luck and are beyond their control, it seems unjust that some but not others with the same type of disorder would have access to a particular treatment for it. This situation would also conflict with the ideal of providing healthcare to allow all affected people fair equality of opportunity over a lifetime (Daniels, 1985, 2008). This is significant given the lifetime burden of disease from depression, anxiety, and other forms of mental illness. Lack of access to effective treatment is an obstacle to equal opportunity for people with diseases in general and mental illness in particular.

Publicly funded healthcare systems have limited resources and cannot provide all forms of care to all people who need and could benefit from it. Mental disorders are among the most costly conditions to treat. This is especially the case in children, but it also applies to adolescents and adults. NFB can be time-consuming for patients and more labor intensive for clinicians than prescribing antidepressant, antipsychotic, or anxiolytic drugs. This can make it more costly for patients if their health insurers do not pay for the sessions and for clinicians if they are not reimbursed for providing the service. NFB is more widely available in countries with a higher percentage of private healthcare compared with public insurance, such as Medicaid and Medicare in the United States. Yet private insurers are selective about the services for which they pay. Just because the technique is available in some countries but not others does not mean that where people live gives them an advantage in access to healthcare. Furthermore, because no drugs are involved in NFB, the pharmaceutical industry would not be interested in funding large clinical trials to test the efficacy of the technique, which has been questioned by many neurologists and psychiatrists. If a therapy such as NFB were effective for a large number of patients with neurological and psychiatric disorders, then in principle health policy should include it among covered treatments. But policymakers would give it lower priority than drug therapy in allocation decisions about psychiatric treatment for the reasons I just cited. I discuss a different set of social justice issues regarding access to DBS in Chapter 4.

## Conclusion

There is considerable variability in responses to psychotropic drugs for the treatment of psychiatric disorders. This reflects differences in people's brains, as well as how these disorders change their brains over time. In some disorders, drugs that improve some symptoms may exacerbate others. This may occur in the mixed states of bipolar depression. An antidepressant that regulates depressive episodes may increase the risk of manic episodes and the rate of mood cycling in some individuals with this disorder. It can be challenging to use these agents to alter some neural circuits and neurotransmitters while leaving others intact. Suboptimal or poor responses to psychopharmacology may be the result of targeting monoamines rather than other types of neurotransmitters. Studies have shown or suggested that drugs acting on GABAergic or glutaminergic pathways may be more effective in controlling diseases of the brain and mind. There is a need for newer-generation antidepressant and antipsychotic drugs. Despite this need, since 2011 all major pharmaceutical companies have stopped or markedly reduced their investment in psychopharmacology.

Alternatively, techniques using electrical stimulation can modulate neural circuits while avoiding the delayed, nondiscriminating, and often debilitating side effects of psychotropic drugs. Many research and clinical neuroscientists describe ECT, TMS, tCS, and TI as noninvasive, in contrast to invasive DBS and neural ablation. Yet any form of neuromodulation is invasive in a broader sense because it causes changes in neural activity. Rather than distinguish between invasive and noninvasive neuromodulating techniques, it is more accurate to distinguish between more and less invasive techniques. The main ethical issue regarding all of these treatments is not the degree of invasiveness as such. Instead, the issue is whether they involve a favorable benefit–risk ratio for patients. Psychiatric researchers, clinicians, patients, and research subjects have to consider the potential for positive and negative outcomes in administering or undergoing interventions in the brain.

I explored the possibility of pharmacological blockade of reconsolidation of pathological fear memories implicated in anxiety, panic, and PTSD. In addition, I described which patients would be more likely to benefit from ECT and speculated that the side effect of retrograde amnesia may be a consequence of an otherwise therapeutic mechanism. In discussing TMS and tCS, the main ethical concern is that people using these techniques may believe that they entail little or no risk and use them without professional supervision. When not used properly, repeated electrical pulses activating the cortex may cause adverse neural and mental effects. To protect individuals who use them, these techniques need to be regulated by the coordinated action of device makers, psychiatric organizations, and government agencies.

In my discussion of noninvasive psychological treatments, I outlined the circumstances in which nondeceptive and even deceptive use of placebos could be justified in clinical psychiatry. Depending on certain features of patient–physician interaction, a psychiatrist can prescribe a placebo to relieve symptoms without undermining trust or respect for patient autonomy. This action can also be consistent with the physician's obligations of beneficence and nonmaleficence. In NFB, the patient rather than a drug or device can modulate brain function and relieve symptoms through her psychological response to brain activity visualized on EEG or fMRI. The success of NFB depends on how well the practitioner trains the patient and how well the patient learns through this conditioning to use the technique. NFB is more likely to benefit patients with moderate symptoms amenable to this conditioning and less likely to benefit patients with severe symptoms. Any risk of harm is associated more with patient expectations than with alteration of neural processes.

Less invasive neurostimulation techniques are limited in their ability to control major psychiatric disorders. They may not be specific enough in targeting dysfunctional neural circuits. They may have transient effects, or may not penetrate to subcortical regions of the brain. Direct surgical interventions in these deeper regions may be the only way to modulate circuits and ameliorate symptoms. These interventions include the most invasive forms of neuromodulation—DBS and neural ablation. I discuss some of the ethical, social, and broader philosophical questions raised by psychiatric neurosurgery in the following two chapters.

# Chapter 4

# Psychiatric neurosurgery

The drugs and techniques discussed in the preceding chapter often fail to modulate neural dysfunction or relieve symptoms in severe psychiatric disorders. A significant percentage of these disorders remain refractory to most treatments. Up to 20% of patients with MDD remain resistant to antidepressant and other therapies (Holtzheimer and Mayberg, 2011, p. 2), and 40–60% of patients with OCD fail to respond to pharmacotherapy (SSRIs) and psychotherapy (CBT) (De Ridder, Vanneste, Gillett et al., 2016). In addition, "10%–30% of patients with schizophrenia have little or no response to antipsychotic treatment" (Mikell, Sinha, and Sheth, 2016, p. 917). The incidence of treatment-resistance in AN may be just as high. Due to the mixed manic and depressive symptoms in BD I and II, drugs that improve depressive symptoms may increase the risk of mania and the rate of mood cycling. Clinical trials on ketamine and its effects on glutamate receptors have shown that it can induce rapid positive responses in subjects with depression. Still, further research will need to determine whether this and other experimental drugs can effectively treat depression and other psychiatric disorders.

The current consensus in psychiatry is that major psychiatric disorders are neurodevelopmental disorders involving abnormalities in brain circuits or nodes within these circuits (Insel, 2010, p. 188). In a recent editorial, Brian Harris Kopell and Jonathan Rasouli endorse this position: "As our collective knowledge of the mechanisms behind the human thought process and behavior continue to evolve, we are learning that psychiatric disorders are not simply ailments of abnormal neurotransmitter metabolism. In fact, conditions such as major depression and obsessive-compulsive disorder may actually be due to abnormal neural signaling and brain circuitry. As neurosurgeons, our ability to harness, manipulate and tap into these pathways through neuromodulation techniques such as deep brain stimulation open new frontiers into their treatment" (2016, p. 248). Dysfunctional connectivity in these circuits generates the psychopathology in schizophrenia, MDD, OCD, BD I and II, GAD, and other disorders. Although an imaging-based focus on circuit-level mechanisms does not explain the etiology of these disorders, it can help to explain the underlying pathophysiology. It can also help to explain why psychotherapy and psychopharmacology are often ineffective in treating them. If the underlying pathophysiology occurs at the circuit level, and if the circuits are dysfunctional, then altering neurotransmitters alone may not be sufficient to restore normal neural and mental function. Directly targeting and modulating these circuits may be more effective in controlling these disorders and ameliorating symptoms. While rTMS and other less invasive stimulating techniques have more focused effects than psychotropic drugs, they may not penetrate to structures below the cortex, such as the amygdala, ventral striatum, and midbrain. This is where much of the dysregulation implicated in severe psychiatric disorders occurs. Due to these limitations, many of these disorders remain resistant to these interventions.

This is the rationale for psychiatric neurosurgery. Unlike structural neurosurgery, such as resecting brain tumors or clipping cerebral aneurysms, psychiatric neurosurgery is a type of functional neurosurgery (Lozano and Lipsman, 2013; Hariz, 2016). It modulates dysfunctional cortical and subcortical neural circuits mediating motor and mental functions by electrical stimulation or by ablating discrete areas of neural tissue. DBS and neural ablation are experimental and investigative interventions for psychiatric disorders that have failed to respond to other treatments. While neurosurgeons and psychiatrists often describe stimulating techniques as "neuromodulation" and lesioning techniques as "neuroablation," both are different forms of neuromodulation. Stimulating nodes in dysfunctional neural circuits or altering tissue in these circuits can restore function in them. In Chapters 1 and 2, I cited imaging studies confirming correlations between neural circuit dysfunction and symptoms of psychiatric disorders. In this chapter, I analyze and discuss neuroscientific and ethical aspects of the most invasive neuromodulating techniques to correct dysfunction and improve symptoms. Psychiatric neurosurgery modulates neural circuits so that they are neither overactive nor underactive. In this way, it can improve sensorimotor, cognitive, emotional, and volitional functions.

Psychiatric neurosurgery entails greater risks than less invasive brain interventions because it more directly alters brain structure and function. In addition to the risk of intracerebral hemorrhage, seizures, infection, and edema, there is also a risk of neurological and psychological sequelae from this type of surgery, some of which may be permanent. These risks have to be weighed against the potential benefit from undergoing psychiatric neurosurgery, as well as the risk of continued poor quality of life and suicide from living with a chronic treatment-resistant condition. What makes benefit–risk assessment in psychiatric neurosurgery ethically problematic is that, for many patients, it may be their only remaining treatment option. Because of this, they may not fully consider the risks associated with the procedure. In addition, the disorders for which psychiatric neurosurgery is indicated can impair the cognitive capacity necessary for informed consent to participate in psychiatric neurosurgery research.

After tracing the history of psychiatric neurosurgery, I outline the differences between neural ablation and DBS, focusing on the potential benefits and risks to psychiatric patients who undergo them. Although ablation has been used primarily for treatment-resistant OCD, the evaluation of the risks and benefits of this technique also applies to other psychiatric disorders for which it might be indicated. The main focus of the chapter will be on DBS and its potential to modulate dysfunctional neural circuits and relieve symptoms in moderately severe to severe forms of major psychiatric disorders. I discuss whether people affected by them have the mental capacity to weigh the reasons for and against DBS and give informed consent to participate in clinical trials testing the technique. I also discuss whether the potential for a therapeutic misconception (TM) among potential research subjects undermines consent to participate in DBS clinical trials. In addition, I examine the technical differences between open- and closed-loop DBS, compare their neuromodulating effects, and discuss how they would affect patients and research subjects. I then discuss the obligations of researchers to psychiatric patients who participate in this research. In the last section and conclusion of the chapter, I explore the therapeutic potential of optogenetics in psychiatry and the use of DBS at an earlier stage of the disease process.

Identifying and modulating circuit-level mechanisms implicated in psychiatric disorders does not provide a complete account of the etiology, pathophysiology, and symptomatology of these disorders. Nor do these mechanisms fully explain the variability of patients' responses to neural ablation and DBS. Circuit-based explanations alone do not capture how these disorders affect people's lives. Avoiding a reductionist model in which mental illness is explained entirely in neurobiological terms, I focus on the probing and modulating functions of psychiatric neurosurgery as one aspect of a biopsychosocial model to explain how these disorders develop, progress, and how they might be treated.

## Three eras of psychiatric neurosurgery

The first form of psychosurgery was trephination. Practiced as long as 5000 years ago in Asia, Northern Africa, Europe, and Central and South America, the procedure consisted in scraping burr holes into the skull. The idea was to expose the dura mater to treat intracranial diseases. But the real advent of ablative psychiatric neurosurgery was in 1888, when Gottlieb Burckhardt removed the left frontotemporal cerebral cortex in six patients diagnosed with psychiatric disease (Dyster, Mikell, and Sheth, 2016, p. 1). Burckhardt hypothesized that localized areas of the cortex were "psychic domains," and that ablating tissue in these areas could cure psychic disease. Later, in the 1930s, Antonio Egas Moniz similarly hypothesized that the prefrontal region of the brain was the "psychic center" of a person, and that "faulty wiring" in this region was the cause of schizophrenia and depression (Wind and Anderson, 2008, p. 2; Lapidus, Kopell, Ben-Haim et al., 2013). Although it was informed by immature neuroscience, Moniz's faulty-wiring hypothesis could be interpreted as a precursor of the current dysfunctional circuit approach to understanding and treating psychiatric disorders. Indeed, growing evidence that white matter deficits occur in many psychiatric disorders in some respects confirms Moniz's hypothesis (Wind and Anderson, 2008, p. 2).

Initially, Moniz and Pedro Almeida Lima injected pure alcohol into the white matter of the anterior section of the frontal lobes. The alcohol destroyed what they believed were hyperactive frontal regions. After concluding that this technique was too imprecise, Moniz developed what he called the "leucotome," a device that could more precisely core white matter tracts in the PFC identified as the source of the faulty wiring and associated psychiatric symptoms. Moniz and Lima performed the first prefrontal leucotomy in 1935. Some patients with affective disorders such as anxiety and depression showed improvement after undergoing this procedure. Results in his patients with schizophrenia were not so favorable, however. Moniz received the Nobel Prize for Medicine in 1949 for his contribution of "immense importance . . . for the problems of psychiatric treatment" (Wind and Anderson, p. 2).

A further development of Moniz and Lima's procedure was the frontal lobotomy performed by Walter Freeman and James Watts from the 1930s to the 1960s. Believing that psychiatric disorders were caused by "excessive emotions" associated with faulty neural connections between prefrontal and other regions of the brain, Freeman used the "ice pick" technique to sever these connections (Freeman and Watts, 1942; Pressman, 1998, pp. 113–139, 316–322). This involved slicing through neural fibers with a metal device. Freeman developed this technique to make lobotomies easier. Instead of making burr holes on the vertex of the skull, he inserted the lobotomy device (the ice pick) through the eye sockets. In this way, nonsurgeons could perform the procedure. Freeman and Watts's goal was to relieve their patients' "mental pain" through surgical means (Freeman and Watts, 1942, p. 794).

Although Freeman's patients did not give what we now know as informed consent, this was not always the practice during this period. Thus, not obtaining informed consent from his patients was not unique to him. There were approximately 50,000 lobotomies performed between 1949 and 1956. The surgical risk was considered acceptable at that time. According to records in the George Washington University archives, Freeman performed lobotomies "on children as young as four years old" (Phillips, 2013, p. 2). Many of his patients had no improvement in symptoms. Some experienced significant physical and mental disability. Although Freeman claimed that a third of these operations were successful, the overall negative professional response to Freeman's procedure and the death of his last patient in 1967 led to the demise of the lobotomy. After he stopped performing lobotomies, Freeman travelled across the United States to record long-term outcomes in his patients (El-Hai, 2005). FDA approval of the antipsychotic drug chlorpromazine in the United States in 1952 marked the end of the second era of psychosurgery. It began a period in which psychotropic drugs became the primary form of treatment of psychiatric diseases. These drugs appeared to obviate the need for surgical intervention in the brain for psychiatric disorders. While response rates vary across difference disorders and patients, psychopharmacology remains first-line treatment for severe forms of them.

The 1950s did not mark the end of ablative neurosurgery. Although only a small number of patients with psychiatric disorders would undergo the procedure, ablative psychiatric neurosurgery continued to be practiced. Two significant developments in the technique from the days of Moniz and Lima, and Freeman and Watts, were more scientifically sound hypotheses about the neurobiological causes of mental illness and more targeted ablation with the introduction of the stereotactic technique in 1947. Thus began the second era of psychiatric neurosurgery. Utilizing this technique, in 1949 Jean Talairach performed an anterior capsulotomy, destroying tissue in a hyperactive anterior limb of the internal capsule (Dyster, Mikell, and Sheth, 2016). He relied on the "Papez circuit" model in hypothesizing that the internal capsule had connections with the limbic system and that disruption of these connections accounted for the psychiatric symptoms in his patients. In 1962, H. Thomas Ballantine performed the first stereotactic bilateral cingulotomy on a patient with comorbid anxiety and depression by destroying tissue in a hyperactive anterior cingulate cortex (Ballantine, Cassidy, Flanagan et al., 1967).

The current third era of psychiatric neurosurgery began in 1987. In that year, Alim-Louis Benabid and coinvestigators used high-frequency electrical stimulation of the central thalamus without ablating neural tissue to control motor symptoms in a patient with PD (Benabid, Pollak, Louveau, Henry et al., 1987). They used the procedure after the patient's symptoms became less responsive to levodopa, and dyskinesias developed as a side effect of the drug. In addition to restoring some degree of motor control, Benabid's procedure resulted in the serendipitous discovery that it could have modulating effects on neural circuits mediating mood and motivation. This led to the subsequent application in the late 1990s and early 2000s of DBS as an experimental treatment for MDD and OCD and an alternative to ablation for the second of these disorders. Advanced stereotactic techniques and structural and functional neuroimaging have improved the precision of both neural ablation and DBS. This has resulted in safer and more effective forms of psychiatric neurosurgery than the procedures of the past (Dyster, Mikell and Sheth, 2016; Hariz, 2016). While the first two eras of psychiatric neurosurgery involved neural ablation, the third era involves both ablation and the more recent and more frequently administered DBS. The history of psychiatric neurosurgery parallels the history of biological psychiatry. Both histories are based on a neurobiological explanation of psychiatric disorders.

## Neural ablation and deep brain stimulation

Neural ablation typically involves creating lesions of 1–2 centimeters or less in brain tissue identified as the source of neural circuit dysfunction. There are three main stereotactic lesioning techniques. Lesions can be produced by radiofrequency ablation. In this procedure, a metal probe is inserted through burr holes drilled bilaterally in the cranium. The tip of the probe is heated to approximately 70 degrees Celsius and deactivates or destroys targeted metabolically overactive neurons. Alternatively, Gamma Knife® radiosurgery (GKR) produces lesions in hyperactive neural circuits by delivering beams of gamma radiation to them from a guiding device placed on the head. With this technique, neurons can be inactivated without the risk of bleeding or infection from intracranial surgery. A more recent experimental lesioning modality is magnetic resonance-guided focused ultrasound (MRgFUS). This technique uses acoustic waves to alter neurons and neural circuits. It can direct higher-intensity waves to ablate tissue or lower-intensity waves to modulate nodes and circuits. One advantage of FUS over TMS and rTMS is that it can penetrate deep brain structures to modulate metabolically hyperactive nuclei without affecting normal neurons and tissue in higher brain regions. This mechanism of action is similar to that of temporal interference.

In contrast to DBS, FUS can penetrate and modulate these structures without intracranial surgery. Imaging allows neurosurgeons to direct ultrasonic waves at a localized area of the brain to within 1 millimeter of accuracy. Some randomized controlled trials of high-intensity focused ultrasound (HIFUS) thermal ablation of the thalamus for essential tremor reduced hand tremor in a significant number of subjects (Lipsman, Schwartz, Huang et al., 2013; Elias, Lipsman, Ondo et al., 2016; Louis, 2016). However, 14% of the subjects in one of the trials had permanently altered sensation (Louis, 2016, p. 793).

Lower-intensity FUS may have application for some psychiatric disorders in modulating dysfunctional neural circuits mediating cognitive-emotional processing without creating fixed lesions. HIFUS may also treat these disorders by ablating targeted tissue in metabolically hyperactive neural circuits. It may not be as accurate a lesioning technique as radiofrequency ablation because ultrasonic waves may not pass easily through bone such as the cranium. This can be a problem for patients with greater skull thickness, which can affect the frequency, specificity, and other properties of the acoustic wave. This occurred in five patients in one of the trials (Elias, Lipsmam, Ondo et al., 2016), for whom FUS could not be delivered to the thalamus (Louis, 2016, p. 793).

Ablative neurosurgery in psychiatry includes (1) anterior cingulotomy, (2) anterior capsulotomy, (3) subcaudate tractotomy, (4) limbic leucotomy (a combination of (1) and (3)), and (4) amygdalotomy (De Ridder, Vanneste, Gillett et al., 2016; Dyster, Mikell, and Sheth, 2016). The two main targets have been the dorsal and rostral anterior cingulate (cingulotomy) and the anterior limb of the internal capsule (capsulotomy). Neurosurgeons use these procedures on a small number of patients whose conditions are refractory to pharmacotherapy and psychotherapy and who are not candidates for, or have not responded to, DBS. Most of the ablation procedures in psychiatry have been performed on patients with treatment-refractory OCD. Because some psychiatric disorders often have a common neural substrate with overlapping or interacting neural networks, some of these procedures—particularly cingulotomy and capsulotomy—may also be indicated in some cases of refractory MDD and GAD. For example, capsulotomy can be a therapy for severe OCD and MDD because both disorders involve dysregulation in the ventral capsule/ventral striatum. In severe cases of PTSD, where propranolol or MDMA has failed, theoretically amygdalotomy could be an intervention of last resort to disable a hyperactive fear memory system. Neurosurgeons are now able to target hyperactive localized regions of the brain with accurately placed lesions. This makes the procedure safer and more effective than it was at the time of Moniz and Lima, and Freeman and Watts.

The results of a study of capsulotomy for refractory OCD published in 2008 showed that the procedure reduced the obsessions and compulsions in a majority of 28 subjects. Yet half of these subjects developed apathy and poor self-control. Follow-up several years after the procedure showed that these symptoms persisted without any resolution (Ruck, Karlsson, Steele et al., 2008). More recent studies of electrolytic cingulotomy and Gamma Knife' capsulotomy for this same disorder have demonstrated more positive results and fewer long-term side effects (Shields, Assad, Eskandar et al., 2008; Sheehan, Patterson, Schlesinger et al., 2013; Sheth, Neal, Tangherlini et al., 2013; Spatola, Martinez-Alvarez and Martinez-Moreno, 2018). Clinical trials testing HIFUS cingulotomy for patients with refractory MDD, capsulotomy for patients with refractory OCD, and limbic leucotomy for patients with refractory AN would determine whether the technique could be a treatment for severe forms of these disorders (Meng, Suppiah, Mithani et al., 2017). GKR and FUS do not require drilling burr holes in the skull. This avoids the risk of infection and hemorrhage from intracranial surgery. Still, this does not rule out the possibility of postsurgical lesion expansion to healthy tissue beyond the ablated tissue. In light of this possibility, GKR and FUS do not entirely avoid the risk of sensorimotor impairment or adverse changes in thought and behavior.

Thanks largely to MRI-guided stereotactic techniques, all three types of neural ablation are more accurate, safer, and more effective than the comparatively crude prefrontal leucotomy performed by Moniz and Lima and the prefrontal lobotomy performed by Freeman and Watts. The main medical and ethical concern with ablation is that the lesion is fixed. Any untoward effects on neural and mental function could be irreversible. There is also the possibility of lesion expansion. For some patients, though, the lesion may only be temporary. Endogenous repair mechanisms in the brain may induce tissue reinnervation. This would be a welcome outcome if it involved restoration of normal brain function (De Ridder, Vanneste, Gillett et al., 2016, p. 244). But the nodes and nuclei in the tissue may just as likely return to their hyperactive state. This may explain the high relapse rate in OCD after lesioning of the nucleus accumbens. This outcome would not be preferable to a fixed lesion. A lesion could be reversible rather than permanent, but the result would not be an elimination or reduction of symptoms. Depending on the incidence or degree of reinnervation after ablation, this possibility "suggests that stimulation might be a better mode of neuromodulation" (De Ridder, Vanneste, Gillett et al., 2016, p. 243). Despite advances in the technique, medical and ethical questions remain about its safety and efficacy, as well as when it would be indicated. Further research is necessary to adequately address these questions.

DBS is a more recent and generally safer form of psychiatric neurosurgery than neural ablation (Barrett, 2017). Instead of creating fixed lesions in neural tissue, DBS electrically stimulates dysfunctional neural circuits and modulates them so that they are neither metabolically overactive nor underactive. The goal of the technique is to ameliorate sensorimotor, cognitive, emotional, and volitional functions impaired by neural circuit dysfunction and disrupted connectivity. DBS creates a virtual lesion by inducing electrophysiological silence in a circuit. Electrodes are surgically implanted unilaterally or bilaterally in an area of the brain identified as the source of the dysfunction. The electrodes are stimulated at varying frequencies and intensities through leads connected to a pulse generator implanted under the collarbone, or in the abdomen. A programmable hand-held device controls the pulse generator. The electrodes deliver continuous stimulation to modulate neural activity in targeted areas. Patients undergoing the implant procedure may be asleep under general anesthesia or awake, as in psychiatric applications. This allows them to report cognitive, emotional, or motor effects to the neurosurgeon.

DBS can be an alternative for patients whose conditions do not respond to psychopharmacology. In fact, as noted, DBS and other forms of neuromodulation have had to fill the therapeutic vacuum left by the lack of development of new psychotropic drugs. DBS is a more focused means of neuromodulation that targets a specific structure in a particular circuit. This can avoid the distributed and nondiscriminating action of psychotropic drugs. These can lead to significant side effects such as weight gain and other metabolic changes that may result in nonadherence. DBS offers the ability to dissociate key brain structures and study them and the motor and mental capacities they mediate in real-time. The technique is also superior to less invasive techniques such as TMS because it can modulate dysfunction in subcortical regions, such as the striatum and midbrain. In addition, the sustained effects of constant DBS may do more to control these disorders than the more transient effects of TMS and psychopharmacology.

One of the first experimental uses of DBS for TRD decreased metabolic activity in the subgenual cingulate (Brodmann area 25). Behavioral changes and PET imaging confirmed that the stimulation improved function in a cortical–limbic circuit and improved depressive symptoms in a small number of patients (Mayberg, Lozano, Voon et al., 2005). A later study showed that bilateral stimulation of the subcallosal cingulate also relieved depressive symptoms in a significant number of the participants (Lozano, Mayberg, Giacobbe et al., 2008). In another study, stimulation of the same brain region relieved symptoms of both unipolar and bipolar depression in some subjects (Holtzheimer, Kelley, Gross et al., 2012). A different clinical trial testing stimulation of the nucleus accumbens relieved anhedonia in participants with no adverse effects (Schlaepfer, Cohen, Frick et al., 2008). DBS trials for OCD have been conducted over a longer period (Nuttin, Cosyns, Demeulemeester et al., 1999; Mallet, Polosan, Jaafari et al., 2008; Greenberg, Gabriels, Malone et al., 2010). A recent study showed that DBS of a metabolically overactive posterior hypothalamus and ventral thalamus decreased aggressive behavior in some patients with impulse control disorders (Micieli, Rios, Aguilar et al., 2017).

These are just some examples of how DBS can restore some degree of motor and mental functions impaired in psychiatric disorders. There are significant risks associated with DBS, however. These include intracranial hemorrhage, edema, and infection from surgical implantation of the electrodes, lead fractures, and neurological and psychological symptoms such as hypomania from imprecise electrode placement or overstimulation (Lozano and Lipsman, 2013; Castrioto, Lhommee, Moro et al., 2014).

In many of the DBS trials for MDD, the effects of the technique take weeks to occur. The latency period of DBS may be similar to that of psychotropic drugs. Yet one study testing DBS of the medial forebrain bundle significantly reduced symptoms in seven patients with treatment-resistant MDD within 7 days of the onset of stimulation (Schlaepfer, Bewernick, Kayser et al., 2013). These differences in response time illustrate the variability in responses to neurostimulation, depending on the extent of brain dysfunction, the selected target, and the fact that DBS has different effects at different time scales (Agnesi, Johnson, and Vitek, 2013). They may also reflect different levels of neuroplasticity among patients undergoing DBS (Crowell, Garlow, Riva-Posse et al., 2015). Responses to DBS for OCD may be delayed because, even when neural circuits are modulated, it takes time for the patient to unlearn pathological behavior associated with the disorder (De Ridder, Vanneste, Gillett et al., 2016). This indicates the role of memory in learning and unlearning pathological patterns of thought and behavior. These processes have both neurobiological and psychological aspects and thus are not entirely determined by neural activity.

As a neuromodulating technique, DBS is superior to ablation in at least three respects. First, assuming that insertion of the electrode does not cause bleeding, it creates a virtual rather than a fixed lesion in brain tissue. This avoids or at least reduces the risk of permanent neurological and psychological sequelae. Second, its effects are generally reversible because the psychiatrist and neurosurgeon can change electrode placement, adjust stimulation parameters, or surgically remove the electrodes from the patient's brain. Third, DBS has both neuromodulating and probing mechanisms of action (Lozano and Lipsman, 2013; Holtzheimer and Mayberg, 2011). By probing the brain and receiving information about brain structure and function from neuroimaging such as diffusion magnetic resonance tractography, PET, and fMRI, neurosurgeons and psychiatrists can identify the neural source of the disorder. This enables them to locate the right targets for electrode placement and activation, as well as to monitor the effects of stimulation. In addition, reports from awake patients undergoing stimulation can shed light on the disordered mental states associated with it. The technique can elucidate different dimensions of the brain–mind relation.

Still, the risks associated with the procedure are a key factor in assessing the consent of research subjects with psychiatric disorders to consent to participate in DBS clinical trials. DBS has been approved as therapy for the movement disorders of PD, essential tremor, and dystonia. It has also been used for epilepsy and impulse control disorders such as Tourette syndrome. Yet except for a humanitarian device exemption for OCD in 2009, it remains experimental and investigational for all other psychiatric disorders. More long-term randomized controlled clinical trials are needed to establish its safety and efficacy in psychiatry. This will require more precise targeting of neural circuits and setting of the frequency and intensity of the electrical current delivered to the brain. Achieving these goals would do more to ameliorate symptoms and prevent neurological and psychological sequelae.

The dual probing and neuromodulating ability of DBS is a further development of Wilder Penfield's technique of using a probe to deliver low-level electric current directly to the temporal lobe. From the 1930s to the 1950s, Penfield used this technique to detect the source of seizures of his patients undergoing awake surgery for epilepsy. While the main goal of Penfield's probing technique was to identify and remove brain regions responsible for seizures in patients with this neurological disorder, he produced maps of sensory and motor cortices, or what he called "functional localization"(Penfield and Rasmussen, 1950; Fried, Katz, McCarthy et al., 1991). These states included autobiographical memories of patients' pasts, which he was able to elicit in some patients by stimulating the temporal cortex.

In his neural mapping and resectioning of tissue in the temporal lobes, Penfield was performing functional and structural neurosurgery at the same time. His cortical stimulation for the treatment of functional brain disorders introduced the modern era of functional neurosurgery. The combination of imaging, intraoperative electrophysiological recording of brain activity, and the effects of electrical stimulation on cortical and subcortical structures has led to a better understanding of the pathophysiology of psychiatric disorders. More generally, it has led to a better understanding of the correlations between normal and abnormal neural and mental states. These procedures allow neuroscientists to study abnormal neural and mental features as a way of gaining knowledge of the relation between the normal brain and mind. They show that investigating and treating psychiatric diseases is not exclusively the domain of psychiatrists but also includes neurosurgeons, neurologists, psychologists, and radiologists. Penfield's combined probing and mapping technique is a good example of overlap among different neuroscientific domains.

A hypothetical and more controversial use of DBS or neural ablation would be to erase pathological fear memories implicated in anxiety, depression, panic, phobia, and PTSD. These would be potentially more effective interventions for erasing these memories than protein synthesis inhibitors or other drugs. They would be more precise than these drugs in targeting the neural source of the memories. These techniques would be indicated when the emotional representation, or trace, of the memory was localized in identifiable neurons and excitatory synapses in the basolateral amygdala of the fear memory system. Functional neuroimaging could confirm metabolic hyperactivity in this region when a patient retrieved the memory. Inactivating the nuclei by creating a virtual lesion with DBS or an actual lesion with HIFUS could remove the memory trace. High-frequency DBS could effectively erase the memory by inactivating the nuclei without destroying neural tissue. This would make it a safer procedure for this purpose than ablation. There is a empirical basis for this hypothesis. One group of researchers found that cigarette smokers with brain damage to the insula, which is associated with conscious urges, were more likely to stop smoking than those without this damage. The injury caused the smokers to "forget" their addiction (Naqvi, Rudrauf, Damasio et al., 2007). Erasing the memory trace in a hyperactive insula with DBS or ablation may be a way of treating refractory addiction. Still, fear and addiction are learned behaviors. Behavioral interventions would have to complement neurostimulation to produce the desired effect.

Inactivating or ablating nuclei associated with a fear memory and erasing the memory trace could resolve the pathological thought and behavior caused by the memory. Lower-frequency DBS or lower-intensity FUS could modulate metabolic hyperactivity. These techniques could have the same effect of attenuating the emotional content of traumatic memory as the drug propranolol (Pitman, Sanders, Zusman et al., 2002; Lonergan, Oliveira-Figueroa, Pitman et al., 2013). They could leave the cognitive content of the memory intact. Yet if they only weakened the memory and did not erase it, then that would leave open the possibility of stimuli reactivating its emotionally charged content. High-frequency DBS or HIFUS could inactivate or destroy the neurons and excitatory synapses within the memory trace and remove it from the brain (Glannon, 2017). This would be an expanded application of DBS to modulate metabolically hyperactive neural circuits in patients with depression. DBS and FUS are much safer than the prefrontal leucotomies and frontal lobotomies of the past. Using these techniques to neutralize or remove the neural source of a pathological fear memory by creating a virtual or actual lesion in the critical circuit would have the same goal of relieving patients' mental pain.

There are questions about whether inactivating or destroying neurons within the fear memory trace would have expanding adverse effects on adjacent neurons and synapses regulating normal memory mechanisms. Not all fear memories are maladaptive or pathological. Many are necessary to respond appropriately to environmental threats and thereby promote adaptability and survival. This can be a problem with the distributed and nondiscriminating effects of a protein synthesis inhibitor. While the action of DBS or FUS would be more precise than that of a drug, it is unclear whether these techniques could be precise enough to affect only the localized nuclei in the basolateral amygdala constituting the memory trace. Slightly off-target DBS or ablation could inactivate or destroy not only the nuclei associated with the problematic memory but also nuclei associated with other memories. The aim of targeting the neurons and synapses of the fear memory would be to remove it permanently from storage in the amygdala. Yet any irreversible effects on neurons and synapses mediating normal fear and positive emotional and spatial memories could harm persons by impairing their ability to navigate the environment. It is also possible that this intervention could erase episodic memories and disrupt the psychological connections constituting one's autobiography. It could disrupt the integrity of the self. This underscores the importance of specificity and selectivity in all forms of psychiatric neurosurgery. As in some cases of ablation for OCD, the nuclei in the amygdala targeted by DBS or FUS could become reinnervated and not be "erased" after all. This would not be a welcome reversible effect of these techniques.

It is important to emphasize that the amygdala is involved in all emotions, not just fear. The emotions may not be traceable to a particular memory of a particular experience. Stimulation of the amygdala for PTSD or a neurological disorder such as tinnitus, for example, may induce crying in a patient without any external stimulus. It might result in a nonspecific emotional response without any link to any specific memory (De Ridder, in correspondence).

Following a view about DBS held by many, I have claimed that, unlike most cases of neural ablation, the effects of neurostimulation are generally reversible. "Generally" implies that the effects are reversible in many but not all cases. There is some evidence that DBS induces anatomical changes in the brain. In one study, stimulation of the fornix resulted in changed volume in this region and the hippocampus (Sankar, Chakravarty, Bescos et al., 2015). Neurosurgeons and psychiatrists do not know whether this or other changes would be temporary or permanent, or whether they would be beneficial or harmful. It is also possible that this technique could alter synaptic connectivity and neural signaling in ways that may not become apparent until much later. It would be difficult to predict what these changes might be or how they might affect patients' mental states and capacities. Still, DBS allows more control than ablation over the neuromodulation process. The neurosurgeon probing and targeting the dysfunctional areas while the electrodes are stimulated can regulate the neural and mental effects of stimulation. Under local anesthesia, the patient is awake during the procedure and can respond to questions to report and confirm these effects. Parameters can be adjusted after the initial implantation and stimulation in response to patients' reports and what PET or fMRI display about brain function intraoperatively and postoperatively. In cases of serious sequelae, neurosurgeons can remove the electrodes from the brain. Adverse effects from stimulation may be reversible.

Stimulation alone does not cause all adverse effects. Bleeding that occurs during implantation can have devastating consequences in the brain that could be permanent. Although changes in the brain from neural ablation are more likely to be irreversible than changes from DBS, ablation can be less costly and impose less of a postoperative burden on the patient. There is no need for device monitoring, parameter adjustment, battery and lead replacement, and the time involved in these and other aspects of follow-up. But the permanence of lesioning in most cases of neural ablation is significant, as is the possibility of lesion expansion. As I explain later in this chapter, replacing open-loop with closed-loop DBS may provide decisive reasons for preferring electrical stimulation to neural ablation among patients who are candidates for both procedures.

Many researchers define a successful outcome of psychiatric neurosurgery in terms of symptom relief. A meta-analysis shows that lesioning of the anterior limb of the internal capsule has had a successful outcome in 50–70% of patients with OCD, and that electrical stimulation of this region has had a successful outcome in 50% of patients with this disorder (De Ridder, Vanneste, Gillett et al., 2016, p. 243). Overall, only 30–40% of patients with different psychiatric disorders respond to neurostimulation. Among other factors, this may be due to the genotype of the patient and polymorphisms in dopamine and other neurotransmitter transporter genes (De Ridder, Vanneste, Gillett et al., pp. 242–243). Failed or incomplete responses are a more fundamental problem than delayed responses. While, on balance, stimulation may be a safer form of neuromodulation than ablation, it is not always effective in treating severe forms of these disorders. From an ethical perspective regarding the weighing of benefit and harm, there may be unavoidable trade-offs between efficacy and safety. Each of these interventions may relieve symptoms, but at the cost of some neurological and psychological sequelae.

The differences between DBS and neural ablation as the most invasive forms of neuromodulation are also pertinent to ethical issues regarding perception of risk and informed consent of research subjects to participate in research testing these techniques. The greater risk of ablation compared with stimulation has to be assessed together with the benefits. For some patients, ablation may be more beneficial overall than stimulation. A sufficient number of prospective randomized controlled clinical trials comparing the short- and long-term benefits and risks of the two procedures are necessary to determine which intervention is more effective in treating refractory psychiatric disorders. Differences in people's brains and the fact that some patients may not be candidates for ablation or DBS complicate a straightforward answer to this question. Intuitively, the greater risk in ablation compared with stimulation may suggest that the former is the treatment of "last resort" (Pressman, 1998). This may lead many patients to prefer stimulation to ablation. Patient perceptions may influence a decision to undergo one procedure rather than the other. Joshua Pepper, Marwan Hariz, and Ludvic Zrinzo claim that "the current popularity of DBS over ablative surgery for OCD is not due to nonefficacy of AC (anterior capsulotomy) but possibly because DBS is perceived as more acceptable by clinicians and patients" (2015, p. 1028.). Similarly, Sabine Muller, Rita Riedmuller, and Ansel van Oosterhout claim that "from a mere medical perspective, none of the procedures is absolutely superior; rather, they have different profiles of advantages and disadvantages. Therefore, individual factors are crucial in decision-making, particularly the patients' social situation, individual preferences and individual attitudes" (2015, p. 1; Christen and Muller, 2018).

For patients who have not responded to other interventions, there may be equally justifiable reasons for participation in clinical trials testing neural ablation or DBS. Differences among patients' brains can determine who would be more likely to respond to these techniques, as well as who would be candidates for either or both of them. In light of these factors, the research question of whether electrical stimulation is more effective in controlling symptoms than ablation may be decided only on a case-by-case basis. If a patient is a candidate for both DBS and neural ablation, the patient's informed preferences regarding issues such as long-term follow-up may play a significant role in these decisions. Ultimately, assuming that subjects are exposed to an acceptable degree of risk and are competent to understand the design and goals of the research, participation in a DBS or neural ablation clinical trial can be ethically justified. Nevertheless, there are many questions about consent to undergo experimental procedures in psychiatric neurosurgery. As DBS is a more common form of this research than ablation, I will focus on it in discussing these questions.

## Consent to participate in psychiatric neurosurgery (deep brain stimulation) clinical trials

Psychiatric neurosurgery research is more invasive and entails more risk than psychopharmacology, ECT, or TMS. This seems to make it more ethically problematic than less invasive psychopharmacology research. Yet DBS may be the only remaining option for patients with severe treatment-resistant conditions. As a matter of justice, the idea that these patients are worse off than other patients with treatable conditions generates a moral imperative to allow them to participate in psychiatric neurosurgery research that might lead to treatments for severe mood and other psychiatric disorders (Nugent, Miller, Henter et al., 2017). The relation between research and therapy in psychiatry is complex, and distinguishing them is often not a straightforward issue. Many DBS trials are "doubly innovative" and may test both safety and efficacy in the same phase or in overlapping phases. They could be described as combined phase I/II trials. The fact that DBS targets the neural source of thought, decision-making, personality, and behavior presents ethical challenges for researchers enrolling and monitoring patients as research subjects in clinical trials testing this technique. Insofar as neural ablation involves greater risks, the ethical challenges in protecting research subjects undergoing this technique from potential harm may be even greater.

When a psychiatric disorder has been chronically resistant to psychopharmacology, psychotherapy, or other interventions, the severity of the disorder may impair the patient's cognitive and emotional capacity to understand the reasons for and appreciate the risks in a psychiatric neurosurgery clinical trial. This could impair his capacity to consent to participate in it as a research subject. Informed consent requires a certain degree of decisional capacity, which depends on a certain degree of cognitive-emotional processing mediated by cortical, limbic, and subcortical brain regions. Psychiatric disorders are associated with impaired function in one or all of these regions, which can impair cognitive-emotional processing, decisional capacity, and thus the capacity to give informed consent to undergo an experimental intervention in the brain.

Risk is proportional to invasiveness. In neuromodulation, the more invasive the procedure is, the higher is the risk. Higher risk requires a higher degree of competence or decisional capacity to understand this risk in deciding to undergo a brain-altering technique. The duration and persistence of symptoms in these disorders may cause patients to have unrealistic expectations about participating in these trials and believe that they will likely benefit from them. Some may have a TM about the research. At the same time, these trials provide the opportunity for psychiatric patients to participate in studies that could yield knowledge of disease pathology and lead to safe and effective therapies for them and others suffering from mental illness. Psychiatrists and neurosurgeons conducting this research are obligated to inform potential research subjects of the risks of undergoing DBS or ablation and to explain the scientific rationale of the research and design of the trial. Information about risk would include data from other trials, including not only data about improvement in symptoms but also all neurological and psychological sequelae. In a randomized placebo-controlled trial, this would involve explaining why some subjects are assigned to the control arm receiving a sham procedure. Whether researchers duly discharge their duties of nonmaleficence in protecting research subjects from harm and respecting their autonomy will depend on how they design and monitor clinical trials and whether they obtain valid informed consent from these subjects.

There are technical differences between competence and capacity (Jonsen, Winslade, and Siegler, 2010, p. 65–73; Beauchamp and Childress, 2012, Chapter 4). Competence is a legal concept decided by courts. If a person is deemed incompetent, a court will assign a guardian to make decisions on the person's behalf. Capacity is the mental ability to process and understand information and make decisions based on the information. A physician, often a psychiatrist, determines whether a patient has the capacity to make informed decisions about participating in research or receiving treatment. Both competence and capacity involve the ability to make choices that are in one's best interests. These two concepts are often used interchangeably in the bioethics literature (Appelbaum, 2007, p. 1834), and I will follow this practice in discussing ethical issues in psychiatric research.

Paul Appelbaum and Thomas Grisso state, "the legal standards for competence include the four related skills of [1] communicating a choice, [2] understanding relevant information, [3] appreciating the current situation and [4] manipulating information rationally" (1988, p. 1635; Appelbaum, 2007; Grady, 2015). Skills 2–4, especially 4, are relevant to assessing a patient's capacity to give informed consent to participate and continue participating in a psychiatric neurosurgery trial. Dysfunction in cortical, limbic, and subcortical circuits targeted by DBS may interfere with the ability to process information and thus the capacity to give informed consent (Fins and Pohl, 2016, pp. 19–20). In psychiatric disorders, dysfunction in the neural *source* of this capacity may interfere with the mental *resources* necessary for consent (Appelbaum, Grisso, Frank et al., 1999).

The mental impairment caused by these disorders comes in degrees. Retaining a sufficient degree of decisional capacity may be enough for one to consent to participate in psychiatric neurosurgery research. Being cognitively and emotionally impaired to some degree does not necessarily undermine the capacity to rationally process information about DBS or neural ablation. Whether one has a sufficient degree of capacity will depend on the degree of impairment, which can be determined by a psychiatric assessment of the patient considering becoming a research subject. In addition to decisional capacity, ethical justification of participation in these trials rests on weighing the risks of a brain intervention against the unremitting psychic harm from treatment-resistant psychiatric disorders. This weighing can justify first-in-human and proof-of-principle studies, as well as more advanced testing where nontherapeutic and therapeutic goals may collapse into each other. Cognitive and emotional impairment as such does not imply that a potential research subject is incapable of understanding the purpose of the research. Nor does it imply that he lacks the capacity to appreciate the risks of enrolling in a clinical trial (Dunn, Holtzheimer, Hoop et al., 2011; Lipsman, Giacobbe, Bernstein et al., 2012). If a patient with a psychiatric disorder approaches a researcher about participating in a research study, and the patent's competence is in question, a clinical psychologist or psychiatrist not directly involved in the patient's care or the study can confirm whether the patient has enough decisional capacity to make a rational and voluntary decision to become a research subject.

When a patient lacks a sufficient degree of capacity to understand the goals of and appreciate the risks in research, in some cases a family member may be allowed to give proxy consent (Buchanan and Brock, 1990, Chapters 2, 4). But the patient's lack of capacity would make him a vulnerable research subject. Because of this, there could not be more than minimal risk, and there would have to be clear evidence that participating in the research was in the patient's best interests. The research could lead to a better understanding of the etiology and pathophysiology of the disorder and possibly more effective interventions for individuals like the patient afflicted with the same disorder. Depending on the design and outcome of the study, the patient-subject may benefit from an experimental intervention. In these cases, the proxy may have a better understanding of the patient's condition than the patient himself, given the degree of mental impairment caused by the disorder. The proxy may conclude that it would be in the patient's best interests to participate in the research and consent on their behalf. This may occur in DBS or TMS studies for AN, for example. When a disorder is ego-syntonic, as is AN, the patient's lack of insight into or denial of having the disorder may leave him without the motivation to participate in research, much less have the capacity to consent to participate in it. But lack of motivation does not mean that the patient could not subsequently benefit from being a research subject.

Some have questioned whether the capacity threshold for consent to undergo DBS for mood disorders should be higher than it is for movement disorders (Synofzik and Clausen, 2011). This question does not hinge on the question of whether DBS has received FDA approval or still is experimental. Rather, the question hinges on differences in the primary symptoms of mood and movement disorders, as well as how these differences influence decisional capacity. In PD, dystonia, or essential tremor, impaired motor function is the primary symptom. Cognitive and emotional capacities are either intact or impaired to a lesser extent. In contrast, cognitive and emotional impairment is the primary symptom in MDD, GAD, and OCD. Still, these differences do not support a universal claim about decisional capacity based on the type of disorder at issue. Differences in sensorimotor, cognitive, emotional, and volitional capacities and impairment between neurological and psychiatric diseases are differences of degree rather than kind. They overlap to a considerable extent. Sensorimotor impairment is the defining feature of PD, though it may not be the only impairment. In Chapter 1, I cited studies showing that some patients with this disease develop cognitive impairment before motor impairment (Foltynie, Brayne, Robbins et al., 2004). Accordingly, the *disorder* should not determine the level of decisional capacity necessary for consent. Instead, consent should be based on a determination of *capacity* itself. Given variability among symptoms, capacity can be assessed only in individual cases.

All applications of DBS can alter neural circuits mediating motor and mental functions, and all involve the same or similar risks. Thus, there is no decisive reason for different competency thresholds for neurological and psychiatric disorders regarding mental competence to consent to participate in DBS research. Nevertheless, a higher capacity threshold may be required for participation in neural ablation clinical trials compared with DBS trials because the potential harm from irreversible effects of lesioning implies a greater degree of risk.

In psychiatric disorders, the disease process itself would not necessarily preclude an accurate estimation of the risk of undergoing DBS. A person with one of these disorders may retain enough cognitive and emotional capacity to meet the criteria of informed consent. These would be ego-dystonic disorders, where the patient's awareness of having the disease and understanding the purpose of research can justify trial enrollment. In ego-syntonic disorders, the lack of this awareness and understanding may indicate the lack of the capacity to consent (Lipsman, Giacobbe, Bernstein et al., 2012, p. 109). The question of informed consent may not even arise if patients completely lack insight into their mental disorder. They are not motivated to seek medical help, much less to participate in an experimental psychiatric neurosurgery clinical trial. The cognitive and volitional impairment in ego-syntonic disorders may prevent patients from consenting to be research subjects. Ego-dystonic disorders may present a different problem. The severity, chronicity, and treatment-resistance of the disorder may cause desperation in a patient wanting to enroll in a clinical trial. As in other refractory medical conditions, some patients with severe MDD or OCD may disregard their well-being and fail to adequately appreciate or even ignore the risk of participating in research (Elliott, 1997). Desperation for symptom relief may interfere with a rational assessment of risk. They may perceive DBS as a final opportunity for symptom relief and have unrealistic expectations about benefiting directly from an investigative study. These expectations may be more likely in DBS and neural ablation than in pharmacological or psychological interventions because some patients may believe that the technique will get at the "root" of the problem (Lipsman, Giacobbe, Bernstein et al., 2012, p. 108). This may be more problematic in an ablation study if the subject believes that the investigators will not merely get at the root of the problem but "root it out" by creating a fixed lesion that could erase the source of the disease.

This perception is an example of the potential power of brain-based explanations of thought and behavior. These can be misleadingly reductive in suggesting that psychiatric disorders can be explained entirely in terms of localized dysfunction in neural circuits, or nodes within these circuits. It fails to appreciate the fact that, while psychiatric disorders are disorders of the brain, they are not just disorders of the brain. They also involve other biological and psychological and environmental factors. Although a dysfunctional neural circuit, or dysfunctional connectivity between circuits, is the proximal or direct cause of the disorder, factors outside of the brain can influence neural dysfunction as distal or indirect causes. These causes are not detectable by imaging showing changes in brain activity before and after electrical stimulation. Distal causes have a longer duration than proximal causes and may have a broader range of physiological effects in the brain. Both types of causes are necessary to account for psychiatric disorders. However, when the chronicity of a disorder results in treatment-refractory changes in the brain, effectively it has become entirely brain based.

In addition to influencing a potential research subject's perception of risk, beliefs about an experimental procedure eliminating the cause of the disorder could make him susceptible to psychological harm. This would be in addition to what he already has experienced from the symptoms and functional limitations of the disorder. He could be harmed if the outcome of the trial failed to meet his expectations. In this respect, the treatment-resistance of the disorder, and how it shapes his hopes and expectations, could make a psychiatric patient a vulnerable research subject (Ford, 2009; Bell, Racine, Chiasson et al., 2014). Still, being vulnerable does not automatically preclude one from having enough cognitive and emotional capacity to consent to participate in psychiatry research.

When the ability to process information and make rational decisions based on this information is in question, some form of third-party assessment can confirm that a person has, or lacks, a sufficient degree of this ability to consent to participate in the trial. A clinical psychologist or psychiatrist not directly involved in the patient's care or the research study could confirm that the potential research subject had or lacked the requisite mental capacity to make a rational and voluntary decision to agree or decline to participate in it. The third party could use MacCat-T or MacCat-CR assessment tools for this purpose (Grisso, Appelbaum, and Hill-Fotouhi, 1997; Lipsman, Giacobbe, Bernstein et al., 2012, p. 109).

Any sense of vulnerability associated with misperception or underestimation of risk by research subjects in psychiatry cannot be separated from an objective assessment of risk associated with the intervention itself. Despite being a more focused means of neuromodulation than psychopharmacology or ECT, the risks of DBS are greater than the risks in less invasive interventions. According to 2012 data, these include a 2–3% risk of intracranial hemorrhage, a 5–8% risk of infection, and a 0.4% risk of death during the surgery (Lipsman, Giacobbe, Bernstein et al., 2012, p. 109). There may also be postoperative complications. A number of individuals receiving DBS for both neurological and psychiatric disorders have developed impulsivity, personality changes, hypomania, and mania. Most of these side effects have resulted from overstimulation of targeted circuits or unintended stimulation of nontargeted circuits. While the incidence of adverse effects will not be eliminated, more precise design and stimulation of circuits at the right frequency and intensity put DBS within an ethically acceptable standard of risk. These ethical assessments must be informed by weighing the risk *with* DBS against the risk of suicide and continued poor quality of life *without* DBS when the disorder has not responded to other interventions.

As noted, in some cases where patients have ego-syntonic disorders and lack sufficient capacity to consent, some family members or other caregivers may want to enroll them in a clinical trial. They may not be motivated by the patient's best interests, but instead by the burden of caregiving, and the physical and emotional fatigue they experience from the patient's chronic treatment-resistance. They may be desperate for any intervention that would ameliorate the patient's symptoms and relieve their own burden. This could generate another sense of vulnerability if the patient relied on others in making decisions on their behalf about enrollment in research. It would be an exception to the permissibility of proxy consent. If the cognitive capacity of potential research subjects is impaired to the extent that they cannot consent to participate in research, but not so impaired that they cannot assent, then the capacity they retain may not be enough to reduce pressure from surrogates in influencing decisions about trial enrollment.

Even if the patient was involved in discussions about enrollment, the combination of surrogate pressure and the inability to make these decisions on their own could further diminish their autonomy. This situation would warrant protecting these potential research subjects from undue influence or coercion from proxy decision-makers. It would recommend the involvement of a social worker in addition to a clinical psychologist and a psychiatrist not involved in the study to assess the patient's cognitive capacity and general state of mind. These professionals could assess whether the patient's decisional capacity was so impaired as to allow proxy consent to enroll in a psychiatric neurosurgery clinical trial. They could also assess whether the proxy's motivation was appropriate and whether it was what the patient would have wanted.

## The therapeutic misconception in psychiatric neurosurgery

The severity, chronicity, and treatment-resistance of a psychiatric disorder may contribute to a TM about neural ablation and DBS (Appelbaum, Roth and Lidz, 1982; Lidz, Appelbaum, Grisso et al., 2004). This misconception consists in the conflation of the distinct goals of research and therapy. It involves a belief in a relatively high probability of direct benefit from participating in research. The potential research subject may have unrealistic expectations in believing that he will directly benefit from being in a research study. He may fail to understand that the main purpose of research is to gain scientific knowledge of the experimental intervention. Failure to understand the design of a randomized controlled clinical trial and that he may be randomly assigned to the control rather than active arm of the trial may reinforce this belief. The fact that many psychiatrists conducting research also treat patients and thus have dual roles as investigators and clinicians may incline a potential research subject to misunderstand the differences between research and therapy. The agents in this relationship are not simply researchers and research subjects but clinician-researchers and patient-subjects. This may blur the distinction between conventional and investigational interventions in the brain.

This phenomenon is not limited to situations in which the psychiatrist is both the patient's treating physician and the researcher recruiting her for research into a novel intervention. It can also occur when the treating psychiatrist makes a referral to a neurosurgeon and a different psychiatrist conducting a DBS or neural ablation study. The patient may mistakenly infer that she is being transferred from one therapeutic setting in the psychiatrist's office to a different therapeutic setting in the clinical trial. What may increase the likelihood of the TM is that some DBS trials are doubly innovative (Lipsman, Giacobbe, Bernstein et al., 2012, p. 110). These trials may not neatly separate the goals of establishing the safety and efficacy of the technique in distinct phases of distinct studies but aim to test both of these endpoints in the same study. "Efficacy" in the description of the study would refer to the type and extent of neural and psychological responses to the experimental intervention. Yet some subjects may misinterpret this term to mean that they will likely experience symptom relief from participating in the study.

As in assessments of a prospective research subject's mental capacity to give informed consent to participate in psychiatric research, a medical professional not directly involved in the research could help to disabuse subjects of the idea that an experimental intervention is a form of therapy. A member of the research team other than the principal investigator could emphasize the main nontherapeutic goal of the trial when interviewing the patient prior to enrollment (Christopher, Appelbaum, Truong et al., 2017). This could reduce the probability of the subject identifying the research as therapy and the researcher as therapist. It would not entirely prevent the TM, however. This belief is a function of a complex set of cognitive and emotional attitudes such as expectation and hope, which are not indicative of mental impairment. Having a TM about the probability of benefiting from participating in a clinical trial does not imply impaired capacity to understand the information presented by the researcher to the patient about the design and purpose of the trial. It would not necessarily interfere with the capacity to consent to participate in the trial. The TM may lead one with the capacity to distinguish research and therapy to fail to exercise it. Alternatively, a patient may distinguish them, but her motivation for participating may be based on the hope that she will benefit. In either case, a potential research subject could have a TM while meeting the criteria of informed consent. The motivation could be separable from and not interfere with a rational assessment of the information presented to her by the researcher.

This claim is supported by a recent study conducted by Scott Kim and coinvestigators. The aim of the study was to determine whether the TM influenced the decision of 90 patients with advanced PD to enroll in sham surgery-controlled neurosurgical trials (Kim, De Vries, Parnami et al., 2015). Although there are differences between primary movement disorders such as PD and disorders of cognition and mood such as OCD and MDD, motivational factors in trial participation between these types of disorders are relevantly similar. Kim and colleagues divided subjects into three groups based on three distinct motivations: (1) those who participated because of a belief in therapeutic benefit, (2) those who participated because of invitations from their own doctors as researchers, and (3) those who participated for altruistic reasons. The investigators state that "60% had primarily therapeutic motivation and 44% had their own doctor as the site investigator, but neither were generally associated with increased TM responses" (Kim, De Vries, Parnami et al., 2015, p. 391).

The results of the study indicate that a patient may understand the purpose of a trial and meet the criteria of informed consent while being motivated to participate in it because he believes that he will or may benefit. The study illustrates the need to distinguish the subject's motivation to participate in a clinical trial and his understanding of the information about it presented to him by the investigator. Hope and expectation of benefit from an experimental study do not necessarily distort one's judgment about its main purpose of generating scientific knowledge about a functional neurosurgical technique. Motivation and understanding are separable but not mutually exclusive. Having the first does not necessarily preclude the second. The TM is not an example of cognitive dissonance. Rather, the cognitive-emotional content of desire, hope, and expectation is different from the cognitive content of understanding. One can understand that a clinical trial has a primary nontherapeutic purpose yet believe that one will benefit without clouding this understanding. This would include knowledge that the subject may be randomly assigned to either the active or control arm. Retaining this understanding could minimize the risk of psychological harm if participating in a trial failed to relieve the patient's symptoms.

A TM by itself would not be sufficient grounds for excluding a competent patient from participating in research. One can make this claim even if the potential subject knows that the probability of benefit is only 1%. It may be rational to participate on this basis when the patient's condition has been refractory to all other interventions. This assumes that the patient's hope for relief does not interfere with the capacity to process information about the trial. In particular, being motivated by a desire or hope for therapeutic benefit does not necessarily cause a potential research subject to ignore risk. On the contrary, in the study by Kim and coinvestigators, subjects motivated by the prospect of therapeutic benefit, rather than altruistic reasons or the recommendation from their treating physician, were more sensitive to risk. They were also more likely to provide the correct rationale for why a sham arm was necessary to counter the placebo effect. The results of this study run counter to what many have claimed about the undermining effect of the TM on informed consent. If the belief in benefit from a trial does not distort the patient's capacity to process information presented to him and to make a reasoned decision based on this information, then he can meet the criteria of consent.

## Consent to expanding applications of deep brain stimulation

When DBS modulates dysfunctional neural circuits, it can make a psychiatric disorder amenable to CBT. CBT can also facilitate and augment positive effects of DBS (Mantione, Nieman, Figee et al., 2014). These treatment modalities are not mutually exclusive but can combine to produce more beneficial outcomes than what either of them could produce on their own. This combined therapeutic strategy can ameliorate symptoms in MDD, OCD, and GAD. There are some indications that CBT can alleviate the reduced motivation, anhedonia, flat affect, and reduced attention in some patients with the negative symptoms of schizophrenia (Grant, Huh, Perivoliotis et al., 2012). Most available evidence indicates that most patients with either positive or negative subtypes of this disorder do not respond to this technique. Antipsychotic drug therapy is still first-line treatment. As noted in the introduction to this chapter, though, 10–30% of patients with schizophrenia have little or no response to antipsychotic treatment, including atypical antipsychotics (Mikell, Sinha, and Sheth, 2016). For those who do respond to typical or atypical antipsychotics, extrapyramidal and metabolic effects can be significant and cause cardiovascular disease, diabetes, or nonadherence. The history of psychosurgery shows that neural ablation for schizophrenia has been a failure. DBS has been the focus of current research in neurosurgery for schizophrenia (Mikell, Sinha, and Sheth, 2016).

One of the difficulties in clinical trials for this disorder has been recruiting enough research subjects to conduct them. This may be due to questions about patients' capacity to consent to participate in research and whether adequate protections would be in place for them. Two DBS trials for treatment-refractory negative symptoms of schizophrenia are in the process of recruiting subjects at The Johns Hopkins University Hospital (Baltimore, MD, USA) and the Hospital Santa Creu i Sant Pau (Barcelona, Spain) (ClinicalTrials.gov, 2017a and NCT02377505). One study application from a team at the Centre for Addiction and Mental Health in Toronto, Canada, was withdrawn in 2015 when no participants were enrolled (ClinicalTrials.gov, 2017b). It will be some time before data on outcomes of DBS for schizophrenia are available. Ideally, neurostimulation would control the waxing and waning of psychosis in positive symptoms and improve cognition, mood, and motivation in negative symptoms.

Like bipolar depression, schizophrenia presents challenges for investigators exploring new therapies because there are two distinct types of symptoms resulting from dysfunction in distinct neural pathways. Positive symptoms in schizophrenia are associated with hyperdopaminergic activity in mesolimbic pathways. Negative symptoms are associated with hypodopaminergic activity in mesocortical pathways (Castle and Buckley, 2015, p. 15). Stimulating one pathway may reduce one set of symptoms but increase a different set. Even when a pathway is not overstimulated, expanding effects of the stimulation could adversely affect another pathway. This has occurred in some cases of DBS for PD, where stimulation of the motor circuit in the basal ganglia has affected limbic and associative circuits. There is no fundamental difference in weighing potential benefits and risks of neurostimulation in schizophrenia and PD.

Nevertheless, schizophrenia may pose a unique problem for informed consent to participate in functional neurosurgery research. It is not clear whether different types of cognitive and emotional impairment with the different sets of symptoms would preclude the capacity to process information about experimental interventions and make an informed decision to undergo them. Although the positive and negative symptoms are generally dissociable, they may overlap in some cases, and patients may have symptoms of both subtypes. This could exclude the possibility of treating these patients with neuromodulation, since knowing whether the technique was effective would rule out stimulating more than one circuit or node at a time. Yet if the circuits and pathophysiology of the two forms of schizophrenia were dissociable, then it is unlikely that overstimulation of the circuit associated with mood and motivation would induce delusions and hallucinations, despite the risk of hypomania and mania. In that case, there would be no compelling medical or ethical reasons for excluding patients with the negative form of schizophrenia from participating in a DBS trial targeting the relevant circuit.

A particular challenge in considering DBS for schizophrenic patients with positive symptoms is that some may not welcome the implantation of electrodes in their brains. In schizophrenia with paranoia, patients often claim that they have devices implanted by others to control them. In these cases, implanting electrodes would only confirm their paranoid beliefs. Patients would not understand the reasons for this procedure, which could exacerbate the psychopathology. Schizophrenic patients with paranoia should be excluded from DBS research.

In the absence of this or other exclusionary conditions, DBS could modulate hyperdopaminergic activity in the dysfunctional mesolimbic network in schizophrenia and relieve positive symptoms (Mikell, Sinha, and Sheth, 2016). It could also modulate hypodopaminergic activity in the dysfunctional mesocortical network and ameliorate negative symptoms. In addition, it might modulate glutaminergic signaling in prefrontal areas associated with cognition and mood. With precise delivery of electrical current at the right frequency to the dysfunctional node or nodes in this network, DBS theoretically could be a form of neuromodulation for both subtypes of the disease. It is questionable whether any of the three current ablative techniques could be a viable option for schizophrenia. Depending on the proximity of nodes within the mesolimbic circuit, it is not clear whether creating a lesion in one node would re-establish balance between inhibitory and excitatory activity in this circuit or other adjacent circuits to which it projects.

Research into the application of DBS for schizophrenia is a recent development. Many longitudinal randomized controlled clinical trials need to be conducted to determine the safety and efficacy of this neuromodulating technique for this disorder (Soares, Paiva, Guertzenstein et al., 2013). Anhedonia, avolition, and flat affect would not necessarily undermine the mental capacity necessary for consent to participate in DBS research for the negative subtype of schizophrenia. It would depend on the extent of the patient's cognitive impairment. Delusions and hallucinations would seem to make an affected person unable to consent to participate in research for the positive subtype. Here too, though, it would depend on how cognitively impaired the person was.

Temporary discontinuation of antipsychotic medication would be necessary to accurately assess the efficacy of neuromodulation for schizophrenia. Depending on when the drug was discontinued and the duration of its effects in the brain, this could cause a return of ego-syntonic delusions and hallucinations. It could cause the loss of the cognitive capacity necessary for consent to participate, or continue participating, in a psychiatric neurosurgery trial for this disorder. A determination of cognitive capacity may be difficult in these cases because the subject's psychotic and nonpsychotic states may wax and wane. But if they retained enough capacity to assent to being enrolled in the trial and had some input in the discussion about whether or not to be enrolled, then proxy consent from a substitute decision-maker might be permissible. Enrollment in a phase I trial or a doubly innovative phase I/II study may offer these patients an opportunity to contribute to research that could yield a better understanding of the pathophysiology of schizophrenia. It could be followed by advance-phase trials possibly leading to new therapies. These could be superior to antipsychotic medication in controlling or relieving symptoms and avoiding the serious side effects of antipsychotic drugs.

Justification for enrollment of a patient with the positive symptoms of schizophrenia as a subject in a DBS trial would require a clear sense that it is what the patient would have wanted if he had retained the requisite degree of mental capacity to decide on his own. This could be based partly on comments by the patient during lucid moments while on antipsychotic medication. It is reasonable to assume that any individual whose debilitating cognitive symptoms had not responded to drug therapy, or had experienced adverse effects from it, would want to participate in research that might lead to treatments with fewer or no side effects. If a surrogate based a decision about enrolling a cognitively impaired patient in a clinical trial on this assumption, and if the researchers conducting the trial closely monitored the patient, then proxy consent for enrollment in such a trial could be ethically justified. This would depend on the patient's attitudes about having electrodes implanted in her brain. If she did not want them, then a substitute decision-maker would have to respect this desire and not enroll her in the research. The patient's negative attitude about implants, the risk of the procedure, and the lack of data on positive outcomes would rule out proxy consent.

In cases where proxy consent was permissible, monitoring and follow-up might be difficult. If the trial were placebo-controlled, then the investigators would temporality discontinue antipsychotic medication. Even in the active arm, the patient's symptoms might not respond to electrical stimulation. He could experience a relapse. If there were a return of severe symptoms, then this could leave the subject without the capacity to communicate his experience to the investigators. He may also lack sufficient insight into his condition and fail reality testing. A full complement of a study psychiatrist, neurosurgeon, clinical psychologist, and social worker would be necessary to ensure adequate protection of the patient-subject. Given the complex set of medical and ethical factors in this research, it would be appropriate to conduct DBS trials for the positive subtype of schizophrenia only after the technique had been tested for the negative subtype. The similarities between the symptoms of MDD (impaired mood and cognition, anhedonia, and avolition) and the negative subtype of schizophrenia, and the fact that the same or similar neural circuits would be targeted, suggest that the same ethical standards for consent and risk in DBS research that apply to the first condition would also apply to the second.

While patients with ego-syntonic delusions and hallucinations may not have enough cognitive capacity to consent to participate in this research on their own, in principle it seems unfair to exclude them from research on these grounds. Fairness requires equal consideration of equal claims of need. In principle, all individuals living with the burden of any treatment-resistant psychiatric disorder should be allowed to participate in research that might subsequently benefit them and others with the same disease. Because those with positive symptoms of schizophrenia have as much of a burden of functional disability as others with MDD, OCD, GAD, or the negative subtype of schizophrenia, it would be unfair to exclude them from research because they do poorly in reality testing and have little insight into their disorder. Excluding those with severe cognitive impairment who lack the capacity for even a minimal understanding of the research would be justified. But those with moderate impairment who retain some insight into the disorder and who could assent should be allowed to participate in research through proxy consent of a family member or caregiver. This would assume that research participation is consistent with the patient's wishes and best interests. It can be difficult to know what these interests are in patients with paranoia or other psychotic states. Participation in research also presupposes that researchers provide adequate protection of these subjects in monitoring their behavior during the trial and ensuring that they are not exposed to more than minimal risk.

Another psychiatric disorder that presents challenges for informed consent to functional neurosurgery is AN. This disorder affects mainly adolescent and young adult women. Some men are also affected by AN. The disorder is associated with dysfunction in the somatosensory and reward systems that impairs cognitive and affective processing about the body. Possibly because the dysfunction becomes more hardwired in the brain in this disorder compared with others, many individuals with AN fail to respond to antidepressants and anxiolytics. Results of a phase I DBS trial involving six women with treatment-refractory AN were published in 2013. Although one patient suffered a seizure from the neurostimulation, the overall positive outcome supports the hypothesis that, on balance, it can be a safe procedure for the most severe forms of this disorder (Lipsman, Woodside, Giacobbe et al., 2013). A 1-year follow-up of a second DBS open-label trial for the same disorder showed sustained improvement in affective symptoms among 16 patients who enrolled in the study (Lipsman, Lam, Volpini et al., 2017).

Many people with AN do not retain enough insight into their disorder to recognize the need for treatment. If they are given standard therapy but do not respond to it, then they may not have enough cognitive and emotional capacity to consent to participate in a clinical trial testing an experimental intervention such as DBS (Maslen, Pugh, and Savulescu, 2015). This can be problematic when patients are adolescents. The combined effect of natural immature frontal lobe development and the disorder may preclude the capacity for consent. This cognitive impairment may also explain why many people with this disorder fail to respond to CBT. Severe AN can be categorized as an ego-syntonic disorder. In moderate to moderately severe forms, the complexity of the bodily and neural factors influencing the patient's mental states can make it difficult to categorize AN as a purely ego-syntonic or ego-dystonic disorder. It can be difficult to ascertain whether there is incongruity between what the patient actually believes about herself and her body and what she wants to believe. Specifically, it may not be clear that she realizes how harmful her thought and behavior is to her. Depending on the extent of the disconnection between their perception of their body and its actual state, these patients may at most have the cognitive capacity to assent to being a subject in a research study. In that case, a parent could give proxy consent to enroll their daughter or son in a trial.

Treatment for AN is effective when it restores normal information processing about the body. When the disorder is treatment-resistant, participation in research that might lead to effective treatment can be justified. In severe cases, this may only be possible with proxy consent. Persuading an adolescent with the disorder to become a research subject may be challenging, especially if she is emotionally immature. Even if the patient were capable and willing to discuss reasons for and against her participation in research, persuading an adolescent to enroll in a clinical trial without clear therapeutic benefit may be difficult to justify. Nevertheless, when conventional therapies have not been effective, and when participation in research involves only minimal risk, parental proxy consent to enroll their daughter or son in a research study may be consistent with the patient's best interests.

Parents would have to understand that the purpose of a phase I trial for AN was not therapeutic and not expect their daughter to experience a rapid remission of symptoms. Reasonable expectations by parents about the purpose of the research would be necessary to prevent psychological harm to her. This could be the outcome if the lack of a positive response to the experimental intervention frustrated the parents by not meeting their expectations about such a response. They may express this frustration in negative interaction with their daughter after the trial had ended. If interviews determined that the disorder was ego-syntonic for that patient, then she might not recognize its severity or even the fact that she had it. The patient would fail to recognize the reasons for research into neuromodulating techniques (Abbate-Daga, Amianto, Delsedime et al., 2014; Widdows and Davis, 2014). She may lack the capacity to assent to participate in research. In that case, parental substitute decision-making may involve not just persuasion but coercion. Forcing a person into a clinical trial would not be in her best interests and would violate her negative right to noninterference. It would invalidate proxy consent. In addition, it could undermine any remaining feeling of control of her body, which the disease already had impaired to a significant degree. These considerations show, not just how psychiatric disorders can impair cognition, but also how they can limit proxy consent.

There are similar problems with informed consent to undergo rTMS as an experimental technique for AN. Here too, a potential research subject may not sufficiently appreciate the rationale for investigating the safety and efficacy of this technique (Coman, Skarderud, Reas et al., 2014). There is a significant difference between DBS and rTMS as experimental forms of neuromodulation. Generally, the greater risk entailed by the more invasive DBS would require a higher level of decisional capacity than what would be required for the less invasive rTMS. Yet if the ego-syntonic nature of the disorder impaired the patient's capacity to understand the reasons for research and to consider risk, then there would be no significant ethical difference between the two techniques regarding the level of capacity for consent. The patient would fail to meet the criteria for consent to participate in research for both rTMS and DBS. There *could* be a significant difference between these techniques regarding proxy consent. The greater risk in DBS would require clear evidence that the proxy was acting in the patient's best interests and that participation in research was what the patient would have wanted. If the patient's interests were unclear, then participation in research would have to be consistent with the interests she had before disease onset and full-blown development of symptoms.

One explanation for why this disorder is particularly intractable is that it involves dysregulation in a distributed network involving the somatosensory cortex and the reward system (Titova, Hjorth, Schioth et al., 2013). For this reason, ablating tissue in a node of a dysfunctional reward system of a patient with AN would probably not reduce symptoms. More importantly, the likely irreversibility from even one lesion would make it difficult to justify allowing proxy consent in which a decision to destroy even a small amount of neural tissue was made not *by* but *for* the patient. Although DBS would seem a more justifiable intervention for this disorder than neural ablation, there is a distinctive risk associated with DBS. Emaciated patients are deficient in subcutaneous fat. This could increase the risk of infection from implantation of the pulse generator under the collarbone or in the abdomen. It may also affect the stability of the generator.

The question of what constitutes benefit in psychiatric neurosurgery research involves more than the distinction between the potential for positive physiological or psychological effects in particular subjects. It involves more than the question of whether the intervention is therapeutic in ameliorating symptoms and thus should be construed broadly rather than narrowly. Some institutional review boards and Research Ethics Boards may define "beneficial research" as research conducted with a therapeutic hypothesis. Most studies intend to generate scientific knowledge about a disease and potential treatments for it. Some studies rest on both nontherapeutic and therapeutic hypotheses. The goal may be to determine the safety and efficacy of an intervention and help the patient, though they may not have the latter result. This applies to what I have described "doubly innovative" phase I/II trials testing both safety and efficacy. These trials are distinct from nonbeneficial research in which there is no therapeutic goal. Proof-of-principle and phase I trials focusing on safety in traditional medical research fall within this category.

Enrolling a patient as a subject in a trial intended to test DBS as a treatment for AN could be beneficial in different respects. This may occur even if the study does not directly result in symptom relief for the patient-subject. The results of the trial could lead to a better understanding of the pathophysiology of the disease and more effective treatments for the AN patient population. These treatments could ameliorate symptoms or even resolve the disorder for the patient. Enrollment in a clinical trial could also benefit the patient psychologically by making her aware of contributing to this research. Still, this would depend on whether the disorder was ego-dystonic or ego-syntonic and how the patient perceived her disorder.

Although DBS has improved sensorimotor, cognitive, affective, and volitional capacities for many patients with psychiatric disorders, questions remain about its efficacy. This technique has been effective in controlling movement disorders. These involve a smaller number of neural targets than mood disorders. It is more difficult to modulate both motor and mental functions in psychiatric disorders. A number of trials for MDD have yielded positive results. However, the more recent BROdmann Area 25 DEep brain Neuromodulation (BROADEN) study of DBS for depression sponsored by St. Jude Medical was discontinued after initial disappointing results (Underwood, 2015). St. Jude stated in a letter that it decided to stop the trial before completion because the probability of a successful outcome was only 17.2%. Tractography showing abnormalities in subcallosal cingulate white matter confirmed this as an appropriate target. But the actual effects of DBS on depressive symptoms failed to meet expectations. Ninety participants were randomly assigned to active or sham stimulation between April 2008 and November 2012. Lead author Paul Holtzheimer spells out the findings: "Both groups showed improvement, but there was no statistically significant difference in response during the double-blind, sham-controlled phase" (Holtzheimer, Husain, Lisanby et al., 2017, p. 839). Equally significant, "28 patients experienced 40 serious adverse events, eight of these (in seven patients) were deemed to be related to the study device or surgery" (2017, p. 839).

The outcome of this study is one example of a problem for neuromodulation in general. Most open-label studies of DBS demonstrate a very promising effect. Yet this effect often fails to occur in placebo-controlled trials. The outcome of this study also underscores the difficulty of identifying and modulating the dysfunctional nodes of the circuits implicated in MDD. It underscores the necessary precision of electrode placement and optimal stimulation frequency. Advanced imaging may not always enable psychiatrists and neurosurgeons to locate the right targets, which can vary depending on the subtype of depression at issue and the level of metabolic hyperactivity in the targeted regions.

An earlier study by Helen Mayberg and coinvestigators produced more positive results in the same region of the brain (Mayberg, Lozano, Voon et al., 2005). The difficulty in replicating effects of DBS in the same or adjacent circuits illustrates that brain-based models for treating depression with electrical stimulation are far from perfect. Variable results from these studies are indicative of the heterogeneous nature of depression. Results may depend on the timing of stimulation and how it affects neural oscillations in targeted regions. Major depression has multiple causes, and different people with this disorder may have different degrees of neural and mental dysfunction. For these reasons, research subjects may or may not respond, or may respond to varying degrees, to different interventions in the brain. If they respond to DBS, then there may be less than a 50% reduction in symptoms. The results of the BROADEN study might also suggest that this and other psychiatric disorders cannot be explained entirely in terms of dysfunctional neural circuits. Failed studies like this one indicate the limitations of DBS as a treatment for psychiatric disorders. They highlight the need for more advanced versions of the technique or novel neuromodulating techniques with different mechanisms of action.

## Open-loop versus closed-loop devices

Some of the suboptimal responses and adverse events in DBS studies may be attributed to mechanical features of the open-loop devices (OLDs) used in most applications of the technique. In OLDs, there is no information feedback from the neural output of the stimulator to stimulation input and no mechanism for the electrical frequency to adjust to changes in the brain. The output quantity has no effect on input. Electrical impulses are delivered unidirectionally and independently of any feedback. The system is "open loop" in the sense that the implanted pulse generator constantly delivers invariant, preprogrammed stimulatory pulses without adjustment of these pulses. They are not sensitive and do not respond to the unique and dynamically fluctuating characteristics of the disease state in the brain. Stimulation parameters are programmed into the device and held constant until the next programming session. This occurs regardless of changes in the neural environment (Foltynie and Hariz, 2010).

The main technical disadvantage of OLDs is that the lack of sensing feedback signals prevents the system from automatically correcting errors in the parameters of stimulation frequency, intensity, and pulse duration. These errors can interfere with the intended neuromodulation. The only way of knowing about device malfunction or suboptimal function is from a subjective report from a patient when symptoms emerge or re-emerge. Device programmers and clinicians can then confirm that the device is the source of the problem and make the necessary adjustments. This approach is far from optimal because it is time-intensive, observer dependent, and limits the battery life of the pulse generator. Any adverse effects may be immediately detectable in movement disorders. But cognitive and emotional symptoms from device malfunction in a psychiatric disorder may take weeks or even months to appear. Aberrant neural activity may be more difficult to modulate the longer the aberration goes uncorrected. This could prevent research subjects in doubly innovative or advanced-stage trials from receiving maximal benefit.

In closed-loop devices (CLDs), information is fed back from changes in neural activity to the stimulator. This allows adjustment of the frequency, intensity, and duration of the electrical current (Santos, Costa, and Tecuapetla, 2011; Hebb, Zhang, Mahoor et al., 2014; Potter, El Hady, and Fetz, 2014). This makes CLDs preferable to OLDs by increasing the probability that the targeted neural circuits are neither overstimulated nor understimulated. They appear to provide a safer and more effective means of stimulation by providing a greater degree of precision in regulating neural network oscillations. CLDs may overcoming the design and operational flaws in OLDs, making diseases of the brain more amenable to the neuromodulating effects of DBS. By using algorithms that allow the device to respond to changes in the brain as they occur in real time, a CLD can be a form of "smart" DBS. Neurostimulation is tailored to the unique activity in each person's brain (Grahn, Mallory, Khurram et al., 2014; Reardon, 2017).

In addition to reducing side effects, the more precise stimulation of CLDs can extend the battery life of the pulse generator. It may also reduce the probability of lead fractures, which can result in open or short circuits in the device. Most commercially available DBS systems using OLDs are still nonrechargeable, and battery depletion requires replacement. The longer battery and lead life with CLDs would benefit patients by significantly reducing the frequency of time-consuming travel to research centers or clinics for battery or lead replacement (Grahn, Mallory, Khurram et al., 2014). The cost of these replacements is more burdensome than the time required to replace them. Battery replacement surgery may cost anywhere from US $20,000 to $50,000 (Underwood, 2017). Burdens of time and cost could contribute to nonadherence to device monitoring, and some patients or research subjects may fail to keep appointments. This could interfere with the successful completion of a clinical trial or defeat the therapeutic purpose of the technique in a clinical setting. Rechargeable batteries in pulse generators could avoid the replacement problem in OLDs. Still, this would not resolve flaws in the feedback of information from the brain to the device.

Given these limitations of CLDs, Peter Grahn and coauthors point out that "existing clinical programming and stimulation paradigms are poorly suited to cope with the dynamic and comorbid nature of most neurological disorders." They emphasize the need for "dynamic feedback systems that can continually and automatically adjust stimulation parameters in response to changes within the environment of the brain" (Grahn, Mallory, Khurram et al., 2014, p. 2). The need is greater in psychiatric disorders, where positive and negative effects of electrical stimulation in the brain and the cognitive, emotional, and volitional states it mediates are typically not immediate but delayed. Overstimulation or understimulation that remains uncorrected for an extended period could exacerbate rather than ameliorate impairment of these states.

CLDs could influence debate on the comparative risks and benefits of neurostimulation and neural ablation. Let us assume that a patient with a psychiatric disorder would be a candidate for both procedures. Ablation is generally faster, more cost-effective, and requires considerably less postoperative management than DBS. These are all relevant considerations regarding patient adherence to device monitoring and follow-up. They are also important in light of the mandate to control healthcare costs. Recent reviews of the literature on these two procedures suggest that anterior capsulotomy may be as effective as DBS for treatment-refractory OCD (Greenberg, Gabriels, Malone et al., 2010; Greenberg, Rauch, and Haber, 2010; Pepper, Hariz, and Zrinzo, 2015). A preference for neurostimulation over ablation in treating this disorder may not be due entirely to differences in efficacy. Instead, the preference may be due to the perception that neurostimulation does not involve destruction of neural tissue.

However, the fact that any effects of overablating tissue, or ablating the wrong area of tissue, are permanent is significant. The risk of untoward irreversible effects of these errors on thought and behavior, such as apathy and cognitive impairment, is a persistent problem that even more advanced forms of lesioning might not avoid. If CLDs reduced the time and costs associated with postimplantation monitoring with OLDs, if they could respond rapidly to information received from the brain, and if any of their unintended effects were reversible and did not destroy neural tissue, then closed-loop DBS would be preferable to ablation.

Devices that automatically adjusted to changes in the brain would obviate the need for external monitoring and eliminate the burden of having to undergo regular parameter adjustment in the research or clinical setting. They would also be more versatile in modulating both metabolically hyperactive and hypoactive circuits, unlike ablation, which is typically indicated for hyperactive circuits. This could result in a more favorable perception of DBS compared with ablation. There may be cases in which lesioning may modulate a hyperactive circuit more effectively than stimulation. On balance, though, CLDs may offer the safest and most effective means of neuromodulation for psychiatric disorders.

Nevertheless, closed-loop systems raise some concerns. Focusing exclusively on objective electrophysiological and neurochemical measures of brain activity may ignore the subjective aspect of having a neurological or psychiatric disorder. Paying too much attention to the device could fail to appreciate the patient's unique experience of having a disorder and its effects on her conscious mind. It is persons, not neural circuits, who have and suffer from diseases of the brain and mind. Attention to the mechanical properties of a device implanted in the brain cannot meet the medical, psychological, and social needs generated by these disorders. There may not be a strict correlation between the neural dysfunction detected by the device and a patient's symptoms in every psychiatric disorder. Even with real-time feedback from neural activity to the device, imaging or electrophysiological recording may not detect subtle abnormal changes in the brain manifesting in the mental and behavioral characteristics of neuropsychiatric disorders (Glannon and Ineichen, 2016).

While in many respects CLDs may be superior to OLDs in sensing neural activity, in a particular respect they are limited in their capacity to sense activity in limbic circuits regulating emotion. Alik Widge and Chet Moritz point out that "The largest barrier to closed-loop limbic stimulation is not hardware or control algorithms; it is sensing. Despite extensive investigations, there is no electrophysiologic signature that closely or reliably tracks the symptoms of any known mental disorder" (2016, p. 231). This could make the claim that CLDs could be a form of "smart" DBS premature. The precision of a CLD presupposes that the practitioner knows how to set or adjust the stimulation parameters to what the device senses. Yet what needs to be sensed may not be known. Subjective reports of sensorimotor, cognitive, affective, or volitional impairment from patients and research subjects undergoing neurostimulation for psychiatric disorders may be the most reliable indicators of abnormalities in brain regions mediating physical and mental capacities.

In gaining a better understanding of psychiatric disorders, feedback from outputs to inputs at a brain-systems level should supplement rather than supplant feedback from patients and research subjects to clinicians and investigators at an interpersonal level. How a patient experiences and reports symptoms, how the medical professional responds to the report, and how the patient responds in turn to the professional are all critical components of the therapeutic process. These psychological responses may influence whether symptoms persist or resolve. This is especially the case in psychiatric disorders characterized by different types and degrees of motor and mental impairment. CLDs may enable therapeutic responses by modulating aberrant neural activity, but the device cannot completely account for these responses or changes in a patient's mental content before and after neurostimulation.

Moreover, CLDs are not immune to malfunction. Imprecise programming of the device, lack of sensitivity to changes in neural activity, or technical failures may result in inappropriate responses to alterations in brain circuitry from electrical stimulation. Although these problems may be less likely to occur in CLDs than OLDs because of the feedback mechanism built into the device, they would be possible nonetheless. Since CLDs run more automatically, any adverse effects might be observed later than they would be with OLDs. This could allow a longer period of neural dysregulation. Constant monitoring would be necessary to alert the user of the device of any technical problems. There may be differences in neural correlates in chronic versus acute or subacute stages of disease. This may involve varying levels of neural activity that the stimulator has to sense, which may affect how the stimulator responds to it. While closed-loop stimulation has been tested in some human subjects with neurological disorders, the research is at a very early stage for psychiatric disorders. It will be some time before data are available to confirm whether CLDs could control symptoms more safely and effectively than OLDs.

## Researchers' obligations

A critical advance in the ethical justification of psychiatric neurosurgery has been greater protection of human subjects undergoing the procedure. This protection has resulted from the establishment of an infrastructure for research ethics in medicine in general and psychiatry in particular. The *Psychosurgery Report* and Recommendations in 1977 was included in the *Belmont Report* of the US National Commission for the Protection of Human Subjects of Biomedical and Behavioral Research in 1978 (Belmont Report, 1978). The three ethical principles for research spelled out in *Belmont* were respect for persons, beneficence and justice.

Psychiatrists conducting research on DBS or neural ablation have three main obligations. First, they have an obligation to design and conduct clinical trials to generate scientific knowledge about the safety and efficacy of the experimental intervention. Second, they have an obligation to fully inform research subjects (or their surrogates) of the purpose, design, and risks of participating in these trials and obtain consent from them based on this information. Third, they have an obligation to ensure that the benefit of participation outweighs the risk. "Benefit" should be construed broadly, consistent with my earlier definition, and "risk" should be within a reasonable professional standard. The second and third obligations overlap to some extent because the long-term effects of stimulating and altering deep structures in the brain are largely unknown. While pointing out this uncertainty to potential research subjects is a necessary part of the process of obtaining informed consent, it is not clear *how* researchers should present this information to subjects. Short-term benefit in the form of symptom relief in days, weeks, or months following stimulation has to be weighed against the risks of surgery and neurological and psychological sequelae that may occur later from chronic stimulation. Reassuring potential research subjects that they will be closely monitored for any unanticipated effects during a trial may be the most reasonable way for researchers to discharge their duty of nonmaleficence.

These obligations might not seem fundamentally different from the obligations of researchers in other areas of medicine (Emanuel, Grady, Crouch et al., 2008). The researcher's obligation to provide a subject with a reasonable benefit–risk ratio in the clinical trial may be stronger in functional neurosurgery for mental disorders than for movement disorders because of the broader range of effects on thought and behavior. The goal of these interventions is to gain a better understanding of the pathophysiology of psychiatric disorders, ameliorate symptoms, and restore motor and mental function. Yet they may result in unwanted changes in personality, cognition, mood, and motivation. For many patients, these side effects could be worse than pain or other physiological changes resulting from other experimental interventions for other medical conditions. A particular concern about personality change is that it could alter the identity of the subject. I will discuss this further in Chapter 5. The important point for present purposes is that a subject may undergo a personality change but retain the cognitive capacity to make an informed decision to participate and continue participating in a trial. A change in identity does not entail impaired capacity to consent, at least not according to the Appelbaum–Grisso definition. Deleterious effects on thought and behavior go beyond the capacity of a subject to process and make decisions based on information presented to her by the investigator. However, if consent includes not only information processing but also the cognitive and emotional capacity for interests, then stimulation that altered a person's mental states could alter her interests. These might include an interest in continuing to participate in a trial.

The distinctive nature of the risks in psychiatric neurosurgery and the magnitude of the harm from the actualization of these risks suggest that the ratio of benefits to risks in psychiatric neurosurgery should be higher than it is in other areas of medical research. Still, the risks associated with DBS (and even neural ablation) can be ethically justified when a psychiatric disorder is refractory to all other treatments and causes prolonged poor quality of life. More precise mapping and electrophysiological recording of brain function, and more precise stimulation, cannot eliminate the risks in psychiatric neurosurgery. But they can reduce the risks to reasonable levels. Research subjects in randomized placebo-controlled trials for new psychotropic drugs may be exposed to some risk if they are assigned to the control arm and have medication withdrawn during the trial. Assuming that the withdrawal is for a reasonable and safe period, however, they can be adequately protected. This is not an issue for functional neurosurgery trials if the condition of subjects in both active and control arms is resistant to pharmacological treatment.

I have claimed that the TM does not mean that a potential research subject lacks sufficient capacity to consent. A patient expressing an interest in participating in a clinical trial may have an expectation to benefit driven by a desire and hope of symptom relief without this impairing his capacity to understand information about the trial. Researchers and their teams have an obligation to try to disabuse potential subjects of the TM if they suspect it from the interview. Yet failure to do this does not mean that a subject participates without giving valid informed consent. If the potential subject has and retains the TM despite the efforts of the investigator or other members of the research team, then this alone would not be sufficient grounds for excluding the person from the trial. Provided that researchers do not trade on the TM in the way they present information about a trial to ensure adequate enrollment, they are appropriately discharging their duty to inform.

If the principal investigator allowed a suspected TM to influence how they presented the information, then they would fail to discharge this duty. They would also fail to respect the patient and potential research subject as an autonomous agent with the right to receive accurate information about a procedure. They would be violating Kant's Categorical Imperative to treat potential research subjects not merely as means for generating scientific knowledge but also as ends in themselves. Subjects are rational decision-makers acting in their best interests and with the right not to be harmed (Kant, 1785/1964). Surrogates could also be motivated by the TM in giving proxy consent to enroll a noncompetent patient as a research subject in a clinical trial. This would invalidate consent only if the desire or hope for symptom relief interfered with their ability to understand the design and purpose of the trial. Researchers could reduce the likelihood of a surrogate TM depending on how they explain the purpose of the trial to them.

I have also claimed that there is no decisive reason for different competency thresholds of consent for potential subjects to participate in DBS research for neurological and psychiatric disorders. Yet researchers' obligation to disclose known and especially unknown risks of these studies for psychiatric disorders may be stronger than it is for movement disorders. While the underlying mechanisms of DBS are still not well understood, the effects of the technique in PD are more predictable and less difficult to control than they are in MDD or OCD. The targets for movement disorders such as PD are typically the subthalamic nucleus and globus pallidus interna. The targets for MDD and OCD involve a larger number of neural circuits. They include the subgenual cingulate white matter, ventral capsule/ventral striatum, nucleus accumbens, medial forebrain bundle, rostral anterior cingulate, and subthalamic nucleus. These circuits mediate not just sensorimotor but also cognitive, emotional, and volitional functions.

Moreover, while the effects of stimulation in PD and other movement disorders are often immediate, the effects of stimulation in MDD, OCD, and other psychiatric disorders are often delayed. This latency, the larger number of targeted circuits, and the greater variability in symptoms make it more difficult to predict what the effects of DBS might be for psychiatric disorders than for movement disorders. These factors present challenges for investigators in preventing adverse effects. Even when DBS ameliorates symptoms, researchers cannot underestimate the short- and long-term neuropsychological impact of altering the brain. They must include the uncertainty surrounding this impact when they discuss the potential risks of the technique with potential research subjects prior to enrolling them in a trial.

Randomized controlled clinical trials in psychiatric neurosurgery include sham surgery in the control arm (Galpern, Corrigan-Curay, Lang et al., 2012; Holtzheimer, Husain, Lisanby et al., 2017). In a sham-controlled DBS trial, a stereotactic frame is placed on the heads of controls, burr holes are drilled in the cranium, and an incision is made in the collarbone or abdomen. But there is no implantation of electrodes or pulse generator. In an electrolytic radiofrequency neural ablation trial, burr holes are drilled in the cranium of controls, but no brain tissue is ablated. In a GKR ablation trial, a Gamma Knife' is placed over subjects' heads, but no gamma beams are transmitted through the skull. In a FUS trial, a device is placed above controls' heads, but no ultrasonic waves are transmitted to the brain. Unlike DBS and electrolytic ablation, subjects in the control arm of GKR or FUS sham-controlled trials are not exposed to the risks to which those in the active arm are exposed. There is no incision in the body or cranium, no tissue is lesioned, no neural circuits are altered, and subjects do not receive any radiation.

A randomized placebo-controlled clinical trial of DBS or ablation with a sham control would be more scientifically robust than a trial without it. This may be the only way to demonstrate that either of these procedures is effective. This would require testing the techniques against placebo responses. These responses to drugs have been statistically significant in some psychiatric disorders, especially moderate MDD. Placebo responses may also occur in neurosurgery, as has been observed in subjects in the sham control arm of surgical trials for PD (Cherkasova and Stoessl, 2014; Ko, Feigin, Mattis et al., 2014). They may occur in psychiatric neurosurgery as well, probably because of subjects' belief in the efficacy of direct intervention in the brain. Despite the scientific rationale for sham controls in neurosurgery clinical trials, some ethicists have claimed that some of these trials are unethical because subjects in the control group are exposed to the risk of infection, edema, and hemorrhage from cranial incisions (Macklin, 1999; Horng and Miller, 2003). Nevertheless, provided that subjects were informed that they would be participating in a randomized placebo-controlled trial with sham surgery in the control arm, they would not be deceived just because they did not receive the stimulation or ablation. Nor would the risk of infection from the burr holes be ethically objectionable because they would be given prophylactic antibiotics, and their condition would be closely monitored.

A study with a delayed start design would probably be the most ethically acceptable. Eventually, each participant would receive an implant and stimulation, but half of the participants would receive placebo stimulation in the first phase. Some or many of the controls would eventually know from their sensory experience that they had not received the active intervention. This knowledge could influence placebo responses and complicate a comparative assessment of the active versus the sham procedure. This is a limitation in all placebo-controlled trials. Knowing that one was in the placebo control arm of a trial could result in psychological harm if a subject was motivated to enroll by the TM and realized that he would not directly benefit from it. This would not be an issue for the ethical justification for the trial, however, if the subject gave valid informed consent to participate in it.

A more ethically contentious issue in functional neurosurgery research is weighing the risks to which subjects in the active arm of a trial are exposed against the potential benefit to subjects in the control arm. There is also the issue of weighing this risk against the potential benefit to patients with the same psychiatric disorder who do not participate in the research. This issue pertains not only to the more invasive neural ablation and DBS but also to the less invasive GKR, FUS, and TMS. Outside of doubly innovative trials testing both safety and efficacy in the same phase, the risk–benefit ratio applies to different cohorts and extends over time. Subjects in an active arm of a trial may subsequently benefit if the research demonstrates that the intervention is safe and effective. Would this future therapeutic possibility justify exposing them to the risks associated with the trial?

Commenting on a double-blind sham-controlled trial of fetal tissue transplantation for PD in the 1990s, Rita Redberg points out that "the institutional review board believed that the risk of sham surgery had to be weighed against the greater risk of mistakenly believing an invasive procedure to be useful because of its placebo effect" (2014, p. 892). She notes that "had there been no trial including sham surgery, many Americans with Parkinson's disease might be receiving craniotomies for only a placebo benefit" (2014, p. 892). The critical point is that "sham interventions are ethical when the benefits of information from a sham-control trial exceed the risks of using an intervention not shown to be more therapeutic than a sham" (Redberg, 2014, p. 893). Further, "without careful use of non-therapeutic controls, we may be submitting millions of Americans to harm from risky, invasive procedures without benefit" (Redberg, 2014, p. 893). The potential and actual harm is not limited to Americans but applies globally to all people with neurological and psychiatric disorders undergoing functional neurosurgery.

The outcome of the BROADEN trial testing subcallosal cingulate DBS for depression supports Redberg's position. The fact that this trial showed no statistically significant difference in benefit between active and sham stimulation and resulted in a significant number of adverse events among participants underscores the importance of sham controls for answering the research question of the efficacy of a technique. It also underscores the importance of designing sham controls to reduce the incidence of adverse events not only in active but also in control arms of a trial. Placebo responses to sham surgery can complicate establishing the efficacy of an experimental treatment for neurological and psychiatric disorders. Because these responses are typically short term, long-term studies could neutralize or cancel the confounding effects of placebo responses in answering the critical research question. Interestingly, some patients with PD have experienced long-term motor improvement from sham surgery. Mariya Cherkasova and A. Jon Stoessl note that investigators could identify presurgery activity in a neural circuit associated with placebo responses (2014). This could help to identify placebo responders and reduce placebo-related variance in functional neurosurgery trials. If similar confounding effects of placebo responses to a sham procedure occurred in psychiatric neurosurgery trials, then a course of action like the one recommended by Cherkasova and Stoessl could be applied to these as well.

Despite the outcome of the BROADEN study, data from many DBS trials indicate that the technique has considerable therapeutic potential for a range of psychiatric disorders. Whether outcomes of the technique improve will depend on a better understanding of the pathophysiology of these disorders from advanced imaging and electrophysiological recording of brain activity. This may enable more precise identification and stimulation of dysfunctional neural circuits. Whether the risk–benefit ratio in DBS for psychiatric disorders is ethically acceptable must be assessed not only research subjects in particular trials but also with respect to different groups of subjects in many trials over time. Like other areas of medical research, psychiatric neurosurgery research is a diachronic enterprise. Accumulated knowledge from meta-analyses of how the technique alters brain function will determine whether neurosurgeons and psychiatrists accept DBS as a safe and effective form of neuromodulation,

RESEARCHERS' OBLIGATIONS | **177**

It is instructive to apply these considerations to neural ablation clinical trials. Subjects in the control arm of such a trial would be exposed to less risk than those in the active arm. Subjects undergoing actual rather than sham ablation would be exposed to the highest risk among all experimental brain interventions. Having what could be a permanent lesion in the brain would be significantly different from the reversible effects of DBS. This seems to involve an unfair distribution of risk among subjects undergoing these distinct procedures, despite the fact that they have the same neuromodulating purpose. Nevertheless, questions about justifiable risk have to be framed by the rationale for ablation trials, which is to investigate the therapeutic potential of the technique for treatment-refractory psychiatric disorders. Some degree of risk is ethically acceptable, especially if this intervention is the only one that could modulate dysfunctional neural circuits and restore some degree of motor and mental functions. The greater risk in neural ablation research can be justified if the subject is not a candidate for DBS, the condition is refractory to all other treatments, and the source of the disorder is a localized hyperactive circuit that can be precisely targeted.

GKR and HIFUS may seem more ethically acceptable forms of ablation than electrolytic radiofrequency ablation because they do not require intracranial surgery and thus are less invasive. Still, the effects on targeted neural tissue could be the same in all of these interventions. Assuming that researchers obtain informed consent from subjects, do not expose them to unreasonable risk, and closely monitor their condition during the trial and with long-term follow-up, they discharge their duties of respect for patient autonomy and nonmaleficence. At the same time, they discharge their duty to generate scientific knowledge about the pathophysiology of psychiatric disorders and potential therapies for them.

Device makers funding DBS trials for psychiatric disorders have an obvious interest in demonstrating that their product can modulate dysfunctional neural circuits. This has the potential to create a conflict of interest for researchers investigating how DBS alters the brain and mind of subjects if the manufacturer influences the design of the trial and the interpretation of its results. The potential conflict is greater if the researcher is a shareholder in such a company. Policies must be in place to prevent or reduce the probability of conflict by ensuring the scientific integrity of the trial and unbiased interpretation of results. More generally, device-maker interests should be compatible with the interests of psychiatric patients in experiencing symptom relief and improved quality of life (Fins and Schiff, 2010; Curfman and Redberg, 2011; Fins, Schlaepfer, Nuttin et al., 2011; Ineichen, Glannon, Temel et al., 2014). I discuss this issue further in Chapter 5.

## Optogenetics

A novel neuromodulating technique that may have greater therapeutic potential than neural ablation or DBS for psychiatric disorders is optogenetics. This technique uses light-sensitive proteins (opsins) that conduct electricity to control activity in neurons and neural tissue. Neurons are genetically modified to express light-sensitive ion channels. Exposing neurons to light can activate or inhibit electrical activity in the brain (Deisseroth, Etkin, and Malenka, 2015). Although there are important differences among psychiatric disorders in the contribution of genes to brain function and dysfunction, all of these disorders involve multigene effects. In optogenetics, inserted genes are not disease-related but make neurons light sensitive. These could be inserted in neurons in brain regions associated with specific mental disorders.

The main theoretical advantage of optogenetics over traditional DBS is that the latter form of neuromodulation is nonspecific in influencing both excitatory and inhibitory neurons. Optogenetics can selectively activate excitatory glutaminergic or inhibitory GABAergic neurons and be more specific in modulating neural functions. Because it acts on a broader range of factors in the pathophysiology of psychiatric disorders, optogenetics may be more effective in regulating this balance than temporal interference. It has better spatial resolution and is a more focused means of neuromodulation than DBS. In addition, it has considerable temporal precision, making it superior to the delayed and distributed effects of psychopharmacology. Another positive feature of optogenetics is that opsins have the potential to regulate the balance between excitation and inhibition in neurons for an extended duration. In this regard, it may be at least as effective as continuous DBS.

As Sarah Jarvis and Simon Schultz describe the technique: "Manipulation of neural activity can be achieved via the insertion of light-sensitive proteins (opsins) that act as ion channels or pumps into a neuron's membrane and are preferentially controlled by photons of different wavelengths, providing temporal control on the order of milliseconds" (2015, p. 1). The combination of "specificity for targeting neuronal populations, activation flexibility due to the range of opsins available, and excellent spatiotemporal control" (2015, p. 3) provides optogenetics with a degree of precision lacking in DBS and "a more finely targeted alternative to traditional neuromodulatory treatments" (2015, p. 2). Jarvis and Schultz point out that "optogenetics exploits its ability for altering neural activity with high temporal precision. By using short, well-timed pulses, it is possible to not only induce short-term plasticity but also induce long-term potentiation . . . and the possibility of reprogramming circuits" (2015, p. 3). DBS may induce neuroplasticity when initiated at an early stage of the disease process. FUS may be able to deliver growth factors into atrophied brain regions by opening the blood–brain barrier (BBB). But neither of these techniques appears to have the same neurogenerative potential as optogenetics.

One potential application of optogenetics in psychiatry would be to erase fear memories associated with PTSD, anxiety, and panic disorders. As discussed earlier, because these disorders are traceable to a memory of a traumatic or disturbing experience, in principle removing the memory could resolve the disorder. In one study, researchers used this technique to weaken a fear memory in mice (Kim and Cho, 2017). The researchers activated the fear memory in the amygdala by generating a high-pitch tone. They were able to identify the memory trace in this brain region by observing activation in the neurons and synaptic connections constituting the trace as the mice responded to the sensory cue. The light was able to selectively stimulate and inactivate only the neurons and synapses constituting the fear memory trace. The greater neuromodulating precision of optogenetics compared with DBS could overcome the problems of localization and selectivity in memory erasure. If its effects were highly specific, then it could erase a maladaptive or pathological memory while leaving normal adaptive fear and episodic memories intact. In these respects, optogenetics could become an effective treatment for some psychiatric disorders.

Thus far, optogenetics has been used only in animal models. A number of problems would have to be addressed before the technique could become a viable alternative to DBS in treating major psychiatric disorders. Optogenetics involves interactions between genes and neurobiology, which involves a higher level of complexity in different aspects of neural mechanisms than genetics or neurobiology alone. Maintaining these interactions between excitation and inhibition may be difficult to control. It would require identifying the optimal opsin for a given neural target, as well as determining optimal neuron–opsin combinations within a particular neural circuit. In versions involving an implantable fiber-optic light source, the procedure would be "highly invasive" (Jarvis and Schultz, 2015, p. 6). Research subjects in an optogenetics study could be exposed to greater risks than those in a DBS study. Implantable optogenetics would require "both manipulation of genetic material as well as the subcranial placement of devices to provide optimal activation" (Jarvis and Schuktz, 2015, p. 6). The procedure would entail a risk of both adverse events from overstimulating circuits, and adverse events from manipulating genes. The compounded risk in optogenetic clinical trials would require researchers to provide even greater protection of research subjects than in DBS trials.

A critical question is how safely and effectively opsins could be delivered into a targeted brain region. The history of gene therapy is replete with experiments that have failed because of problems with viral vectors intended to deliver genes to specific sites in the body. This should serve as a cautionary tale for the development and application of this novel technology. There would be less reason for concern, though, if the genes involved were not disease-related. An external light source is a less invasive and less risky alternative to implantable forms of optogenetics. But this has limitations. Scattering of the light by bone and tissue could prevent it from penetrating to deep brain structures. An implantable system could prevent or minimize light scattering, but it would entail greater risk. Jarvis and Schultz further point out that there must be a uniform spread of light over a targeted area of tissue (2015, p. 5). The illumination must cover the targeted area but not be so focused as to cause tissue damage from overheating. As with the sound waves in FUS, the intensity of the light in optogenetics would have to be high enough to have a neuromodulating effect on dysfunctional circuits, but not so high as to damage adjacent functional circuits and healthy tissue.

In addition to the risks associated with placing and activating a device in deep neural structures, optogenetics would involve the manipulation of genetic material in the brain. This would involve the risk of losing control of transcription and growth factors regulated by genes. It is unclear how researchers could prevent the potential for uncontrolled proliferation of these factors. These two separate risks from separate sources would provide greater challenges for investigators in ensuring the safety of human subjects undergoing this experimental procedure than with less invasive temporal interference or more invasive DBS. Also, because its mechanism of action seems to make it more effective in regulating excitatory neurons than inhibitory ones, the application of optogenetics could be limited to psychiatric disorders with hyperactive circuits. On a more positive note, the potential to activate neuroplastic and neurogenerative processes suggest that the technique could have an important role in countering the pathogenesis and neurodegenerative effects of chronic psychiatric diseases. This could make optogenetics not only a neuromodulating technique but a neurogenerative one as well.

Optogenetics is very much at an early stage of research and development. It will be some time before it moves from animal models to first-in-human trials. Many questions about the neurophysiological effects of the technique need to be addressed. Jarvis and Schultz claim: "From the challenges of opsin delivery to the difficulties in optically driving neurons with implantable devices, applying optogenetics outside of research remains a remote possibility in the foreseeable future" (2015, p. 8). In addition to neurophysiological questions, there are many ethical questions about the potentially beneficial and harmful effects of the technique on research subjects and patients. These need to be addressed before optogenetics could become a safe and effective form of neuromodulation, and possibly neurogenesis, for psychiatric disorders.

## Conclusion

A significant percentage of severe psychiatric disorders do not respond to pharmacotherapy, psychotherapy, and less invasive forms of neuromodulation such as ECT and TMS. In these cases, psychiatric neurosurgery may be indicated as a means of controlling and ameliorating symptoms. Psychiatric neurosurgery is a form of functional neurosurgery consisting in the modulation of dysfunctional neural circuits underlying mental dysfunction in psychiatric disorders. The two main forms of psychiatric neurosurgery are DBS and neural ablation. Current stimulating and ablating techniques are safer and more effective for patients than techniques of the past because of advanced stereotactic neurosurgical methods and more precise recording, mapping, and targeting of brain activity.

Both ablation and neurostimulation remain experimental and investigational procedures. More randomized, double-blind, placebo-controlled clinical trials are needed to establish the safety and efficacy of these interventions for psychiatric disorders. These disorders can impair the mental capacity necessary for reasoning and decision-making. But decisional capacity comes in degrees, and many patients have enough of this capacity to give informed consent to participate in psychiatric neurosurgery research. The TM does not necessarily interfere with a subject's capacity to consent because understanding the design of a clinical trial and the hope of benefiting from it may be compatible regarding the motivation for participating in DBS or neural ablation clinical trials.

More ethically challenging are expanding applications of these neuromodulating techniques to conditions such as schizophrenia and AN. The extent of cognitive impairment in these disorders may preclude the decisional capacity for consent. In some cases, allowing a surrogate to give proxy consent to the enrollment of a patient in psychiatric neurosurgery research can be justified. Ethical justification of direct and proxy consent also depends on a reasonable risk–benefit ratio of participating in a trial. Benefit must be assessed in terms of not one cohort at the time of a trial but among different cohorts in many trials over a longer period. The fact that experimental psychiatric neurosurgery can directly alter thought and behavior seems to require a higher level of decisional capacity for consent to participate in trials testing these techniques than in other areas of medicine. Yet the severity and treatment-refractory nature of these disorders, and the potential of the research to yield new knowledge leading to new therapies, may justify allowing less strict criteria for consent. This could allow more patients to participate in research from which they and others with these disorders may subsequently benefit.

The fact that the effects of DBS are generally reversible and that those of neural ablation are generally irreversible entails greater risk in the latter procedure. This seems to place a higher standard of mental capacity on patients being considered for a neural ablation study. It also means that investigators have a stronger ethical obligation to protect these research subjects from harm than in DBS or indeed any other area of medical research. If proxy consent is allowed, then surrogates must display a high level of understanding of the technique and the goals of the trial to ensure that they are acting in the subject's best interests. Investigators must strike a medical and ethical balance between allowing patients the opportunity to participate in research while protecting them from harm.

Although it can relieve symptoms, there is no conclusive evidence that DBS can reverse the pathophysiology of neurological and psychiatric disorders. Closed-loop systems using algorithms to detect neurophysiological signals regulating mood and motivation may be more effective than open-loop systems in controlling symptoms. But it is questionable whether they can alter underlying disease mechanisms.

Results of some studies of DBS for PD indicate that initiating the technique in younger patients at an earlier disease stage may produce greater benefit than initiating it in older patients at a later stage (Schuepbach, Rau, Knudsen et al., 2013; Woopen, Pauls, Kory et al., 2013; Abramowicz, Zuccotti, and Pflomm, 2014). There are some indications that earlier brain stimulation for PD could enhance neuroplasticity and activate endogenous repair and growth mechanisms in the brain. These effects might occur in later disease stages as well. They could slow the progression of PD and Alzheimer's disease. It is also possible that DBS could induce these mechanisms when used for psychiatric disorders. Initiating neurostimulation soon after disease onset might prevent abnormal neural development and subsequent neurodegeneration. This could create an obligation for psychiatrists to administer the technique at the first sign of disease. Still, the potential benefits and risks associated with DBS would have to be weighed against the potential benefits and risks of less invasive interventions typically used before DBS. Researchers would have to determine whether a technique currently investigated for advanced treatment-resistant psychiatric disorders should replace or complement first-line treatment.

A study of patients with moderately advanced PD found that they "did not seem to endorse earlier implementation of DBS, and they considered that it should be the last resort when really needed" (Sperens, Hamberg, and Hariz, 2017, p. 1). This attitude reflected their concern about the risks of the procedure, which outweighed their beliefs about its therapeutic potential. This could weaken the claim that researchers have an ethical obligation to offer DBS earlier in the disease process. It could present a conflict between patients' autonomy and researchers' obligations of beneficence and nonmaleficence. Waiting until the disease was advanced could limit the therapeutic potential of the technique. Yet researchers have an ethical obligation to respect the autonomy of competent patients in making decisions about receiving therapy and participating in research. If the risks were the same at earlier and later times, then informing patients that earlier administration of DBS potentially could be more effective than later administration could change their attitudes. It could reassure them that participating in this research could be in their best interests. This may be the case both for patients with movement disorders and those with cognitive and mood disorders. This would depend on whether electrical stimulation of the brain was indicated as an alternative to first-line treatment.

FUS and optogenetics are hypothetical interventions for psychiatric disorders. Optogenetics has considerable therapeutic potential because it can modulate both gene expression and functional connectivity in the brain. HIFUS and diffusion tensor-guided linear accelerator radiosurgery may eventually replace standard forms of neural ablation (Kim, Sharim, Tenn et al., 2018). FUS has additional therapeutic potential beyond its role in neuromodulation and neural ablation. While protecting the brain from harmful molecules, the BBB also prevents the delivery of drugs that could treat brain disease because the drugs consist of molecules that are too large to penetrate it and enter the brain. The ability of FUS to open the BBB could allow delivery of drugs to modulate amyloid-beta metabolism in the brain implicated in Alzheimer's disease (Bu, Xiang, Jin et al., 2017; Lipsman, Meng, Bethune et al., 2018). Implantable ultrasonic devices may also be used for more efficient delivery of chemotherapeutic drugs to treat different forms of brain cancer (Burgess and Hynynen, 2014; Horodyckid, Canney, Vignot et al., 2017). FUS might allow the infusion of trophic factors to promote neuroplasticity and induce neurogenesis. It might reverse pathogenesis in brain regions atrophied by the effects of chronic psychiatric disorders. It may even be possible to do this in adolescent brains and prevent the development of full-blown disease. Although they are still at a very early stage of research, optogenetics and FUS could revolutionize therapy for otherwise intractable diseases of the brain and mind by slowing, reversing, and possibly preventing them.

# Chapter 5

# Neuromodulation: Control, identity, and justice

Major psychiatric disorders can impair agency and free will. Dysfunctional neural circuits that ordinarily enable motor and mental capacities impair them and the ability to form and execute action plans. The combination of structural and functional brain imaging and patients' behavior can confirm connections between neural and mental dysfunction. Less and more invasive interventions in the brain can modulate these circuits and the motor and mental capacities they mediate. When psychopharmacology and other interventions in the brain are ineffective, functional neurosurgery can re-establish normal or near-normal levels of brain function. In the most severe cases, DBS and neural ablation can liberate patients from psychopathology by modulating neural circuits stuck in a repetitive pattern of disordered information processing. These most invasive brain-altering techniques can restore some degree of flexible thought and behavior and adaptability to the environment. They can restore varying degrees of agency and free will. In its continuous modulating effects on dysfunctional neural circuits underlying disordered mental states, DBS can be described as a "pacemaker for the brain" or a "prosthesis for the will" (Glannon, 2018).

Some would claim that persons undergoing DBS are no longer the source of their mental states and actions. The device implanted in their brains regulates what they think and do. The person and her conscious mind seem to have no causal role in restoring autonomous agency and free will. While DBS is the most common invasive form of neuromodulation, implantable wireless devices in optogenetics may generate the same concern because of their direct effects in the brain and indirect effects on the mind. Indeed, not just implanted devices but any device that alters neural and mental functions may cause some to question the claim that neuromodulation can enable people with major psychiatric disorders to control their thought and behavior. Something other than the person seems to be in control.

The neural implant in DBS does not replace the person as the source of her actions. On the contrary, by restoring the motor and mental capacities impaired by these disorders, DBS can restore some degree of autonomous agency and free will. There is shared control between the device and the person in whom it is implanted and activated. Still, there is a question of whether a patient with a device implanted in her brain has a moral and legal responsibility to use it in certain ways. This raises the related question of whether it is fair to hold the person to what seems like a higher standard of responsibility than a person who does not need a device to maintain normal brain function.

Some may also express concern about the effects of neuromodulation on the psychological connectedness and continuity that constitutes personal identity. Even when it relieves symptoms of psychiatric disorders, it may not be clear that a technique that causes changes in these psychological relations benefits the person who undergoes it. Neither DBS nor neural ablation necessarily causes substantial changes in one's identity. Although these techniques may cause changes in one's psychological properties, when its effects are salutary the technique does not alter but restores identity by restoring the connectedness and continuity of the psychological properties disrupted by these disorders. Rather than transforming them into different persons, DBS restores the premorbid selves that psychiatric patients had before the onset of their symptoms. When restoration of autonomy and identity in these patients requires continuous neuromodulation, this presupposes continuous access to the technique. Many patients may not have this access, which raises additional ethical issues about social justice (Fins and Pohl, 2016).

## Restoring control

Recall that the *DSM-IV-TR* mentions an "important loss of freedom" as one of the defining features of mental disorders. Loss of freedom is equivalent to loss of control of thought and behavior. By modulating dysfunctional neural circuits, DBS and other techniques can restore some degree of sensorimotor, cognitive, emotional, and volitional capacities and thereby restore some degree of this control. Studies have shown that neuromodulating techniques can have these effects in MDD, OCD, GAD, and BD. It is also possible to produce these effects in AN, PTSD, and schizophrenia.

Assessing the restorative effects of DBS for OCD and addiction, De Ridder and coauthors claim that the technique "gives them the freedom to engage in other aspects of life, and having more thoughts, not being hijacked anymore by an all-overwhelming thought and urge to obtain the substance of abuse. In other words, it liberates them to have more control over their thoughts and actions" (De Ridder, Vanneste, Gillett et al., p. 242). By modulating dysfunctional circuits consisting of the anterior cingulate cortex, nucleus accumbens (NAc), and the anterior limb of the internal capsule, and re-establishing the balance between negative and positive feedback of information in the brain, DBS can restore "flexible behavioral adaptations" (De Ridder, Vanneste, Gillett et al., p. 242). Martijn Figee and coinvestigators have observed a similar outcome in a DBS study of patients with OCD targeting the NAc (Figee, Luigjes, Smolders et al., 2013). Stimulation of the NAc reduced hyperactive connectivity between this region and the PFC. Combined with decreased prefrontal low-frequency oscillations, the stimulation reduced symptoms in some patients. With the obsessions reduced or eliminated, the patient does not feel the need to engage in compulsions as a compensatory strategy. He does not feel overloaded by unnecessary motor, cognitive, and emotional demands and no longer feels stuck in an unremitting cycle of intrusive thoughts and unwanted actions. Neuromodulation can restore free will to patients with this disorder by allowing unconscious brain processes mediating motor and cognitive functions, such as procedural memory, to operate as a matter of course. They no longer have to worry about or feel paralyzed by their lack of trust in these processes. The technique can re-establish the patient's trust and self-confidence in these automatic functions and enable flexible and adaptive behavior.

A comment by Nir Lipsman and Andres Lozano on DBS for OCD further elucidates how the technique can restore some degree of control in people with this disorder:

> OCD is marked by both a thought (anxiety-generating obsessions) and a motor component (anxiolytic compulsions). Critically, DBS for OCD aims to reduce anxiety by targeting limbic structures rather than addressing the action components of the condition by targeting motor structures. A reduced *drive* to engage in time-consuming and disabling compulsions, which the patient realizes are disproportionate, is the desired outcome. If patients feel unable to control their compulsions secondary to paralyzing anxiety that *compels* them to act in a pathological fashion, DBS provides them with control by inhibiting their anxiety. Here too, as in PD and depression, the ability to act in accordance with one's wishes is enhanced by DBS. (Lipsman and Lozano, 2015, p. 199)

In this way, DBS can restore the patient's autonomy over his motivational states and actions. It can enable the patient to have the mental states he wants to have and for these states to move him to act in accord with his considered desires and intentions. Autonomy or free will in normal circumstances is a graded capacity reflecting a complex interaction of neural, psychological, and environmental factors. For people who have lost some or much of this capacity from psychiatric disorders, DBS may restore it to varying degrees. Complete restoration of normal neural, motor, and mental functions may not be possible in most cases. This may depend on the severity of the disorder. It may also depend on whether the patient is a candidate for the technique and how the brain responds to neuromodulation. Restoring these capacities to levels approximating premorbid levels may enable patients to achieve a reasonable degree of functional independence.

Electrical stimulation of a metabolically hyperactive subgenual cingulate can restore some degree of function in cognitive and emotional components of the will in a subtype of MDD (Mayberg, Lozano, Voon et al., 2005; Lozano, Mayberg, Giacobbe et al., 2008). In a different subtype of this disorder, DBS of the ventral tegmental area of the mesolimbic dopamine reward system can restore some degree of function in motor and volitional components of the will (Schlaepfer, Bewernick, Kayser et al., 2014). More speculatively, high-frequency stimulation of metabolically hyperactive neurons and synapses in the basolateral amygdala could inactivate the nuclei constituting a pathological memory trace and effectively erase it. Equally speculative, DBS might be able to reduce the delusions that patients in psychotic states construct as a maladaptive compensatory strategy to make sense of abnormal perceptions and thoughts. The compulsive behavior of people with OCD is a similar maladaptive compensatory response to their obsessions. DBS would reduce these behaviors by re-establishing normal connectivity and information integration and processing in thalamocortical and corticocortical circuits. This could relieve the cognitive load on the patient by obviating the need for strategies such as "double bookkeeping." DBS neuromodulation of nodes in the auditory cortex might also reintegrate information in this and other regions to which it is connected and reduce the incidence of auditory hallucinations. It might restore normal alignment of perceptions with the patient's body and external world and restore normal beliefs, intentions, and effective agency.

More generally, modulation of circuits mediating cognitive-emotional processing could restore patients' capacity for insight into their disorder and provide reasons for adhering to this or other treatments. In these and other respects, in a wide range of neurological and psychiatric disorders DBS can restore brain function and the motor and mental capacities that constitute free will. However, the salutary effects of this technique may be limited in many cases. This may depend on whether the neural dysfunction is more localized in specific circuits or more distributed across broader neural networks.

The neuromodulating effects of DBS on neural circuits can re-establish and sustain optimal levels of neural function, preventing extremes of deficit and excess, or hypoactivity and hyperactivity. They can re-establish and sustain optimal levels of motor and mental functions. Overstimulating targeted circuits at too high a frequency, or inadvertently stimulating normal circuits, may cause a different psychopathology. This can have equally disabling effects on the will as the effects of the disorder that is treated. It can undermine rather than restore control. In PD, for example, electrical stimulation of the subthalamic nucleus or globus pallidus interna can resolve hypodopaminergic activity causing motor, cognitive, and emotional inhibition. But imprecise stimulation or overstimulation of these brain regions may induce hyperdopaminergic activity resulting in disinhibition and compulsive or addictive behavior (Frank, Samanta, Moustafa et al., 2007; Castrioto, Lhommee, Moro et al., 2014). The ethical implications of altering brain circuits in terms of trade-offs between benefit and harm have been documented in reports from PD patients experiencing motor symptom relief but also neurological and psychological sequelae (Muller and Christen, 2011; Christen, Bittlinger, Walter et al., 2012). Not all psychological effects are the direct result of stimulation. In one study, researchers found that patients' assessment of tremor severity in PD and essential tremor was predictive of depression following DBS (Achey, Yamamoto, Sexton et al., 2018). Nevertheless, the direct psychological effects of the technique can be significant.

Physical and emotional effects of stimulating the subthalamic nucleus or globus pallidus interna can be difficult to dissociate because the basal ganglia include motor as well as limbic and associative circuits in close proximity to each other (De Long and Wichmann, 2012). There is considerable overlap between these circuits, with afferent inputs and efferent outputs regulated by the same neurotransmitter—dopamine. This is one example of how the neural correlates of the motor and mental capacities necessary for agency are not localized to a single brain region but distributed over broader networks. These regions may not be functionally segregated. In DBS for GAD and MDD, overstimulation of the NAc in the reward circuit may reduce anxiety and improve mood but also cause hypomania or mania. The outcome would be a different type of mood disturbance. To prevent these adverse events, more precise electrode placement, and targeting and stimulating circuits at the right frequency could sustain optimal levels of oscillations in targeted circuits without adversely affecting others. This can be challenging because of the connectivity between circuits and the ways in which they interact in projecting to and from each other. This is the main respect in which CLDs could be superior to OLDs for psychiatric disorders. They could provide real-time critical feedback between stimulating input and brain output in maintaining optimal levels of activation, connectivity, and oscillations among neural circuits within these circuits.

## Who or what is the agent?

Even if DBS can modulate the neural circuits implicated in psychiatric disorders and ameliorate symptoms, some may be concerned that the restoration of motor and mental functions comes at too high a cost. The concern is that a mechanical device implanted in the brain controls a person's behavior completely outside of her conscious awareness. It suggests that she is not the author or source of her mental states and actions. Despite the overlap between neurological and psychiatric disorders, this concern is greater in psychiatric disorders because of greater impairment in mental than motor functions. Mental functions form the core of free will and personal identity. How can a person act freely and remain the same person if something other than his own brain and mind is controlling how he thinks and what he does? The concern may be greater with CLDs than OLDs because the former provide a higher level of mechanistic and automatic control of brain processes than the latter. Who or what is the agent behind one's thought and behavior? Are our actions really our own? Are they entirely the products of normally functioning neural circuits or devices that restore dysfunctional circuits to normal function?

Concern about neuromodulating techniques undermining control is unfounded. Instead, they can restore the motor and mental functions associated with behavior control and thereby restore autonomous agency and free will. They can also restore the mentally healthy selves that existed before the onset of mental illness. Some neuroscientists may divide neural implants into those that *replace* or *substitute* for a dysfunctional part of the brain and those that *supplement* or *support* it. DBS falls within both categories. It replaces abnormal electrical signaling with regular electrical current and supports the activity of dysfunctional brain circuits (Lipsman and Glannon, 2013, p. 466). The technique substitutes for these circuits because continuous activation of the device is necessary to restore normal function. Any substitution or replacement is only partial, because in most cases other neural circuits to and from which dysfunctional circuits project are functionally intact.

Still, the idea of any type of brain implant altering thought and behavior seems anathema to the ideas of autonomy and responsibility for our actions. These concepts presuppose that our actions do not result from causal routes that bypass our mental states as the direct causes of our actions (Mele, 1995; Davidson, 2001a, 2001b, 2001c). To be autonomous and responsible for what they do, agents must act from their "own mechanisms, which cannot be formed by pills, *electronic stimulation* of the brain or brainwashing" (Fischer and Ravizza, 1998, p. 236, emphasis added; Bublitz and Merkel, 2013). Being morally responsible for one's actions excludes "severe manipulation of the brain, hypnosis and the like" (Fischer and Ravizza, 1998, p. 53). Shaun Gallagher claims that, "if my bodily movement is determined by something other than my own reflective thought, then it is an involuntary movement but not an action" (2006, p. 110). If one accepts these views, then it seems that, as a neural prosthetic, DBS undermines the conscious control of thought and behavior necessary for autonomous and responsible agency. A mechanism other than the person's own normally functioning brain and mind is doing all of the causal work.

In PD, dysfunction in the basal ganglia can interfere with the ability to perform voluntary bodily movements. In MDD, OCD, and GAD, dysfunction in corticolimbic pathways can interfere with the ability to form and carry out intentions in mental acts, such as decisions, and physical acts, such as bodily movements. These and other disorders limit or preclude agency by limiting or precluding the critical sensorimotor, cognitive, emotional, and volitional capacities. DBS can restore some degree of autonomous agency by modulating the neural circuits implicated in these disorders, improving these capacities, and thereby enabling control of the actions that we want or do not want to perform. When DBS functions properly, it enables a person with any of these disorders to control her thought and behavior. There is shared control between the device and the person in whom it is implanted and activated (Glannon, 2014, 2018).

Control of decisions and actions presupposes that conscious mental states have some causal role in them. The fact that DBS operates outside of the patient's awareness and without any apparent conscious contribution from her seems to eliminate the conscious agent from this process. It is not enough for persons to be basic agents to control their behavior. They must be autonomous and as such the authors of their actions. The actions must be their *own*. If a person's neural and mental states are modulated by DBS, then it seems that their actions are traceable to an artificial source. One might conclude that the device rather than the person regulates how she thinks and acts (Klaming and Haselager, 2013). Regarding one of the moral implications of DBS as a neural prosthetic, Jens Clausen asks, when behavior is caused by a brain–mind machine, "Who is responsible for involuntary acts?" (2009, p. 1080). The "brain–mind machine" would be any device implanted in the brain that alters neural and mental processes. The "involuntary" acts would be those resulting from processes caused by the device. Presumably, the acts would be involuntary and outside of a person's control because they were not initiated by the person's conscious mental states. One could not be responsible for actions that were not one's own. We need to assess whether these actions would be truly involuntary and thus not autonomous.

In ego-dystonic disorders such as MDD (without psychosis) and OCD, the patient has impaired autonomy because of the incongruity she experiences between the mental states she wants to have and the pathological mental states she actually has. Patients retain insight into their condition, interpret symptomatic mental states as imposed upon, or alien, to them, and yearn to rid themselves of these states. The state of knowing that they have a disorder and the motivation to seek treatment for it is a sign that they retain some degree of autonomy. This is absent in those with ego-syntonic disorders who experience no such incongruity, cannot recognize reasons for treatment, and may even resist it. If the neuromodulating effects of DBS can reduce the patient's internal conflict between pathological and healthy mental states, then they can increase the patient's autonomy impaired by the disorder (Meynen, 2010, 2012, 2015). If DBS enables a patient with an ego-syntonic disorder to understand that she has a disorder and recognize reasons for seeking and adhering to treatment, then it can restore the patient's autonomy in this respect as well. The degree of restoration may be greater in an ego-syntonic disorder because of the degree of the initial cognitive impairment indicated by the patient's lack of insight into her disorder. Yet, as I pointed out in Chapter 4, ego-syntonic disorders may preclude the cognitive and motivational capacities necessary to understand the need for treatment. This could include DBS and thus rule out any therapeutic and restorative potential of the technique.

The claim that control of thought and behavior is necessary for free will and responsibility does not imply that it must be complete control. It does not imply that each event in a sequence of events resulting in an action must be within the conscious content of the agent's mental states. Provided that the person can freely form motivational states, endorse them as her own, and translate them into actions by activating the device, she can act freely and responsibly. The fact that the device facilitates this translation at an unconscious level does not undermine the will of the person operating the device. Besides, as I pointed out in the discussion of the role of consciousness in OCD in Chapter 2, being too conscious and trying too hard to control behavior can result in a psychopathology causing one to lose control. There is no complete conscious control of thought and behavior in healthy brains and minds. Flexible, adaptive behavior presupposes that unconscious processes constrain consciousness in many respects.

I also emphasized in Chapter 2 the need to distinguish constraint at the neural level from constraint at the mental level. Mental constraint in the form of impeded initiative, fearful anticipation of the future, or general cognitive impairment may be symptomatic of psychopathology. Failure of some brain regions to constrain or inhibit others to which they are functionally connected may result in neural hyperactivity manifesting in the subjective experience of constraint or inhibition in the inability to perform desired actions. It could also manifest in feeling compelled to perform actions involuntarily. Some degree of constraint or inhibition at the neural level is necessary for a person to feel free from the subjective experience of constraint, inhibition, or compulsion at the mental and bodily level. Lipsman and Lozano express this idea in their claim that the modulating effects of DBS on hyperactive circuits can provide OCD patients with control "by inhibiting their anxiety" (2015, p. 199). More precisely, by sending accurate information about the world to the PFC, the thalamus constrains this region and prevents it from becoming hyperactive and sending distorted information to the striatum and limbic structures. This ensures that these regions do not become hyperactive or hypoactive. At the conscious mental level, this type of constraint prevents the experience of anxiety.

In impulse control disorders and addiction, a normally functioning PFC fails to inhibit the reward system and prevent it from become hyperactive. This hyperactivity drives the impulsive and addictive behavior. In these and other psychiatric disorders, unconstrained neural activity at different levels in the brain can become hyperactivity resulting in pathological thought and behavior that interferes with autonomous agency. Some degree of constraint by subcortical on cortical regions, and vice versa, and some degree of constraint by unconscious on conscious processes, and vice versa, is not only compatible with but necessary for behavior control. Control of thought and behavior requires these types of constraints at different levels of interacting neural and mental activity.

This is consistent with Feinberg's and Spence's conceptions of constraint. Higher- and lower-level processes in the brain interact with each other in a series of re-entrant loops to promote homeostasis within a human organism and its ability to adapt to the external milieu. Normal signaling of information about the world by the thalamus to the PFC enables this region to constrain the striatum and limbic areas in preventing anxiety-generating obsessions and compulsions. There is a disruption of this signaling in OCD. Normal functional connectivity among cortical and subcortical neural networks is necessary for these control-enabling constraints. Constraint is a property of optimal levels of neural processing enabling optimal levels of mental processing necessary for voluntary action.

An actual case of a patient with a psychiatric disorder treated with DBS illustrates this point. It also casts suspicion on the idea of stimulating neural circuits to enhance motor and mental functions by trying to raise them above optimal levels. A patient with a history of GAD and OCD became less anxious and experienced improved mood and motivation after receiving continuous, bilateral, electrical stimulation of the NAc. He told his psychiatrist that he wanted to feel even better and asked him to increase the frequency of the electrical current from the stimulator. This caused him to feel "unrealistically good" and "overwhelmed by a feeling of happiness and ease" (Synofzik, Schlaepfer, and Fins, 2012, p. 32). Despite the euphoria, he retained enough insight into his condition and enough cognitive capacity to know that the elevated mood and motivation could cause him to lose control of his thought and behavior. He expressed fear that his euphoria would "tilt over," and that his anxiety would return. Accordingly, he agreed with his psychiatrist to lower the frequency to the initial level that modulated the critical neural circuits and restored mental and motor functions. This case shows that trying to enhance these functions above optimal levels could disturb the equilibrium that DBS had restored and result in cognitive, emotional, and volitional states that would be as maladaptive and pathological as those caused by the disorder itself. Consistent with the concept of neuromodulation, there are limits to the extent to which DBS can improve motivation and mood. Given the risks of stimulating beyond a certain level, Marwan Hariz insists that "neuromodulation should not be allowed to become neuromanipulation" (Hariz, 2014, p. 324).

The fact that DBS operates outside of a person's awareness does not undermine but instead supports behavior control and free will by modulating dysfunctional neural circuits that generate and sustain mental states and actions. Electrical stimulation of a dysfunctional frontal–limbic–striatal circuit in MDD or frontal–thalamic–striatal/limbic–frontal circuit in OCD, for example, may restore not only some degree of normal neural function but also the phenomenology of being in control of motor and mental functions (Melloni, Urbistondo, Sedeno et al., 2012; Figee, Luigjes, Smolders et al., 2013; De Ridder, Vanneste, Gillett et al., 2016). Like the cognitive state of a person with an implanted cardiac pacemaker, the subject's implicit knowledge that electrodes are implanted and activated in her brain does not figure in the explicit content of her awareness. As an enabling technique, DBS does not interfere with but allows the formation and translation of unconscious intentions in motor skills and conscious intentions in effective decision-making.

Most normal brain processes are not transparent to us. We have no direct access to the afferent neurons that transmit information from the peripheral nervous system to the CNS. Nor do we have direct access to the efferent neurons that transmit information from the CNS to the peripheral nervous system. Afferent and efferent systems underlie our unconscious motor plans, and we only experience the sensorimotor consequences of these plans. It does not matter whether these consequences are produced by a natural or artificial system. Provided that a neuromodulating system such as DBS connects in the right way with the neural inputs and outputs that regulate thought and behavior, it allows the subject to initiate and execute action plans. It allows the subject to control how he thinks and acts. By ensuring that one has the thoughts one wants to have and performs the actions one wants to perform, DBS is not an "alien" system that hijacks one's neural and mental functions. Instead, when the device operates safely and effectively, the person in whom it is implanted can identify with it as her own, as an extended feature of her brain. The electrodes are an extension of the person's brain in the sense that they are an adjunct or supplement to neural circuits that have become dysfunctional (Glannon, 2014, 2018). Although it is not implanted in the brain but under the collarbone, the pulse generator that activates the electrodes and the leads connecting them are extended features of the person's brain in this same sense. These interconnected devices ensure that the brain generates and sustains normal mental states when it cannot do this on its own.

We can make this same claim regardless of whether neuromodulation is from an OLD or CLD. Differences in *how* these devices modulate brain function are not as important as the fact *that* they have modulating effects on the brain and re-establish normal mental function. Restoration of autonomy in a person with a psychiatric disorder, or the degree to which it is restored, does not depend on the invasiveness or noninvasiveness of the procedure as such. Invasive systems consisting of devices implanted in the brain can affect brain function more directly than noninvasive systems located outside of the brain and cranium. Because of the implant in the brain, the first type of system entails greater risk, which has to be weighed against the potentially greater benefit compared with other treatments. Regarding the restoration of autonomy, there is no significant ethical difference between invasive and noninvasive systems if both modulate the relevant neural and mental functions to the same degree. Sabine Muller and Henrik Walter claim that neuromodulation requires some revision of the concept of autonomy because it can influence the neural basis of autonomy (2010). DBS can restore normal function of neural circuits, the mental states associated with autonomy, and thus autonomy itself. There is no need to revise the concept of autonomy because of the restorative effects of neuromodulation but only to examine how this technique produces them.

It is instructive to compare DBS with NFB to further clarify how neuromodulation can improve motivation and mood. The main difference between DBS and NFB is that DBS has no learning effect. As described in Chapter 3, NFB is a form of learning through operant conditioning. The visual feedback the person receives from information about the brain displayed on EEG or fMRI enables her to modulate aberrant brain activity. NFB appears to promote autonomy more than DBS because the modulation of neural circuits and mental states results not from an implanted device but the mental activity of the subject (Linden, Habes, Johnston et al., 2012; Schermer, 2015). Activity at conscious (expectation) and unconscious (conditioning) mental levels produces salutary changes at the neural level, which improves symptoms.

NFB is an example of brain–mind and mind–brain interaction. This technique does not require any devices placed on the head or implanted in the brain to cause changes in neural networks. Brain recording or imaging can display neural activity to which the person responds by altering her psychological processes and in turn physical processes in her brain. Neurophysiological measures do not have a direct causal role in modulating neural or mental function. The person and her mental states do this without any aid from an artificial device placed on the head or implanted in the brain. NFB confirms mind–brain interaction and nonreductive materialism. The content and causal efficacy of the person's mental states and actions involve more than activity at a brain-systems level. In contrast, in DBS the device produces effects at both brain- and mental-systems levels without any participation by the subject. The subject does not appear to have any causal role in changing the brain and mind, regardless of whether this involves open- or closed-loop systems.

This does not mean that a person with a device implanted in her brain has less control and is less autonomous than a person who uses NFB as a neuromodulating technique. It is the psychiatric disorder and the underlying brain disease rather than the neural implant that impairs autonomy or free will. Balanced activity between interacting conscious and unconscious mental and neural processes regulates thought and behavior. When operating safely and effectively, DBS regulates neural functions and mental and physical capacities impaired by diseases of the brain. Being a "passive recipient" of the effects of DBS without any conscious participation from the person does not imply that he has no control of his behavior. Although it operates outside of conscious awareness, by restoring function in dysfunctional neural circuits and associated mental states the device does not replace but supports them. It does not eliminate the person as the source or author of her actions. Instead, it enables voluntary and effective agency by restoring the functional integrity of the neural circuits mediating the relevant capacities. DBS can improve decision-making by combining its neuromodulating action with the endogenous action of functionally intact neural circuits.

What matters for behavior control is not whether restoration of motor and mental functions results from an artificial device or one's own psychological responses to information about the brain. Rather, what matters is that the technique modulates and restores function in the critical neural circuits. DBS can liberate some patients from the psychological burden imposed on them by diseases of the brain. The shared control between the person and the implanted device is not fundamentally different from the shared control between a mentally healthy person's conscious mental states and naturally occurring unconscious processes in her normally functioning brain.

Lower-frequency electrical stimulation over an extended period could retrain the brain's lower-frequency electrical activity, modulate dysfunctional neural circuits, and relieve symptoms even after the device had been turned off. This occurred in two patients participating in a study of DBS for dystonia

(Cheung, Zhang, Rudolph et al., 2013). The effect may be possible in psychiatric disorders as well, though it could be the exception rather than the rule. Most studies indicate that neurostimulation alone may not be sufficient to restore normal motor and mental functions in refractory psychiatric disorders. Additional interventions may be necessary to achieve a therapeutic goal. DBS can modulate the dysfunctional neural circuits implicated in MDD, OCD, and other disorders to make symptoms amenable to CBT (Mantione, Nieman, Figee et al., 2014). The bottom-up modulating effects of DBS on subcortical regions and their projections to limbic and cortical regions enable the top-down modulating effects of subjects' psychological responses to CBT on cortical activity. Although the subject's mental states may not have as direct a role in modulating brain activity as in NFB, the combination of DBS and CBT to control symptoms is an example of interacting neurobiological and psychological dimensions of a holistic rather than dualistic model of mental health and mental disease. Focusing exclusively on a neural circuit model can overlook variability in patients' responses to DBS, as well as how complementary interventions can enhance these responses. It can overlook the extent to which these other interventions can contribute to improved behavior control.

Two patients with depression suffering from anhedonia and avolition may experience improvement in their symptoms from electrical stimulation of the NAc. Even if fMRI or PET showed the same general pattern of neural activity before, during, and after stimulation, one of these patients may be more successful in forming and executing intentions to act. It is plausible to assume that the difference between these patients may be attributed at least partly to the greater mental effort that one of them puts into trying to act. While the modulating effects of DBS in the NAc are necessary to restore some degree of free will for both patients, the greater success that one of them has in exercising her will cannot be accounted for entirely by quantitative measures of activity in this brain region. Something more than modulation of neural circuit dysfunction is necessary to explain the release from motor and mental paralysis. Physiological and psychological processes are both necessary to explain any restoration or improvement in the person's agency. This is an example of how a device implanted in a person's brain does not eliminate her as the source of her actions.

## A burden of control?

I have explained how there is shared control between a person with a psychiatric disorder and a DBS device to modulate neural dysfunction. The ability to turn the stimulator on and off is one component of this control that lies entirely with the person in whom it is implanted. The decision to inactivate and then reactivate the device indicates that at least some of the person's behavior involves conscious deliberation and decision-making. Among other reasons, this is necessary for a person with this brain implant to pass through airport security without triggering alarms. How a patient operates, or fails to operate, a neurostimulating device can have moral and legal implications. Cognitive control presupposes that the person who turns off a stimulator knows when to turn it back on. It also presupposes that he knows that doing this is necessary to resume modulation of motor, cognitive, emotional, and volitional functions. Retaining this cognitive capacity while the stimulator was off would be necessary for him to retain control through a period in which there were no neuromodulating effects from the device.

The greater degree of behavior control this possibility offers him appears to generate an obligation that he would not have if he did not have a psychiatric disorder and a brain implant to regulate it. He would have an obligation to keep the device on to prevent self-harm and harm to others. If he lost control of his motor and mental capacities after turning it off, then arguably he would be morally and criminally responsible for outcomes involving harm to others. He could be responsible both for negligence in failing to turn the device back on and for the consequences of this omission. If he willfully refused to turn it back on, then he would be responsible for this action and its consequences. Because of its critical role in controlling thought and behavior in treatment-refractory psychiatric disorders, a person with a DBS system in his brain would have an obligation to use it in a way that did not entail any risk of harm. Assuming that he had the necessary level of competence, he would be cognitively able to consider these scenarios before implantation of the device, as well as when it was activated. The issue is not whether mental impairment from a psychiatric disorder is a mitigating factor or excuses patients from moral and criminal responsibility for their actions. Rather, the issue is whether patients can be responsible for operating a device that restores their mental capacities.

These considerations need to be framed by the more general point about the connection between options for action and behavior control. Presumably, the more options one has, the more control one has over how one thinks and acts. This does not necessarily follow. Sometimes having more options can be disabling by causing cognitive overload and interfering with the executive capacity to form or complete action plans. Too many options may reduce rather than increase control. Having some limits on choices may be more of a blessing than a burden if these limits facilitate focused attention resulting in effective agency.

Even if it is reasonable to claim that operating a neurostimulating device on one's own is not unduly burdensome, there is the question of whether it would be fair to hold people operating it to a higher standard of behavior control than those without a psychiatric disorder who do not need it. Why should a device necessary to restore normal function in an unhealthy brain generate an obligation to use it in a way that would not apply to people with healthy brains? I will return and respond to this question following discussion of two hypothetical cases.

Suppose that the patient in the case of DBS-induced euphoria could operate the DBS device on his own without close monitoring by his psychiatrist. Suppose further that he increased the frequency and intensity of the electrical current to feel even better. He did this when his mental states were within a normal range. This would ensure that his action was voluntary. If this caused dopaminergic hyperactivity in the NAc and reward circuitry, and the resulting euphoria and impaired rationality led to reckless driving of a motor vehicle that killed another driver, then he would be liable to the charge of criminal negligence causing death. The outcome was causally sensitive to his action. He would not have acted as he did if he had not increased the frequency and intensity of the stimulation. He would be responsible for his subsequent actions and their consequences because, when he voluntarily increased the stimulation, he had the cognitive capacity to foresee a probable harmful outcome. This assumes that the operation of the device at an optimal level restored this capacity from the impairment caused by the psychiatric disorder. The cognitive control he exercised at the earlier time would transfer to the later time when he lost his capacity to reason about which actions to perform or refrain from performing. Because control entails responsibility, the patient's responsibility for his actions and their consequences would also transfer from the earlier to the later time. The harmful outcome of his reckless driving fell within the known risk of becoming euphoric. He could have prevented it by not increasing the stimulation.

This analysis of this hypothetical variant of the actual case provides a response to the question raised by Clausen about *who* could be responsible for behavior caused by a brain–mind machine. Because the patient can control whether and to what extent his brain is stimulated, and control entails responsibility, he can be responsible for what he does with the stimulator and its consequences. It does not completely control his behavior but enables shared control between him and the stimulator. He has enough control in activating or deactivating the device to be responsible for what he does or fails to do.

On the other hand, one could argue that the person would not be fully responsible for the consequence because the manufacturer of the device could have programmed it to limit the level of electrical stimulation it could deliver to the brain. One could sustain this argument even if the disordered mental states and criminal act were foreseeable. The manufacturer could have ensured that, once the stimulation reached an optimal level, it would not be possible for the user to increase it. Assuming that roughly the same level applied to all patients with a particular disorder, the manufacturer could have programmed it into the stimulation parameters. Given the probability of some patients deliberately or inadvertently increasing the electrical frequency and inducing hypomanic or manic states, this could be a reasonable expectation about the responsibility of the device maker. Knowledge of this limitation might cause the patient to feel less in control of her thoughts and actions, which the modulating effects of the device already regulate to some degree. Although this mechanism would ensure control, it could weaken the patient's belief that she shared control of her behavior with the device. Still, any presumed benefit of having more choices over the operation of the device without this limitation would have to be weighed against the potential harm to herself and others from acting on these choices. Having more options does not necessarily result in more effective decision-making. This point applies to those with brain implants and those without them.

The psychiatrist and neurosurgeon who implant and activate the device would be obligated to monitor its function and ensure that the patient was adhering to continuous stimulation. This would be another form of shared control, in this case between the patient and the medical professionals. As in the case of the euphoric patient, the potential for harmful consequences from overstimulation or deactivation could justify not allowing a patient to operate the device completely on his own. This might result in less rather than more control for him. If a patient ignored the instructions of his psychiatrist and increased the frequency of the electrical current beyond an optimal level, or if he deactivated it, then he could be responsible for any harmful consequences of his actions. Again, the transfer of control over time would be the basis for this judgment. The person need not approve of the behavioral changes caused by intentionally increasing the level of stimulation, or turning it off, to be responsible for them. If the stimulation parameters are set within a therapeutic range, then the person can prevent harmful consequences by keeping the device on or turning it back on. In the case of the competent patient with depression and anxiety, he would be responsible for maintaining the stimulation at an optimal level to prevent hypomania or mania and the risk of losing control of his behavior.

Consider the hypothetical case of a competent patient undergoing DBS of the subthalamic nucleus for an impulse control disorder (Moum, Price, Limotai et al., 2012; Micieli, Lopez-Rios, Aguilar et al., 2017). The technique modulates hyperconnectivity between the PFC and the mesolimbic dopamine circuit. This enables the first region to inhibit the second and thereby inhibit impulsivity. The patient could be responsible for keeping the device on to regulate this process.

This would be different from cases in which some patients with PD engage in compulsive behaviors such as gambling, hypersexuality, and uncontrolled anger as a result of DBS overstimulating the limbic circuit of the basal ganglia. In these cases, the behaviors are unintended effects of imprecise stimulation. The question of responsibility would not arise because these effects would be unpredictable and an unforeseeable result of an inadvertent action. However, a competent patient with a DBS implant for an impulse control disorder could be responsible for turning it off and any consequences resulting from this action. A return of hyperactivity in the mesolimbic dopamine system and impulsivity would not result from DBS itself but from the patient deactivating the device. Suppose that the impulsive patient became angry at another person, then assaulted and killed him. Charged with second-degree murder, the accused might argue that she was unable to control her impulse because of hyperactivity in a region of her brain. Because she lacked the requisite cognitive and volitional capacity to control the impulse and refrain from assaulting the victim, she might claim that she was not criminally responsible for the action.

Criminal responsibility for an action generally presupposes cognitive (understanding) and control (volitional) conditions. The first condition says that one must have the capacity to recognize and respond to reasons indicating the wrongfulness of the action (Fischer and Ravizza, 1998, Chapter 3; M'Naghten Case, 1843/1975, p. 217). The second condition says that one must have the capacity to control one's conduct so that it conforms to the requirements of the law (Model Penal Code, 1985, sec. 4.01). Some jurisdictions influenced by the M'Naghten Case have only a cognitive condition for the insanity defense. Other jurisdictions influenced by the Model Penal Code have both cognitive and control conditions. In general, the capacity to recognize and respond to reasons for or against actions involves both cognitive and volitional components. In the case at hand, interaction between reason-mediating prefrontal regions and impulse-mediating limbic regions suggests that cognitive and control conditions might not be separable. The impulse appears to override the agent's rational capacity to restrain it. But presumably she would have the cognitive capacity to know that turning off the device would stop the neuromodulating effects on her dysfunctional prefrontal–limbic network and that she would not be able to restrain the violent impulse. If she had this knowledge and the choice of turning the device on or off, then she might have enough cognitive control over the events leading to the criminal act to be responsible for it. One could make this claim even if the later act was impulsive. Recent research showing that fMRI can predict brain activity associated with knowing states and reckless states in criminal behavior supports the idea that impulsivity as such does not undermine the cognitive capacity to regulate behavior (Vilares, Wesley, Ahn et al., 2017).

An agent may be criminally responsible for an action he is physically unable to resist or prevent at a later time if, at an earlier time, he is cognitively able to foresee that performing a particular action would incapacitate him. As in the case of the patient with DBS-induced euphoria, the patient with the impulse control disorder need not approve of the behavioral changes from turning off the stimulator to be responsible for them. She was able to prevent the criminal act by keeping the stimulator on rather than turning it off at the earlier time. Cognitive control over a sequence of events can make one responsible for an action within that sequence even if the action is an involuntary bodily movement. This requires qualification of the definition of autonomous agency. An earlier voluntary action can make one liable for a later action even if it is involuntary and one does not endorse it as one's own. If one accepts these claims, then self-induced incapacitation by using a neuromodulating device in a certain way may not be an excusing condition for this impaired state and any behavioral consequences of it. Some jurisdictions might consider this type of incapacitation a mitigating condition. It could mitigate a charge of responsibility even if it was traceable to a voluntary action and even if the consequences of the action were foreseeable. But the criminal law is inconsistent on the tracing of later actions and consequences back to earlier actions and omissions, as well as what this implies for criminal responsibility.

As Stephen Morse explains: "An agent will be *prima facie* criminally responsible if the agent acts with the appropriate mental state, *mens rea*, required by the definition of the offense, such as purpose, knowledge, recklessness or negligence. Criminal law typically defines an act as an intentional bodily movement performed by an agent whose consciousness is reasonably intact" (Morse, 2006, p. 399, 2011a, 2011b, 2015). The impulsive action of the agent in my example was not intentional and arguably involuntary. Yet she had the motor, cognitive, and volitional capacity to prevent herself from acting impulsively by keeping the stimulator on, or by reactivating it after turning it off. She failed to exercise this capacity. According to the criteria Morse mentions, she had the requisite *mens rea* to be responsible for a negligent omission and the consequence of impulsively killing another person. She had the ability to prevent herself from being in a situation where she lacked the ability to restrain the impulse.

In the one actual and two hypothetical cases I have presented, the cognitive and motor control the stimulator provides to a person with a psychiatric disorder, and the known probable harmful consequences of not operating it appropriately, constitute reasons for keeping the stimulator on and at an optimal frequency. The device substitutes or compensates for dysfunctional neural circuits and networks that mediate motor and mental capacities in a normally functioning brain. When it functions properly, DBS can provide people with the same control of their thought and behavior as others would have without it. There is nothing unduly burdensome about having to keep the stimulator on, or to turn it back on after turning it off. The fact that there is a device implanted in their brains does not interfere with but sustains their ability to think and act. In this respect, the stimulator itself would not constitute an excusing or mitigating condition. They could be fully criminally responsible for their actions. Nevertheless, the fact that a device is necessary for one to regulate one's actions may at times put one in a difficult position regarding the process of deactivating and then reactivating the device. Some might consider this situation to be unduly burdensome and a mitigating factor regarding the agent's responsibility.

These considerations bring us back to the question raised earlier. Would it be fair to hold a person who needs DBS to control her behavior to what appears to be a higher standard of obligation and responsibility than those with normal brain function who do not need it? The fact that the device is necessary for her to form and execute action plans seems to impose a burden on her not imposed on others without a psychiatric disorder. Why should a device that regulates disordered brains and minds generate an obligation to use it in a certain way that would not apply to people with ordered brains and minds? In jurisdictions where having a brain implant was considered a burden, this could be a mitigating factor in any charge of criminal responsibility for actions or consequences resulting from not operating it properly. Assuming that the patient had the cognitive and motor capacity to know how to operate the device, few if any jurisdictions would consider this an excusing condition. It might even be an aggravating condition, depending on how much control the patient had over the stimulation. Sorting out these legal claims would depend on a better understanding of the mechanisms of action of DBS than what is currently known among researchers and practitioners using the technique.

Another burden of DBS on patients and research subjects is the possibility of "brain-jacking" by hackers violating neural implant security (Pycroft, Boccard, Owen et al., 2016). Third parties could gain unauthorized access to the implanted pulse generator and electrodes through physiological attack vectors and externally disrupt the radiofrequency of these devices. This intervention could not only thwart the intended neuromodulating effects of DBS. It could also cause adverse physiological and psychological events and harm the patient or research subject. This possibility may require them to carry security devices in addition to the implants, which could be unduly burdensome for them. It could also be a disincentive to keeping the stimulator on, leading to nonadherence and a return of psychiatric symptoms. If a person did not have a psychiatric disorder that responded only to this technique, then there would be no expectation or obligation for her to keep the stimulator on and carry an anti-hacking device. This is not an issue for those with healthy brains and minds. Even if they are not held to a *higher* standard, it seems unfair to hold those with a brain implant and an additional security device to the *same* standard of behavior as those without them. This could justify different moral assessments of the actions of those who need this neural prosthetic to regulate their behavior, and those who do not.

A device implanted in the brain, and what one would have to take to ensure that it functioned properly, could be a mitigating factor in judging whether a person with a device was responsible for his actions. This would depend on whether device malfunction was the result of the patient's own negligence, insufficiently considered actions, or external interference. In many cases, it could be difficult to ascertain the source of the malfunction and whether the patient was or was not responsible for it. As in the other cases I have presented, responsibility would depend on the degree of cognitive control the agent had in operating the device. All of the issues I have discussed in this section point to the more general normative issue of determining which mental and behavioral burdens in psychiatric disorders and treatments for them might constitute mitigating or excusing conditions regarding moral and criminal responsibility.

## Identification and personal identity

Autonomous agency for those undergoing continuous DBS depends on the concepts of identification and personal identity. One must identify with the electrodes and pulse generator as enabling devices allowing one to have certain mental states and perform certain actions. In addition, because agency involves future-directed behavior, these devices must sustain the experience of persisting through time as the same individual.

Some patients or research subjects may feel uneasy about continued dependence on a mechanical device to maintain normal neural and mental functions. But there are no rational grounds for this attitude if the device produces a therapeutic response. If neurostimulation ameliorates symptoms and improves the patient's well-being, then it would be mistaken to describe its salutary effects as part of a dependence relation. It would not be the same sense of "dependence" as on an addictive substance. DBS aims to resolve rather than create pathology in motor and mental functions, and it does this by modulating dysfunctional neural circuits. Any feeling of dependence would not be the effect of the device itself but of the patient's attitude about it.

Still, as David Linden notes, the ability of DBS to provide continuous, self-adjusting, long-term modulatory changes may "cause nerve cells to change their spontaneous firing patterns by making different proteins. In this way, they can form cellular 'memories' of the stimulation. As a result, the chronic brain stimulation may become very much a part of the patient's normal neural network" (2014, p. 111). Linden's comment suggests a neurobiological sense of identification, where the device becomes integrated into the patient's brain. This is consistent with the idea of a stimulating device supplementing rather than supplanting brain function. There is also a psychological sense of identification. A patient can identify with the stimulating device if it enables him to have the mental states he wants to have and perform the actions he wants to perform. Symptom fluctuation and disruption of continuity of care from having to undergo periodic parameter adjustment or battery or lead replacement may cause the patient to be more aware of an OLD and its operational imperfections as a threat to his identity. Yet insofar as CLDs avoid these problems and sustain normal neural function, the subject can identify with the device as part of his neural and mental self. He can consider the device as a form of extended embodiment that integrates seamlessly into his brain. What promotes this attitude is that fact that, when the device functions properly, the patient is not aware of it.

A case vignette can help to illustrate the psychological issue of identification in DBS. A 55-year-old teacher with a 25-year history of MDD participates in a clinical trial involving DBS of the subgenual cingulate gyrus. He is randomly assigned to the active arm of the trial and receives continuous, bilateral, electrical stimulation of this brain region. DBS ameliorates many of his symptoms, and he is able to return to work and resume many of his daily activities. Two years into the trial, he begins to experience recurrent episodes of sadness, psychomotor slowing, and feelings of helplessness and despair. These symptoms indicate a relapse of the motor, cognitive, and emotional impairment he experienced before receiving the stimulation. He reports that the change in his physical and mental states occurred suddenly rather than gradually. A psychiatric and neurosurgical evaluation reveals device malfunction due to increased lead impedance. An X-ray confirms this, and the patient is scheduled to have the broken lead replaced. On the morning of the surgery, he is asked about his mood and replies: "I'm nervous about the surgery. But, to be honest, I'm just happy that the problem wasn't *me* but the *battery*" (Lipsman and Glannon, 2013, p. 467).

The concern expressed in the patient's comment is not about *personal identity* but *identification*. He is not disturbed by the idea that the malfunction could alter his mental states and disrupt his experience of persisting through time as the same person. Instead, what disturbs him is the idea that the stimulator could *replace him* as the source of his thought and action. He cannot identify with a device that is alien to his real self, despite the fact that he benefits from it. Because of its functional role in modulating neural circuits underlying his motor and mental capacities, the device seems to introduce a third party that comes between what was a direct connection between his brain and mind before he become ill. The implanted device seems to threaten his belief that he controls how he thinks and acts. His brain function resumes with the new lead and battery, and his symptoms significantly improve. The fact that the modulating effects of DBS occur outside of his awareness and independently of what he believes or does suggests that the device does not merely supplement his agency and will but supplants them. The agent is not the teacher but the brain implant.

There is no rational basis for this concern. The patient can perceive the device as an enabling tool that integrates into his brain, and whose effects integrate into his mind. He need not perceive the stimulator as an alien device that completely replaces the neural and mental processes with which he identifies. By modulating an overactive subgenual cingulate gyrus and re-establishing some degree of cognitive-emotional processing, the stimulation improves his ability to reason, have normal emotions, and make decisions in accord with his interests. The device allows him to have and act on the mental states he wants to have, or those he would want to have in the absence of his depression. Realizing this can help the patient to regain confidence in the belief that he is the source of his thoughts and actions, even if he is not the *only* source but shares it with the device. DBS can restore his cognitive and emotional ability to have a general second-order desire to have particular first-order desires move him to act. In this respect, DBS can restore his autonomous agency and free will.

This interpretation is consistent with the idea of DBS as an intermediary or mediating device operating at the interface of his brain and mind in a way that strengthens rather than impedes agency. The positive neural and psychological effects of neurostimulation enable the teacher to resume engaging in the types of projects in which was engaged before the onset of his depression. By ameliorating his psychiatric symptoms, DBS can ensure that his mental states are the effective springs of his actions and very much his own. Modulation of the subgenual cingulate gyrus releases psychomotor, cognitive, and emotional constraints on the teacher's thought and behavior and restores his feeling of being in control of them. If the symptoms of his depression are refractory to psychotherapy and other treatments and respond only to DBS, then he could not reasonably believe that he could be in complete control of his thoughts and actions without some form of neuromodulation.

Interestingly, the patient probably would not have commented on not wanting to identify with the implant if it had been a CLD rather than an OLD. Because it would be less likely to deplete the battery or result in lead fracture, a CLD could have continued functioning and prevented the return of motor and mental disturbance. Nevertheless, while his comment was driven by malfunction of an OLD, this would not alter the fact that a neuromodulating device was necessary to restore neural and mental functions.

Control depends on which neural circuits and the mental states they mediate are functional or dysfunctional, and the extent to which they are functional or dysfunctional. If one's cognitive and emotional capacities are too impaired for one to form and carry out action plans, then DBS may be able to strengthen these capacities and thereby facilitate decision-making and action. The technique may help to improve these aspects of agency even if it does not completely restore them to premorbid levels. Due to its positive effects on agency, one can identify with the device as integral rather than alien to one's brain and psyche. If a brain implant does not interfere with proprioceptive or somatosensory feedback, then the device can become incorporated into the brain's representation of the body and its relation to the world. It would be consistent with one's experience of oneself as an embodied and embedded subject.

The changes DBS causes in one's neural and mental processes and states raise questions about how they affect one's experience of persisting through time as the same person. A key factor in addressing these questions is whether the changes are nonsubstantial or substantial. Do the changes in mental states before and after DBS occur in the same individual? Or do they occur in distinct individuals? Do these changes indicate a restoration of the premorbid self that existed before the onset of symptoms? Or do they indicate a different set of mental states of a different self? How do these questions influence an assessment of whether a patient benefits from neuromodulation?

Personhood consists in the capacity for conscious mental states. These include self-awareness and awareness of one's surroundings. Personal identity consists in the conditions that make a person persist as the same individual through time. A person can continue to exist while undergoing nonsubstantial changes in these conditions. Substantial changes imply the existence of different individuals before and after they occur. One way of defining the conditions of personal identity is in terms of the connectedness and continuity of psychological states such as desires, beliefs, intentions, and memories (Parfit, 1984, Part II; Schechtman, 1997, 2014; Perry, 2008). These states would have the same origin in a normally functioning brain. Connectedness pertains to relations between and among psychological states over shorter periods, and connectedness pertains to overlapping chains of connectedness holding over longer periods. These psychological relations provide the integrity and unity of the mental states necessary for persistence. Whether a person persists through time as the same individual depends on the degree of psychological connectedness and continuity. When these relations have been disrupted by a psychiatric disorder, does DBS re-establish them? Does the technique substantially change these relations and the person who undergoes it?

Just as psychiatric disorders can disrupt the motor and mental capacities constituting the will, they can disrupt these psychological relations and thus personal identity to varying degrees. The greater the disruption in information integration in the brain, and the greater the disruption in psychological connectedness and continuity, the more disruptive is the effect on identity. Changes in the relations may be substantial, as in recurrent psychosis, and effectively result in a different person. They may be nonsubstantial, as in a change from moderate introversion to moderate extroversion, and occur in the same person. Cases of imprecisely targeted or overstimulated neural circuits causing some PD patients to become impulsive and some MDD or OCD patients to become hypomanic illustrate how DBS may cause substantial personality changes. These changes are usually temporary and reversible from adjusting stimulation parameters. A properly functioning device can resolve pathological states of mind, prevent their recurrence, and restore the psychological unity and continuity that constituted the person's premorbid self. The post-DBS patient would be the same person who existed before disease onset. When the change is from pathological mental states to the normal mental states the patient had before the disorder, there is no substantial change in psychological relations between the earlier and later times and thus no change in personal identity.

When DBS achieves its therapeutic purpose, it may cause personality changes that can result in a difficult period of adjustment for both patients and caregivers. This may occur in a movement disorder such as PD. It may occur more often in psychiatric disorders, since the stimulation would directly affect the neural basis of cognition, mood, and motivation. The patient may not experience discontinuity but re-established continuity between his predisease and post-DBS mental states. Depending on the extent of the behavioral changes before and after the stimulation, the family may not recognize him as the same person. A prolonged period of behavior associated with the disorder may strongly influence how others perceive the patient, how they respond to the changes, and how these factors influence their relationship with him. In these respects, there are similarities between neural and mental changes resulting from neuromodulation and neural and mental changes resulting from cochlear implants and visual prosthetics (Glover, 2006, Part II). There may be a dissocia-tion between how the patient experiences these changes and how the family or other caregivers respond to them.

This requires distinguishing personal identity from relational identity, the re-lations that hold between the patient's mental states and the relations that hold between him and others. It requires distinguishing how the patient experiences changes in his own mental states from how these changes influence interaction between the patient and the family (Christen, Bittlinger, Walter et al., 2012; Synofzik, 2013; Baylis, 2014). The changes in the relations between the patient's mental states before and after DBS are different from the changes in the rela-tions between the patient and caregivers. Personal identity and relational iden-tity may intersect in the sense that the content of one's mental states and one's behavior are shaped by how a person interacts with others. Nevertheless, what matters is whether DBS or other forms of neuromodulation relieve the patient's symptoms and allow him to return to a state of functional independence. The primary concern should be how this intervention affects the patient. How it affects others should be a secondary concern, even if the patient continues to rely on them for care.

Differences in how the patient and caregivers respond to behavioral changes may generate conflict between them. Accordingly, some form of follow-up involving family meetings with a team including a clinical psychologist and social worker in addition to the treating psychiatrist and neurosurgeon may be necessary to help patients and families adjust to these changes. This would include addressing how they might alter the caring relationship. Assuming that the effects of DBS are salutary for the patient and improve his quality of life, it clearly would be preferable for him to adjust to a return of his real self than to continue dealing with the greater challenges associated with living with a mentally and physically disabling disease. When the goal of neuromodulation is to restore normal neural and mental functions, it may be difficult to differen-tiate desired from undesired effects on the psyche and predict how these effects might alter identity (Nyholm and O'Neill, 2016). Potentially adverse changes in behavior and identity have to be weighed against the therapeutic goal of neuromodulation, which is to resolve psychopathology and relieve psychic pain and suffering.

When a neuromodulating technique successfully treats psychiatric symptoms, there may be behavioral changes that are not pathological. They may not be en-tirely salutary, either, and may involve behavior that is different from that of the patient's premorbid self. The psychological relations constituting personal identity hold to varying degrees. In some cases where DBS causes personality change, the technique may not restore the patient's former self but create a new self. Upregulating the reward circuit to relieve anhedonia may cause an extremely introverted patient to become extremely extroverted, or even euphoric. On the other hand, downregulating this circuit to relieve impulsivity could make a patient extremely lethargic. If these outcomes were unpredictable and irreversible, then we would have to ask whether the intervention on balance benefitted the patient. Neuromodulation benefits patients by relieving symptoms and avoiding adverse effects in the brain and mind. Intuitively, normative judgments of benefit and harm should be independent of psychological judgments about identity.

This suggests that a patient could benefit from the technique despite undergoing a substantial change in mental states and thus a change in identity. It raises the question of *who* benefits from the technique if there are two distinct people before and after the neurostimulation. "Benefit" implies that a person is better off than she was before, and this presupposes that the same person exists in the earlier and later states of affairs. How, then, could we evaluate "benefit"? This is not a question that a person suffering from a psychiatric disorder would likely consider when consenting to undergo DBS (Witt, Kuhn, Timmermann et al., 2013; Witt, 2017). His main or exclusive concern would be symptom relief. Yet if a candidate for neuromodulation were told that DBS entailed an unavoidable trade-off between symptom relief and a substantial change of identity, then would she choose to undergo the procedure? Would retaining identity override any improvement in quality of life? Could one's quality of life with a psychiatric disorder be so poor that one would accept the possibility of becoming a different person to improve it?

These are hypothetical questions without definitive answers. Could such an evaluative comparison even be possible if the recipient of the procedure had a qualitatively different set of mental states from the person who consented to it? There is a way of responding to this last question. If a person suffering from a severe psychiatric disorder has an interest in symptom relief, and this relief causes him to become a different person, then he can still benefit from it. His interest in ceasing to suffer would be realized when the symptoms resolve. He can experience this when they resolve, even if this entails a substantial change in his psyche and "he" cannot evaluate what has happened to him after this change. A person who suffered from the symptoms of a disordered brain and mind would no longer have to live with this experience. In severe treatment-resistant psychiatric disorders, identity change resulting from neuromodulation may be the lesser of two evils. There are similarities between this assessment and my discussion of EAS for these disorders in Chapter 7.

# Costs, innovation, and social justice

The ability of neuromodulation techniques to restore some degree of control of thought and behavior for people with refractory psychiatric disorders presupposes that they have access to these techniques. Given the chronic nature of these disorders, effective control of them means that access must not be limited to the duration of a clinical trial. It must be continuous and extend beyond the trial. Control also presupposes that there are adequate protections in place for research subjects from any risk of harm that might befall them from device malfunction. This entails an obligation not only from research psychiatrists and neurosurgeons but from device manufacturers as well. Access and protection both involve strict regulation at professional and policy levels. As discussed in Chapter 4, as a matter of justice, patients with treatment-refractory psychiatric disorders should have the opportunity to participate in research testing neuromodulation techniques that could lead to safer and more effective treatments. This assumes that device makers provide the technology necessary for the research to be conducted. Provision of and access to the technology are also matters of justice. But ethical questions about justice cannot be separated from economic questions about the interests of companies that manufacture neuromodulating devices.

Device makers such as St. Jude Medical and Medtronic sponsor neuromodulation clinical trials in neurology, neurosurgery, and psychiatry. As in medical research sponsored by pharmaceutical companies, sponsorship may lead to a conflict of interest if the company's goal to produce positive results influences trial design and generates bias in the presentation of the results. A more serious potential or actual conflict of interest exists when a researcher testing a device has invested in the company that produces it. These factors can compromise the scientific integrity of the research and adequate protections of patients and research subjects. Actual and potential conflicts of interest justify the need for regulation of these devices (Fins and Schiff, 2010; Fins, Schlaepfer, Nuttin et al., 2011). Yet regulation can be an obstacle to innovation in developing and testing newer and possibly more effective systems for treatment-refractory psychiatric disorders. OLD and CLD versions of DBS are adequate at best. Lack of competition among companies due to a lack of financial and other market incentives may be one reason why there has not been more technological progress in the field of neuromodulation.

Current DBS technology may have realized most of its therapeutic potential. Other than knowing *that* it can modulate hyperactive or hypoactive neural circuits by altering oscillations in these circuits, very little is known about *how* electrical stimulation causes changes in brain function. This limited knowledge highlights the importance of conducting foundational research to gain a better understanding of its underlying mechanisms and therapeutic potential. The advances necessary for this understanding depend on further innovation, research, and development of the technology. This in turn depends on manufacturers getting a return on their investment and remaining competitive in producing devices (Ineichen, Glannon, Temel et al., 2014; Kestle, 2015).

The financial interests of device manufacturers are not always consistent with the mental health interests of research subjects participating in neuromodulation clinical trials. Yet without the device and the manufacturer, investigators could not conduct the research. As part of their economic calculus, manufacturers can determine which studies are worth continuing and which should be initiated or terminated. This can be an obstacle for researchers intending to determine the safety and efficacy of DBS or other techniques if other parties ultimately make decisions about trial design and duration. It can also be unfair to patients who have not responded to psychopharmacology, psychotherapy, or other less invasive forms of neuromodulation.

All persons with major psychiatric disorders have an equal urgent need for treatment. In principle, a just healthcare system should meet these needs by providing safe and effective therapies, or opportunities for research that will lead to them. Clinical trials testing brain implants for only some of these conditions and only some patients can result in unequal access to research yielding scientific knowledge that could eventually benefit many people. Unequal access based on decisions by device manufacturers about which trials to fund could lead to unequal and unfair outcomes for people with the same mental health needs. In practice, though, the ethical imperative for equal access has to be conditional upon the cost of research and therapy for all providers, which can be substantial in the field of neuromodulation. Costs by themselves are not unfair. What may be unfair is when device makers calculate costs to limit access to devices in research or therapy.

There are examples of how costs can unfairly exclude some psychiatric patients from participating in neuromodulation clinical trials. As Emily Underwood points out, "In the United States, companies and institutions sponsoring research are rarely, if ever, required to pay medical costs that subjects incur as a result of their participation" (2015, p. 1187). In some DBS trials lasting many years, Medicare in the United States and private insurance may cover a portion of the costs related to the stimulation system. Some people are financially better or worse off than others due to at least some factors beyond their control. Because genetic, environmental, and other factors that affect the brain and mind are beyond our control, some people are better or worse off than others in terms of mental health through no effort or fault of their own. If those who are worse off in this respect cannot afford to pay the medical costs of participating in a trial, then it would be unfair to exclude them from the trial. Participation would be based on the ability to pay rather than medical need associated with the same disorder. Equal need would be overridden by unequal means of access to the research. It could be unfair to exclude some patients from participating in a clinical trial when this was the only way of determining whether a proposed brain intervention was safe and effective. It could also be unfair to exclude them if they could benefit from the experimental intervention. A universal-payer healthcare system would not avoid this problem because it would not affect the interests of device makers.

If a manufacturer of a DBS device goes out of business and the device is no longer available, then any physiological and psychological benefit a research subject might receive from being in a clinical trial would be temporary. Manufacturers should provide devices to patients who need them. This suggests a long-term commitment, given that major psychiatric disorders are chronic conditions and patients need ongoing medical attention and continuity of care. Yet any idea of an obligation for device makers to make DBS or any other neuromodulating technique available for research is complicated by the fact that they are not healthcare providers. This is despite the fact that providers use these techniques to treat patients. The idea of a device-maker obligation is also complicated because, except for the humanitarian device exemption for OCD, DBS is still experimental and investigational. For this reason, manufacturers would at most have an obligation to provide the device for the duration of a clinical trial, but not beyond it. However, when depression or other disorders are refractory to all other treatments, failing to provide the stimulating device after a trial had ended could deny patients the only available treatment. This is where the line between research and therapy becomes blurred. It would be difficult to claim that St. Jude Medical, Medtronic, or any other device maker had an obligation to provide DBS after the conclusion of a clinical trial in which evidence of safety and efficacy was not clear enough to warrant FDA approval.

The failed BROADEN study sheds light on these issues. Underwood notes that a significant number (44) of the 90 participants in the study wanted to keep their implants (2017, p. 710). Despite the disappointing results, "some patients believe the brain stimulation helped them. More than 30 trial participants reported that they were 'responding' to the treatment—defined as at least a 40% improvement on a standard depression scale—and 19 were in full remission according to that scale" (Underwood, 2017, p. 710). The discrepancy between the actual study results reported by the investigators and research subjects' claims that they responded to the stimulation could be attributed to their belief that this was their last hope of controlling symptoms. This would not generate an obligation for a manufacturer of a neurostimulating system to provide it.

Given that there was no statistically significant difference in outcomes between active and sham stimulation in this study, and given that there was a significant number of adverse events, it would not be unfair or unjust not to continue providing the device to the subjects after the trial had ended. If the trial had provided positive results overall, and if this generated some obligation for the manufacturer to make it available during and after a trial, then the obligation still would be contingent to some extent on the interests of the manufacturer to continue producing it. In that case, the most reasonable course of action for all parties would be for the manufacturer to provide the device at a lower cost.

As explained in Chapter 3, the marked decrease in funding studies of novel drugs by pharmaceutical companies has created a therapeutic vacuum that may have significant negative consequences for psychiatric patients. Initial studies have shown considerable therapeutic potential of ketamine, psilocybin, and MDMA for some psychiatric disorders. But further studies that would confirm realization of this potential need additional funding. Neuromodulation can fill some of this vacuum, though how much it can fill remains to be seen. The availability of stimulating devices for those who might benefit from them involves a unique set of ethical and social issues. If neurostimulating equipment were not available, then replacing batteries or leads or adjusting stimulation parameters would not be an option. The issue could be more problematic for CLD than OLDs if fewer CLDs were available All of these factors could transform a potentially beneficial situation into a harmful one for patients and research subjects.

An earlier example of this in the neural prosthetic industry was the 2001 decision by the company NeuroControl to abandon production of its Freehand device, which could reactivate hands paralyzed from nerve damage (Underwood, 2015, p. 1187). Approximately 250 people who had used the device during and after clinical trials were unable to obtain replacements for the frayed wires in the implants. The same problem can adversely affect psychiatric patients with neural implants for DBS, optogenetics, or other neuromodulating systems. Some companies may inform patients recruited for a trial that medical devices will be available for only a limited time. This could be interpreted as a coercive offer to vulnerable patients with treatment-refractory conditions and no other treatment options. Making potential research subjects agree to participate in a clinical trial in which a device would be available for a limited time could undermine the bioethical principle of respect for autonomy necessary for informed consent. In the United States, former President Obama's Brain Research through Advanced Innovative Neurotechnologies (BRAIN) initiative may lead to additional funding from the National Institute of Mental Health to overcome obstacles associated with the cost of research into neuromodulating devices. With the current administration in the United States, however, there are good reasons for skepticism about the outcome of this initiative.

The basic challenge for neuromodulation in psychiatry is for healthcare institutions to provide patients with access to research leading to applications that will relieve the burden of disease and improve their quality of life. At the same time, there should be economic incentives to promote innovation among device makers resulting in advanced technology that will increase understanding of psychiatric disorders and maximize therapeutic outcomes. These should be complementary rather than competing goals. It is critical to strike the right balance between the interests of patients and research subjects and those of manufacturers. Regulations must be in place to protect patients and subjects from the risk of neurological and psychological harm from brain stimulation. But there should not be so much regulation that it discourages industry innovation in making safer and more effective devices. There is a need for multidisciplinary collaboration among patient and research subject organizations, industry, neuroscientists, and ethics review boards to guide the development and use of neuromodulation for psychiatric disorders. This collaboration is necessary to realize the goal of using this technology to restore behavior control and improve the welfare of people with severely disabling mental illnesses.

## Conclusion

In treatment-refractory psychiatric disorders, DBS can modulate dysfunctional neural circuits and restore sensorimotor, cognitive, affective, and volitional capacities necessary to form and execute action plans. It can restore control by enabling flexible thought and behavior and adaptability to the environment. DBS can allow people to act on their motivational states without compulsion or constraint. It can liberate people with psychiatric disorders from different forms of motor and mental paralysis. In these respects, this form of neuromodulation can restore some degree of autonomous agency and free will. The electrodes and stimulator do not replace the person as the author or source of her actions. They are enabling devices that re-establish the capacity for agency by correcting the neural and mental dysfunction that interferes with this capacity. When DBS functions properly, the shared control between the conscious subject and the device is not fundamentally different from the shared control between the conscious subject and naturally occurring unconscious processes in her normally functioning brain. Instead of considering the neural implant as an alien object, the person can consider it as a device that integrates seamlessly into her brain Moreover, by re-establishing normal neural and mental function, DBS can re-establish the connectedness and continuity of the mental states disrupted by a psychiatric disorder. The technique does not create a substantially different self but restores the patient's premorbid self.

There is the question of whether having a neuromodulating device implanted in a person's brain to control a psychiatric disorder generates an obligation to use it in a certain way. This raises an additional question of whether such an obligation would be unfair to the patient when it would not apply to others who did not need a device to regulate brain function. When a competent patient can operate a DBS system on her own, she may have the cognitive capacity to foresee the probable effects of turning the device on and off. This may entail responsibility for actions performed when the device is off and she may be mentally incapacitated. It is an open question whether having to turn a device on and off at different times would be a mitigating factor regarding responsibility for one's actions or omissions related to the device. There is also the issue of whether manufacturers of DBS or other devices have an obligation to continue providing them to patients and research subjects in clinical trials when this is their only access to treatment for an otherwise treatment-resistant disorder. The interests of device makers and the need for innovation in developing more effective techniques need to be balanced against the welfare of people with major psychiatric disorders.

Even when it modulates motor and mental functions, stimulating the brain alone may not be enough to restore control of psychiatric patients' thought and behavior to predisease levels. Less invasive or noninvasive interventions such as CBT may be necessary complementary interventions to ensure a therapeutic outcome. Social support networks that improve patients' interactions with others can also be critical to improving psychomotor, cognitive, emotional, and volitional capacities. Psychological factors such as the patience, determination, and effort in adhering to device monitoring and continuous stimulation are important in maintaining positive effects of DBS as well. Modulating processes at both neural-systems and mental-systems levels, and positive environmental interaction, are necessary for improving behavior control for people with major psychiatric disorders. The main obstacle to complete restoration of motor and mental functions in these disorders is that, to date, neither electrical stimulation of the brain nor any other intervention has been able to alter their pathogenesis. It is unclear whether earlier application of DBS, optogenetics, temporal interference, or drugs designed to promote neuroplasticity and neurogenesis could do this.

My discussion of neuromodulation for psychiatric disorders extends into the domain of forensic psychiatry. The issue is not whether mental impairment is a mitigating factor or excuses patients from criminal responsibility for their actions. Rather, the issue is whether patients can be responsible for operating, or failing to operate, a device that can restore their mental capacities. Debate about this and related normative questions will increase with expanding uses of neurostimulation. Psychopathy is a disorder that raises a unique set of forensic psychiatric issues. I discuss these issues in Chapter 6.

# Intervening in the psychopath's brain

Psychopathy is a disorder characterized by a combination of personality and behavioral features. These include impaired capacity for empathy, guilt, and remorse and impaired responsiveness to fear-inducing stimuli. They also include impulsivity, aggression, impaired decision-making, and failure to conform to social norms (Cleckley, 1982; Hare, 2003; Glenn and Raine, 2014b). Psychopaths are impaired in both cognitive and affective capacities and in practical and moral reasoning. The *DSM-5* includes psychopathic features as specifiers for antisocial personality disorder (American Psychiatric Association, 2013, p. 765). Psychopathy is a psychiatric disorder in the sense that it involves dysfunctional mental states associated with maladaptive and pathological behavior. Neuroimaging studies have demonstrated that these mental states correlate with abnormal functional connectivity in prefrontal–limbic pathways. Normal function of these neural pathways enables emotional capacities such as empathic responses to others' needs and recognition of harm. It also enables the activation of inhibitory mechanisms in the brain that can prevent or reduce impulsive behavior. Like other psychiatric disorders, the mental impairment in psychopathy is a matter of degree. In addition, like other psychiatric disorders, genetic and environmental factors likely have a role in the etiology and pathophysiology of psychopathy. This disorder has a neurobiological basis. But it is more than a disease of the brain.

One feature of psychopathy distinguishing it from other psychiatric disorders is that it is associated with substantially greater social harm. It appears to involve a higher number of criminal offenders. While not all psychopaths engage in criminal behavior, psychopathy has strong links to criminal behavior. In the United States alone, 20–25% of the prison population would be considered psychopaths as measured by the Psychopathy Checkist-Revised (Hare, 2003; Glenn and Raine, 2014b). There is a stronger association between the cognitive and emotional impairment and criminal behavior in psychopathy than in other psychiatric disorders. Another distinctive feature of psychopathy is that it seems intractable to psychological and pharmacological therapies. The lack of effective treatment rules out admission to a psychiatric care facility as a viable option. Among criminal psychopaths, incarceration is the only way of preventing recidivism and the only means of deterrence. These factors make psychopathy an especially problematic disorder in forensic psychiatry.

Safe and effective treatment that could modify psychopathic behavior could have significant positive outcomes, both for individuals with the disorder and others who are harmed by them. By improving the criminal psychopath's cognitive and emotional capacities and his moral sensitivity, it could rehabilitate him, reduce the risk of reoffending, and provide a humane alternative to long-term incarceration. Given the magnitude of the harm reduction that could result from modulating pathways in the psychopath's brain, it is worth exploring this possibility and its ethical and legal implications for forensic psychiatry. Insofar as this disorder is at least partly brain-based, examining the neurobiological as well as psychological and social features of psychopathy can shed light on different aspects of neurocriminology and neurolaw (Glenn and Raine, 2014a, 2014b; Meynen, 2016).

In *The Mask of Sanity*, Hervey Cleckley distinguishes between two types of psychopath. Primary psychopaths are often socially skilled, intelligent, even charming individuals who display no anxiety in their behavior. Secondary psychopaths are often socially inept and withdrawn individuals displaying high levels of anxiety. What both types have in common is impulsivity and lack of empathy (Cleckley, 1982). These features explain why psychopaths have a diminished ability to consider the rights, needs, and interests of the people they harm. Psychopathic behavior is one of the strongest predictors of violent recidivism. The subpopulation of criminal psychopaths must be distinguished from the general population of people with psychopathic traits. Having these traits does not necessarily result in criminal behavior.

It is possible that psychopharmacology or stimulation of psychopaths' brains could modulate the dysfunctional neural pathways underlying their disordered personality and behavior. This could promote prosocial behavior and reduce the probability of violent aggression. These interventions in the brain could be rehabilitative therapy for psychopaths who have been convicted of criminal offences. More controversially, the interventions might prevent children and adolescents with psychopathic traits from developing full-blown symptoms of the disorder and prevent criminal behavior. Given the large number of people with psychopathy among the human population, the positive social consequences of safe and effective treatment for this disorder would be substantial.

## Sorting out the ethical and legal questions

In considering interventions in the brains of criminal psychopaths to modify their behavior, there are two general questions: one empirical, the other normative. First, which interventions could safely and effectively modulate the critical brain regions to promote prosocial behavior? Second, could these interventions be ethically and legally justified? This second general question is related to more specific ethical questions. Would offering such an intervention to a psychopath convicted of a criminal offence as an alternative to incarceration be coercive and a violation of the right of noninterference in his brain and mind? Would the offer unduly influence his capacity to give informed consent to the treatment? In cases where the psychopath declined such an offer, would it be ethically and legally permissible to forcibly treat him? When a child or adolescent is at risk of developing psychopathy and becoming a criminal offender, would this risk justify intervening in his brain as a preventive measure? Could a parent consent to treatment on their child's behalf? Could forcing a child to take a psychotropic drug be justified?

Offering neuromodulation to a convicted criminal psychopath as an alternative to long-term incarceration would not necessarily interfere with his capacity to make an informed and voluntary decision to accept or refuse it. It would not coerce him into accepting a state of affairs that would make him worse off than he would want to be. Instead, it would enable him to choose a state of affairs that could make him better off than he would be in an incarcerated state. Safe and effective neuromodulation could increase his autonomy by increasing his capacity to respond to reasons and control his violent impulses. The psychopath's autonomy would be constrained in the sense that it would involve a limited number of choices. But he would retain some autonomy if he could freely choose between a brain-modifying intervention and incarceration. In addition, forced treatment might be ethically and legally justified in cases where it promoted positive behavior modification in individuals with a history of violent offences and was more cost-effective than incarceration.

This is significantly different from the ethical and legal question of whether it is justifiable to force medication on people with a psychiatric disorder to make them competent to stand trial (Annas, 2004). In the situation I am considering, the criminal psychopath has already been tried and convicted. Whether offering safe and effective brain-modifying treatment to children at risk of developing psychopathy is defensible would have to be weighed against uncertainty about their future behavior and potential adverse effects of the drugs on their developing brains. Forcing a preventive brain intervention on children might be defensible, but only in cases where they had already committed violent acts of aggression. Whether optional or forced interventions in the brains of those with, or at risk of developing, psychopathy can be justified requires a careful weighing of their rights and interests against the rights and interests of others who may be harmed by them.

One question that has been discussed extensively in the philosophical and legal literature is whether psychopaths have the cognitive and emotional capacity to be responsible for their behavior (Fine and Kennett, 2004; Blair, 2008; Glannon, 2008; Morse, 2008; Glenn, Raine, and Schug, 2009; Cima, Tonnaer, and Hauser, 2010; Glenn and Raine, 2014b; Focquaert, Glenn, and Raine, 2015). I do not engage in this debate here. Focusing on individuals with severe psychopathy resulting in criminal behavior, I assume for the sake of argument that their impaired rational and moral capacities excuse them from moral and criminal responsibility. This motivates the need for interventions that might generate or enhance these capacities, give them more control of their actions, and reduce the risk of them harming others. On the assumption that psychopaths are not responsible and not at fault for their behavior, the justification for incarceration is not punishment but deterrence. The justification for brain- and mind-altering interventions in the psychopath is to improve his rational and moral dispositions. Neurointerventions would be a form of rehabilitative therapy aimed at making the criminal psychopath less likely to engage in additional criminal behavior and more likely to effectively engage in society. If such an intervention achieved its rehabilitative goal, then it would also achieve the related goal of deterrence by preventing recidivism. The main ethical and legal question is whether intervening in and altering the psychopath's brain for a combined rehabilitative and deterrent purpose promotes or interferes with his freedom of thought and whether it can, or cannot, be justified on grounds of protecting the public from harm.

Another question discussed in the literature is whether the psychopath is "mad" or "bad" (Maibom, 2008). The question is whether psychopathy is a mental or a moral disorder, and what this distinction implies for control and responsibility. Risking oversimplification, the basic idea is that if the psychopath is "mad," then she has a mental disorder, cannot control her behavior, and deserves rehabilitation rather than punishment. If the psychopath is "bad," then she fails to exercise the control she has of her behavior and deserves some form of punishment. The dualistic picture implied by this question is unhelpful because there is no straightforward answer to it on either empirical or normative grounds. Psychopathy is a disorder that falls along a spectrum of antisocial behavior. It correlates with different degrees of impairment in cognitive and emotional capacities. There is variability among psychopaths in degrees of mental incapacity and behavior control. A more helpful approach is to avoid raising binary questions about psychopathy that invite binary responses. Instead, the approach should be to examine how brain abnormalities in psychopaths can interfere with the capacity to recognize and respond to moral reasons when they act. Rather than asking whether severe psychopathy is a mental disorder or a moral disorder, it is more appropriate to ask how a neural and mental disorder becomes a moral disorder resulting in harmful behavior and how to prevent it. For criminal offenders with psychopathy, as well as for children and adolescents at high risk of criminal behavior because of psychopathic traits, can brain- and mind-altering interventions be justified for reasons of rehabilitation and deterrence?

I do not consider how the number of offenders with psychopathy compares with offenders with other psychiatric disorders such as schizophrenia or bipolar depression. Pharmacotherapy for these disorders has been effective in many cases when patients adhere to treatment and healthcare providers closely monitor them. In contrast, there are currently no proven treatments for psychopathy. Whether safe and effective treatments become available will depend on a better understanding of the dysfunctional neural circuitry in this disorder, as well as how it shapes the mental content of those affected by it. After describing what is currently known about this circuitry, I explore some potential interventions to modify psychopathic behavior. My focus for the balance of this chapter is on the ethical, legal, and social implications of these interventions.

## Brain abnormalities in psychopathy

Neuroimaging studies have shown that there are structural and functional abnormalities in pathways between the PFC and limbic system in psychopaths' brains (Blair, 2003, 2007a, 2007b, 2008, 2013a; Glenn, Raine, and Schug, 2009; Glenn and Raine, 2014b). The studies have indicated dysfunction in pathways connecting the orbitofrontal cortex, ventromedial/ventrolateral PFC, and amygdala. The PFC receives projections from and sends projections to the amygdala. Ordinarily, there is functional connectivity between these brain regions. The orbitofrontal cortex mediates the emotion of regret, which is critical to counterfactual reasoning in choosing between different courses of action. The amygdala mediates the capacity for responsiveness to fear-inducing stimuli and, together with the ventral part of the anterior cingulate cortex, mediates the capacity for empathy. These structures constitute what Andrea Glenn, Adrian Raine, and Robert Schug describe as the "moral neural network," which is dysfunctional in psychopaths (2009, p. 6; see also Blair, 2007a, 2013b; Glenn and Raine, 2014b). The emotional capacities mediated by these neural circuits enable us to respond to moral reasons for refraining from performing harmful actions. They also enable us to have emotional responses to harmful outcomes of actions and other events.

Many studies provide evidence that moral reasoning involves interaction between cognitive and affective processes (Bechara, Damasio, and Damasio, 2000). They support the view that negative emotions such as fear alert individuals to the moral salience of a situation by causing them to experience discomfort. This influences moral judgments by placing constraints on potentially harmful behavior. Psychopaths are impaired in their capacity for these emotions and thus impaired in their capacity for moral reasoning and decision-making (Decety, Michalska, and Kinzler, 2012).

The psychopath's impaired capacity to respond to moral reasons inclines him to overtly antisocial and criminal behavior in the form of reactive and instrumental aggression. In the first type of aggression, or "impulsive aggression," a frustrating or threatening event triggers an aggressive act without regard for any potential goal. In instrumental, or "proactive aggression," the action is purposeful and directed to a specific goal (Blair, Mitchell, and Blair, 2005; Glenn and Raine, 2009). Bullying is an example of instrumental aggression. James Blair, Derek Mitchell, and Karina Blair note, "there are strong reasons to believe that individuals with psychopathy present with orbitofrontal/ventrolateral frontal cortical dysfunction as well as amygdala dysfunction" (2005, p. 139). These authors further state, "At the core of the model is the suggestion of amygdala dysfunction in individuals with the disorder. This dysfunction gives rise to impairment in aversive conditions for instrumental learning and the possession of fearful and sad expressions. These impairments interfere with socialization such that the individual does not learn to avoid actions that cause harm to other individuals" (2005, p. 139).

Research involving incarcerated individuals with psychopathy further elucidates correlations between frontal–limbic dysfunction and the cognitive and emotional deficits in these individuals. One MRI study showed a reduction in gray matter volume in regions associated with empathic processing, prosocial emotions, and moral reasoning in violent criminal psychopaths compared with normal controls (Gregory, ffytche, Simmons et al., 2012). In a fMRI study, criminal psychopaths exhibited deficits in the ventromedial prefrontal cortex and orbitofrontal cortex in response to pain and distress cues expressed by others (Decety, Skelly, and Kiehl, 2013).

The neurophysiological underpinning of psychopathy is not limited to dysfunctional prefrontal–limbic circuits. Other fMRI studies of this population have shown abnormal functional connectivity in the pathway between the dorsolateral PFC and the ventral striatum in the brain's reward circuit. They have displayed correlations between reduced connectivity in the dorsolateral

PFC–ventral striatum pathway and impulsivity in criminal psychopaths and a greater degree of connectivity in this pathway among those with noncriminal psychopathic traits (Geurts, Von Borries, Volman et al., 2016; Hosking, Kastman, Dorfman et al., 2017). These findings replicate earlier findings of a fMRI study showing hyperactivity in the reward circuitry and maladaptive decision-making in subjects identified as criminal psychopaths (Buckholtz, Treaday, Cowen et al., 2010). These structural and functional brain abnormalities underlying psychopathic behavior may predict more frequent criminal behavior. They may predict which offenders would be more likely to reoffend, and which might be candidates for behavior modification.

## Possible treatments for psychopathy

Ideally, pharmacological or other interventions designed to modulate neural function would improve impulse control and psychological responses to empathy-eliciting stimuli among criminal psychopaths. The goal would be to improve their other-regarding behavior. A better understanding of how dysfunction in neural networks manifests in psychopathic behavior is necessary to inform possible brain interventions for this group. It will be a challenge to achieve this understanding given that psychopathy involves abnormal connectivity in not one but multiple neural circuits. Neuromodulation of the critical circuits is still hypothetical. If a drug or neurostimulating technique could produce these effects in criminal psychopaths, then it could protect the public from harm. It could also rehabilitate and reintegrate the offender into society. The second goal would be a desirable alternative to incarceration for both the offender and the public.

Noninvasive interventions such as CBT may be preferable to invasive interventions such as pharmacotherapy or DBS. They would avoid the risks of intracranial surgery necessary to implant DBS electrodes. They would also avoid the risk of adverse effects of psychotropic drugs on normally functioning neural pathways mediating normal mental states. The general purpose of CBT and other psychotherapies is to enable subjects to reframe their beliefs and other mental states so that they respond appropriately to environmental stimuli. Crucially, though, the efficacy of this therapy depends on the subject's insight into his condition and the reasons for correcting it. Insight is a critical component in the motivation to change one's behavior and produce positive responses from the patient to the therapist's suggestions. Most studies suggest that psychopaths lack the capacity for insight in what is more of an ego-syntonic than ego-dystonic condition. If they fail to recognize that they have a disorder and the reasons for treating it, then the therapeutic potential of this technique may be limited. This would be more likely among adults with the disorder because of a more entrenched pattern of learned behavior. CBT may be a potentially effective treatment for adolescents with psychopathy. Their brains, specifically prefrontal regions, are still developing. Prefrontal–limbic pathways might be amenable to modulation in ways that could promote prosocial behavior. Due to their age, their learned behavior might not be as entrenched in neural circuits as it is in older psychopaths. This might be altered by the modulating effects of the technique.

This is speculative, however, since there are no studies that have established the efficacy of CBT for psychopathy. If this technique were used for this disorder, modulation of the neural circuits, mental states, and behavior of an adolescent with psychopathic traits would depend on the extent to which biological and social factors influenced their developing brains. There is also the question of how effective CBT would be, given that the cognition-mediating frontal lobes of an adolescent are not fully developed. Their brains and minds might not be so amenable to the technique after all. This could limit their capacity for insight and the ability to reframe their thoughts so that they aligned with social norms.

A potentially more promising technique for altering prefrontal–limbic brain activation patterns in psychopathy is fMRI-based NFB. As described in Chapters 3 and 5, subjects modulate their own brain activity by seeing and responding to it on functional neuroimaging or EEG. NFB research using fMRI in criminal psychopaths focuses on the dysfunctional fear network (Focquaert, Glenn, and Raine, 2015). This network includes the orbitofrontal cortex, amygdala, anterior cingulate cortex, and insula. The goal of NFB is to increase neural activity and connectivity in these regions. A more ambitious goal of this technique would be to increase neuroplasticity and neurogenesis to ameliorate reduced volume of these brain regions in psychopaths compared with normal controls.

In one study, Ranganatha Sitaram, Andrea Caria, and Niels Birbaumer have shown that criminal offenders with psychopathy can modulate activity in the left anterior insula through fMRI-based NFB (2009; see also Focquaert, Glenn, and Raine, 2015, pp. 118–119). The results also suggest that this technique might increase synaptic connectivity in the left insula. It would be preferable to psychotropic medication because it could modulate brain and mental function noninvasively through the subject's own psychological response. If it significantly reduced the risk of recidivism, then it would also be clearly preferable to incarceration. But many more clinical trials would be needed before this intervention was proven to be an effective treatment for psychopathy. Besides, the brains of adult psychopaths may be too hardwired to be amenable to NFB. It may not be indicated for younger individuals, either, if their brains are still developing and they lack the cognitive capacity to successfully perform this technique.

Other studies suggest that increasing levels of serotonin in prefrontal areas of the brain can increase subjects' capacity to respond to moral reasons and constrain impulsive behavior. A study conducted by Molly Crockett and coinvestigators showed that the SSRI citalopram increased harm aversion in healthy volunteers (Crockett, Clark, Hauser et al., 2010). They claimed that "these findings have implications for the use of serotonergic agents in the treatment of antisocial and aggressive behavior" in promoting pro-social behavior (2010, p. 17438). Given the connection between antisocial and psychopathic personality types, a drug that could treat the first presumably could also treat the second.

Crockett is more circumspect about the behavior-modifying potential of these drugs in a more recent contribution to a symposium on moral enhancement. She writes, "Most neurotransmitters serve multiple functions and are found in many different brain regions . . . Serotonin plays a role in a variety of other processes [than harm aversion] including (but not limited to) learning, emotion, vision, sexual behavior, sleep, pain and memory, and there are at last 17 different types of serotonin receptors that produce distinct effects on neurotransmission. This intervention . . . may have undesirable side effects, and these should be considered when weighing the costs and benefits of the intervention" (2014, p. 370, 2016). It is not known whether a drug of this class would have similar effects in psychopaths. Further research is needed to know how increasing levels of serotonin in certain brain regions to promote prosocial behavior would affect other brain regions mediating other behaviors. Unlike healthy subjects, psychopaths have dysregulation in dopaminergic and serotonergic systems.

It is unclear whether the effects of an SSRI or other psychoactive drug targeting only serotonergic receptors in the brain would induce or restore normal function in these pathways. Drugs that increased levels of serotonin would be more likely to have this effect in prefrontal cortical areas where this neurotransmitter is more abundant. Given the critical role of an underactive amygdala in psychopathy, it is questionable whether the projections from the prefrontal areas with increased levels of serotonin to the amygdala alone would have the necessary modulating effect on this subcortical structure. Drugs would have to target the amygdala more directly to produce the effect of harm aversion.

Another way of inducing or increasing harm aversion might be to increase levels of oxytocin in the amygdala and other brain regions. This neuropeptide plays a critical role in social cognition (Ross and Young, 2009; Churchland,

2011, Chapter 3). Theoretically, a drug administered intranasally could increase levels of oxytocin in the brain and promote prosocial behavior. This is not equivalent to moral behavior, since prosocial behavior does not imply the capacity to respond to reasons for or against certain actions. But it is a precondition for moral behavior. There are questions about the safety and efficacy of chronic administration of oxytocin. This drug interacts with the HPA axis to inhibit activity in the amygdala. By diminishing the fear response to social stimuli, increasing levels of oxytocin could increase trust and social cooperation. In light of the psychopath's impaired capacity to conform to social norms, this would appear to be a promising therapeutic intervention. The coordinated action of oxytocin and serotonin in the nucleus accumbens of the brain's reward system is required to reinforce social behavior. Studies on the coordinated activity of these systems may lead to the development of treatments for disorders that affect maladaptive and pathological social behavior, including psychopathy. Combing serotonin and oxytocin treatments might incline psychopaths to conform to social norms when they act.

There are at least two problems with oxytocin as a potential therapy for psychopathy. First, recall that psychopaths have an underactive amygdala. This partly explains their impaired capacity for responses associated with fear and empathy. The psychopath does not display an excess but a deficiency of a normal fear response. This deficiency tends to generate and sustain instrumental aggression. Dampening the psychopath's already diminished fear response even further would not promote trust in others but more likely increase her tendency to manipulate them. Oxytocin may enable a psychopath to appear more cooperative. An increase in social interaction would better enable her to use others in achieving her selfish ends. It would more likely exacerbate than ameliorate her instrumental aggression and result in even more harmful behavior. Second, the effects of oxytocin in the brain can be influenced by social factors, and the combined effects of this drug and these factors can influence the expression of psychopathic traits. This may involve altering how one perceives others, which can be a function of the social group to which one belongs. In some cases, social factors can cause oxytocin to promote antisocial rather than prosocial behavior by strengthening a person's bonding and identification with an in-group and perception of those in out-groups as competitors or threats. Increasing levels of oxytocin in the psychopath's brain could reinforce the perceived distinction between her in-group and a competing out-group and increase aggression toward individuals in the latter. In these respects, administering this drug to psychopaths could have harmful social consequences (Bartz, 2016; Bartels, 2012; Hurlemann and Scheele, 2016).

Another concern is that combining serotonin and oxytocin could harm the recipient of these drugs. They could trigger a cascade of adverse neurophysiological events and possibly result in the serotonin syndrome with adverse neurological and psychological effects. Deleterious additive effects of two or more psychotropic drugs could cancel out any presumed salutary effects when the drugs were used separately. Similar remarks apply to altering levels of dopamine. Psychopaths have a hyperactive reward system involving this neurotransmitter. An excess of dopamine in reward circuitry such as the nucleus accumbens/ventral striatum can contribute to impulsivity. A drug that reduced dopamine levels in this system might reduce impulsivity. But it is not known how increasing levels of serotonin and decreasing levels of dopamine could safely and effectively modify the psychopath's behavior. Because dopamine, like serotonin, has many receptors mediating different brain functions, this question can only be answered following the completion of a sufficient number of randomized, placebo-controlled clinical trials involving psychopaths and mentally healthy individuals.

Magnetic or electrical stimulation might be a more effective way of modulating activity in prefrontal areas of the psychopath's brain. Activation of the junction between the right temporal and parietal lobe with TMS in healthy research subjects has been shown to alter their moral judgments (Young, Camprodon, Hauser et al., 2010). One advantage of this technique over psychoactive drugs is that it is a more focused means of neuromodulation. It can avoid many of the side effects of drugs. But the positive effects of this technique are limited, extending only a few centimeters in the cortex and diminishing before the current can reach deeper regions of the brain. These effects may be too weak to influence functional connectivity between the ventromedial PFC and amygdala or the dorsolateral PFC and ventral striatum. The effects of TMS are transient as well. DBS would be more likely to modulate dysfunctional prefrontal–limbic pathways characteristic of psychopathy because it can influence both cortical and subcortical structures in these pathways. Yet because DBS involves intracranial surgery and manipulation of functions deep within the brain, the risks from the surgery or imprecise stimulation are greater than they are for psychopharmacology and TMS.

As psychopathy is not life-threatening and does not involve pain and suffering in the affected person, the risks associated with DBS would make it difficult to justify it as an alternative treatment to TMS or drug therapy for this disorder. In addition, the surgery of implanting the electrodes, pulse generator, and leads, monitoring of patients, and periodic battery replacement of the generator would be prohibitively expensive. While DBS may be more effective than drugs and TMS in modifying psychopathic behavior, the risks and cost of using

DBS for 20–25% of the prison population would not make it a viable therapeutic option for the disorder. On balance, psychopharmacology may be the most reasonable intervention to produce the desired result.

It may be overly reductionist and oversimplified to claim that increasing levels of a neurotransmitter or neuropeptide would make one more empathetic and less impulsive. Human behavior is a function of multiple biological, psychological, and environmental factors, not just neural circuits and neurotransmitters. How and why we act depends on factors both inside and outside of the brain. Nevertheless, psychotropic drugs can alter the mental states and behavior of both healthy subjects and those with different psychopathologies. Because of this, and because of the relatively high percentage of criminal offenders with psychopathy, it will be instructive to examine some of the ethical and legal issues that would arise from interventions in the brains of these offenders to modify their behavior.

## Offering behavior modification

Let us assume that psychotropic drugs would be the most effective means of changing psychopathic behavior. In cases where a psychopath had been convicted of a criminal offence, would the relevant parties be justified in asking him to participate in an experimental study to test a behavior-modifying drug? If a drug were being tested for modifying behavior unrelated to the behavior associated with the criminal offence, then it would be objectionable to ask a psychopath to participate in the study. It would not be objectionable, though, if the experimental drug were being tested for the behavior associated with the offence. Provided that the individual was fully informed of the design and goal of the study and was not exposed to unreasonable risk, he could consent to participate in it. Due to the experimental nature of the study, he would not benefit directly from his role as a research subject. But he can benefit indirectly from participating in the trial. If the drug had been shown to be safe and effective based on the responses of others with the same condition, it could subsequently be given to him and have positive modifying effects on his behavior. If the safety and efficacy of the drug had been established for other conditions and had therapeutic potential for psychopathy, then a sufficiently competent and informed individual could consent to off-label clinical use of a drug for this disorder.

Some might question whether a psychopath would have the decisional capacity to consent to an experimental or even a proven drug to modify his behavior. Psychopaths can respond to practical reasons in their instrumental aggression. Yet their impulsive behavior and limited capacity to foresee the consequences of their actions suggest that they may not have sufficient capacity to consent. Their impaired cognitive and affective capacity for empathy and re-morse makes it difficult for them to engage in counterfactual reasoning about different actions and to imagine outcomes of these actions. But decisional ca-pacity comes in degrees. The rational capacity the psychopath possesses, albeit impaired to some degree, could be sufficient for him to process and understand information about drug-induced behavior modification. It could also be suf-ficient for him to understand the choice between an intervention that could reduce a prison sentence and remaining incarcerated. He could have enough mental capacity to make a rational decision and consent to or refuse such an experimental intervention.

Even if a drug for psychopathy were safe and effective, some would argue that offering it to a psychopathic criminal offender would be coercive. It would pre-clude options for choice and effectively compel him to accept only one course of action. If the drug were offered as an alternative to incarceration at the time of sentencing, or if it were offered to reduce the duration of incarceration, then it seems that the offer would be one that the individual could not refuse. If the offer were coercive, then he could not consent to it. Consent requires that an individual is suitably informed about the proposed intervention and any alternatives, has the cognitive and affective capacity to process and understand this information, and voluntarily chooses to accept or refuse it. Presumably, of-fering therapy in lieu of incarceration would violate the third of these conditions and invalidate consent.

We need to distinguish coercive threats from coercive offers. Some argue that only threats coerce, though not all threats are coercive. Alan Wertheimer claims that a proposal constitutes a coercive threat if it is forced upon an indi-vidual, such that he has no reasonable choice but to succumb to the proposal (Wertheimer, 1987). The proposed psychopharmacological intervention is not a coercive threat in the case at hand because it is not forced upon the psycho-path. Nor is incarceration presented to him as the consequence of refusing the intervention because he is already liable to incarceration as a result of his crim-inal offence.

Lene Bomann-Larsen points out that "The prison sentence is not a threat *made in order to* make the subject accept CNS treatment, but something to which the convict has made herself liable by—*ex hypothesi*—knowingly and willingly breaking the law" (2013, p. 4). The drug is offered to her as a genuine alternative to incarceration. Yet Bomann-Larsen says that this "is surely a coer-cive circumstance, having to choose between staying in prison or undergoing CNS treatment" (2013, p. 4). On the contrary, the fact that the choice is limited to two options does not make it coercive and as such involuntary. This is con-sistent with Harry Frankfurt's claim that someone who is coerced "is *compelled* to do what he does. He has *no choice* but to do it" (Frankfurt, 1988c, p. 36). Others argue that even offers can be coercive. In these cases, the offer prevents the individual from obtaining a situation that would be better for her than the one being offered (Zimmerman, 1981). It causes the individual to accept the less desirable of two states of affairs. But if the alternative to participating in an experimental study of a drug for psychopathy, or taking a safe and effective drug, is incarceration, then it seems reasonable for an individual to accept this to free herself from this restriction on her physical liberty. What is being offered could modify her behavior in a way that would reduce the risk of recidivism, release her from incarceration, and reintegrate her into society. It would make her better off than she would have been without the drug, languishing in prison with little likelihood of rehabilitation (Wertheimer and Miller, 2014).

An offer of a drug to reduce or avoid a prison sentence or as a condition of parole could be coercive or otherwise objectionable if its efficacy was questionable and there was a significant risk of severe side effects from taking it. For many, suffering from adverse physical and psychological effects of a drug without any benefit would be a worse state of affairs than incarceration without the availability of the drug. Experiencing severe effects of a drug would also restrict one's liberty and make one worse off than he otherwise would have been. Coercion involves the imposition of an offer that no one could reasonably refuse. Just because one option is clearly preferable to another, such that a person could not reasonably refuse it, does not mean that the person is coerced into accepting that option and acts involuntarily in accepting it. Indeed, responding to a stronger reason for choosing one option over another is the mark of an informed, rational, and voluntary choice. Acting on a stronger reason does not imply an inability to consider a comparatively weaker reason for choosing an alternative. Also, an individual with the capacity for rational choice may fail to exercise this capacity and make an irrational decision that could still be voluntary. A stubborn refusal to respond to reasons for accepting or refusing an offer is not necessarily the mark of being forced to choose and act in a particular way. Arguments from coercion in the choice between a brain intervention and incarceration are not convincing.

A strong desire to avoid or be released from incarceration would not necessarily undermine one's capacity to process information, deliberate, and make a voluntary choice about whether to accept or refuse a psychotropic drug. An offender may give less weight to any risk associated with the drug because of his desire for a reduced sentence. Together with the fact that the psychopath is impaired in his capacity to represent outcomes of his actions, this may suggest that he cannot adequately assess the benefits and risks of taking the drug. But the capacity to respond to reasons comes in degrees. Although he is cognitively and affectively impaired to some degree, the psychopath may have sufficient capacity to understand and weigh the reasons for and against a CNS intervention and make an voluntary choice to accept or refuse it. If there were questions about whether the psychopath had enough of the requisite capacity, then a psychiatric assessment could establish whether he had or lacked it.

Courts traditionally have offered various treatments to convicted criminal offenders as a condition of release (Chandler, 2013). Evidence that a person has sought or will seek treatment for conditions related to criminal behavior for which he is or will be incarcerated is often considered in the sentencing process. Examples include antilibidinal drug treatment for sexual predators and addiction treatment programs. In the near future, these interventions may also include drugs to modulate impulse control disorders associated with the reactive aggression of the psychopath (Greely, 2008). Some might object that, while not coercive, the fact that release from or avoiding prison is conditional on accepting treatment would severely limit an offender's freedom to choose. Yet by violating the rule of law, the offender has waived his right to liberty and put himself in a situation of constrained choice. If having just two options is the result of criminal behavior, then any constraint implied by the conditional nature of a reduced sentence would not be morally or legally objectionable. Having a choice between incarceration and behavior modification would be preferable to not having *any* choice. We can make this claim when the purpose of incarceration is not punishment but deterrence.

Lack of rational capacity and compulsion are the two standard excusing conditions for actions in the criminal law. Psychopathy does not meet either of these conditions and thus does not qualify as a legal excuse for criminal actions (Morse, 2008). Rather than a mitigating or excusing factor, it is legally considered an aggravating factor in some jurisdictions. It is a risk factor for dangerousness in capital sentencing. Against this view, some have argued that psychopaths are so impaired in their capacity for practical and moral reasoning that they do not act voluntarily in offending and therefore should not be held criminally responsible for their behavior. Accordingly, they do not deserve any form of punishment. Proponents of this position argue that, given the high rate of violent recidivism and unsuccessful attempts to modify criminal psychopathic behavior, incarceration might be justified in order to prevent future harm to others from additional violent offences (Fine and Kennett, 2004). They reject a retributive model of punishing the psychopath based on desert and instead defend a consequentialist model of incarceration based on deterrence. Significantly, this argument does not depend on an answer to the question of whether a psychopath has the mental capacities necessary for free will and moral responsibility (Focquaert, Glenn, and Raine,

2015). Justifying deterrence does not presuppose responsibility or the associated idea of retribution. An offender who lacked the mental capacities necessary for criminal responsibility and did not deserve punishment could still have his liberty justifiably limited by incarceration if he posed a significant risk of reoffending.

Morse points out that, with limited exceptions, "the law does not permit pure preventive detention of individuals solely on the ground that they may pose a risk of harm" (2008, p. 206). Morse also says, "psychopathy is a risk factor for crime, but many might not re-offend despite their mental abnormality" (2008, p. 210). This reinforces the importance of distinguishing people with noncriminal psychopathic traits from criminal psychopaths and the point that having these traits does not imply that they will result in criminal behavior. Yet if an individual has committed criminal offences and is deemed to be at high risk of reoffending, then preventive detention could be justified. The risk of harm would have been actualized in harmful behavior. In cases where a child or adolescent had psychopathic traits, neuroimaging might not clarify the risk of that person engaging in criminal behavior. Any structural or functional biomarkers would not be reliable indicators of risk because their brains would still be developing. Synaptic pruning and myelination in these and other neural pathways would not be complete. Neuroscientists and forensic psychiatrists could not make a definitive judgment about brain function or dysfunction and its association with criminal behavior. More importantly, whether the psychopath was or was not responsible for her criminal behavior would not influence the judgment of whether presenting her with the choice between prison and behavior modification would impair or undermine her ability to choose between them. The purpose of the drug intervention would not be to punish but to rehabilitate her.

There might be a stronger reason for modifying the offender's brain and behavior if she was not responsible. In that case, the intervention would generate or enhance the capacity to respond to moral reasons that she lacked or had only to a limited degree. It would remove two restrictions on her liberty: the brain abnormality preventing her from controlling her behavior; and the prison sentence resulting from this lack of control. Offering an intervention that could make the individual better off in these two respects would not be objectionable. One can sustain this claim if the limited options open to her are a function of a criminal history and a high probability of reoffending. Crucially, the offender would have to retain a sufficient degree of cognitive capacity to deliberate and choose between incarceration and behavior modification while lacking the degree of this capacity necessary for responsibility. Having a higher level of mental capacity and being responsible would make this choice less problematic than if the offender had a lower level of capacity and was not responsible. The capacity to make decisions about brain interventions may be dissociable from the capacity to be criminally responsible for actions. The question would be whether the limited capacity she had would be enough to meet the ethical and legal criteria of accepting or refusing an intervention in the brain, even if she failed to meet the criteria of responsibility. We can assume that it would meet these criteria, at least in some cases. Again, though, a psychiatric assessment would have to confirm this.

Suppose that a sufficiently competent psychopathic criminal offender is informed of the purpose of psychopharmacological behavior modification and is offered it noncoercively as a form of therapy. As such, he has a free choice to accept or decline it. He declines it on the grounds that he does not want any intrusion in his brain and mind. Instead, he accepts a prison sentence or, if he already is incarcerated, a continued sentence. Could the treatment be forced on him despite his objection?

There are legal precedents in the United States for the right of competent patients and prisoners to refuse treatments that alter their thought processes and interfere with their ability to communicate. This right rests on First Amendment protections against forced government intrusion into the mind. For example, in the case of *Rogers v. Okin* (1979), a Massachusetts district court found that competent mental patients had the right to refuse antipsychotic drugs. The court argued that the Constitution recognizes a liberty interest in avoiding the unwanted administration of these drugs, especially when they interfere with freedom of thought. Prisoners also have the right to refuse forced drug treatment on the same grounds. There are different cases in which sexual offenders under supervision have been forcibly prescribed antilibidinal drugs to reduce deviant sexual arousal in order to reduce the risk of harm to others.

The purpose of forced treatment for psychopathy would be to improve the symptoms of a personality disorder and the capacity for practical and moral reasoning and decision-making. Still, this could be described as forced state intrusion into the psychopath's mind and, as such, a violation of his right to noninterference. Even if the psychopath was responsible for his behavior and deserved to be punished by restricting his liberty, he would retain the right to refuse mind-altering treatments. The idea that he has waived his right to liberty by committing a criminal act would not by itself justify forcing treatment on him. He would have the right to refuse being forced into an experimental drug study because of the unknown risk and the right not to be harmed by any adverse effects of the drug. There are no defensible reasons for requiring a person to undergo an intervention that exposes him to any degree of risk. Whether the right to refuse experimental treatment would also apply to a proven safe and effective treatment is debatable. Unless the psychopathy was severe enough to undermine his ability to reason and posed a significant risk of harm to himself, in principle the treatment could not be forced upon him. Although it may seem unreasonable to others, a psychopath may prefer not to take a drug that could alter his personality, despite the fact that it is disordered. Forcing treatment on paternalistic grounds might seem unjustified if he retained some degree of rationality and could make decisions consistent with his best interests. But the state could argue that forcibly altering the psychopath's brain and behavior would be more cost-effective for the criminal justice system and society than long-term incarceration. A behavior-modifying drug would serve the interests of society by reducing the incidence of criminal behavior and the prison population. In addition, it would enable the psychopath to have greater control of his behavior and become a cooperative and productive member of society. Yet unwanted treatment for a person who does not pose a risk of harm to himself or others while incarcerated would seem to violate his autonomy and right to noninterference in his brain.

While courts may recommend offering treatments aimed at modifying brain function and behavior for the sake of mitigation, generally they do not require defendants to accept treatments that present unreasonable risks and unknown benefits. Nevertheless, courts may require a defendant to accept treatments that are experimental if his situation is dire and the new treatment appears very promising in modifying the relevant behavior (Chandler, 2013). But the situation of a person with even severe psychopathy arguably would not be dire. The psychopath would not pose a threat to himself or the public while incarcerated. One objection to forcing treatment on cost-effective grounds is that it would promote the collective interest of society over individual freedom. This objection would have considerable weight if the more expensive approach of incarceration were as effective in reducing harm as the less expensive approach of pharmacologically modifying behavior. Yet because the first approach only serves to reduce the risk of violent recidivism and would not have the same potential to promote prosocial behavior and social reintegration as the second, the objection may not have much weight.

If safe and effective drug therapy were more cost-effective than incarceration in preventing additional criminal acts, then could the interests of society in this form of deterrence override the offender's right to noninterference in his brain? After release from prison, would society's interest in crime prevention through rehabilitation override his right to refuse therapy? The first question depends on whether this right was absolute or conditional, and which conditions would have to obtain in order to justifiably override the right. The second question needs to be informed by the fact that any decision about an intervention could affect two parties: the potential perpetrator of additional crimes whose brain and mind would be altered; and his potential victims whose brains and minds would be altered by his additional criminal acts. One could argue that the offender would have a stronger right against the neurointervention because it would have a direct actual effect on him. The absence of the neurointervention would have only an indirect probable effect on others. The strength of this argument would depend on the predictability of recidivism based on a combination of the offender's previous behavior and brain imaging displaying dysfunction in regions mediating cognitive-emotional processing (Aharoni, Vincent, Harenski et al., 2013; Slobogin, 2013). The predictability and magnitude of the harm to others from a number of offenses might give more weight to intervening in the offender's brain. Perhaps the most defensible claim is that a forced brain intervention without the offender's consent can be justified when it is the all-things-considered least objectionable means of reducing the expected harm the offender would impose on others.

## The freedom of thought objection

It will be helpful to further analyze the argument that forcing violent offenders to undergo psychotropic drug treatment would violate their freedom of thought. On this view, there can be no justification for interfering with a person's cognitive and emotional capacities. This would rule out interventions in the brain that reduced or even eliminated criminal behavior. There is a significant normative distinction between losing one's physical liberty through incarceration and losing one's mental liberty through brain-altering drugs. A person's capacity to think without external interference is the core of dignity, autonomy, and self-determination. The value of these personal properties prohibits any action that would interfere with them. It provides stronger reasons against violating mental liberty than reasons against violating physical liberty. This prohibition holds regardless of social considerations of harm to others.

Some have questioned whether forced neurointervention in a criminal offender could be a logical extension of incarceration (Douglas, 2014). An offender's behavior involves both physical and mental aspects. Presumably, imposing restrictions on both the bodily and cognitive liberty of an offender through incarceration and psychotropic drugs can be justified by the offender's violation of the law. She forfeits her liberty by committing the crime. These restrictions could also be justified by the need to prevent repeat offenses and rehabilitate her. Some commentators separate bodily and cognitive liberty and give more moral and legal weight to the second.

Christoph Bublitz and Reinhard Merkel draw a moral and legal distinction between indirect and direct interventions in a person's thought (Bublitz and Merkel, 2014). They argue that it is morally and legally acceptable to imprison violent offenders as an indirect intervention, but not acceptable to force offenders to take psychoactive substances as a direct intervention. Indirect interventions affect a person's response to stimuli perceived sensually. These are among the effects of being in a prison environment. In contrast, direct brain interventions directly affect one's thought processes. The effects are mental rather than somatic and more significant because they affect fundamental features of the self. In some of their discussions, Bublitz and Merkel do not claim that freedom of thought is an absolute right that can never be overridden by any intervention in the brain. They acknowledge that forced psychiatric interventions on nonautonomous offenders may be morally justified as a last resort when all other treatments have failed (Bublitz, 2014; Bublitz and Merkel, 2014). In other discussions, they suggest that the use of psychotropic drugs on offenders without their consent could not be justified. Their core claim is that nonconsensual brain manipulation "should disqualify as legitimate means to change another's opinion" and that "it would run against the essence of freedom of thought if direct interventions into thought processes were permissible" (Bublitz and Merkel, 2014, p. 53; Bublitz, 2016). These interventions should be prohibited because they violate the offender's right to mental integrity (Craig, 2016).

There are two problems with the stronger position against forced drug intervention. First, it implies that any neurointervention circumvents or undermines the offender's cognitive liberty and autonomous agency. But if the mental disorder that led to the criminal behavior is severe and undermines the capacity to respond to reasons against criminal behavior and make decisions about treatment, then the *disorder* undermines freedom of thought and agency by disabling this capacity. It is not as though the intended modulating effect of the drug disrupts intact neural and mental capacities. On the contrary, by restoring some degree of these capacities in the offender's dysfunctional brain, the drug restores some degree of agency. If brain dysfunction severely disrupts mental processing necessary for mental integrity and cognitive liberty, then there may be no integrity or liberty to violate. Nor does the intervention necessarily circumvent the offender's rational faculties, particularly in cases where these faculties are severely impaired. The intervention is intended to restore his mental capacity and behavior control disrupted by the psychopathology. In addition, the strict separation of mental and bodily integrity can be questioned, since the offender's brain–mind relation is essentially embodied.

Second, the argument against forced drug intervention assumes that altering the brain of a nonconsenting criminal offender always harms and never benefits him. This has to be judged on the reasons for and probable outcome of the intervention. Brain-altering procedures such as a frontal lobotomy or a drug that severely blunted a person's cognitive and emotional capacity would violate freedom of thought by destroying the capacity to think and experience emotions. These interventions would not restore but eliminate the mental basis of autonomous agency. Altering the brain and mind of the character Alex in Anthony Burgess's *A Clockwork Orange* to induce an uncontrollable conditioned nauseous response when thinking about or seeing violent acts would be an impermissible alteration of thought. The interventions in these cases would be impermissible because of their debilitating and dehumanizing effects on the person. Even if they achieved the goal of deterrence, they would do it in a perverse way. The harm visited on these subjects could not be compensated for by any presumed benefit to them, and thus the interventions would be ethically impermissible. These cases are very different from cases in which psychotropic drugs or neuromodulating devices could safely and effectively improve an offender's neural and mental functioning and moral sensitivity.

If a psychotropic drug improved a person's cognitive and emotional capacities and made him responsive to moral reasons for or against certain actions, then the intervention would not undermine but instead would enhance his autonomous agency. The intervention could improve the offender's mental capacities to the point of enabling him to have insight into his behavior and recognize that it was harmful to others and not in his best interests. This insight could provide him with reasons to accept or seek additional drug or other therapy as part of a rehabilitative process. By strengthening an offender's cognitive and emotional capacity and his prudential and moral reasoning, a psychotropic drug could make him better off than he would have been without it. Paternalistic reasons for forced treatment may be justified if the offender lacks insight into his behavior and is unable to appreciate how harmful it is. A psychotropic drug could benefit the offender by providing him with this insight and improving his rational and moral capacities.

Thomas Sobirk Petersen and Kristian Kragh support this position. They ask us to "imagine that, by forcing a violent offender to take certain psychopharmacological drugs that will curb or silence his urge to harm other people, we will actually increase the offender's ability to think more freely and exercise concentration and will-power" (2016, p. 31; see also Ryberg and Petersen, 2013; Ryberg, 2015; cf. Vincent, 2014). Applying this line of reasoning to the hypothetical case of a sex offender, they claim that "such a person may in fact welcome—at least in the long run—the fact that his thoughts have been changed so that he is freer to think about and concentrate on things other than sex" (Petersen and Kragh, 2016, p. 31). In cases of an offender whose criminal behavior is at least partly explained by a pathological state of mind, any form of neuromodulation that could ameliorate the pathology could be justified. It would not interfere with but would restore freedom of thought. Depending on the extent of the pathology, the offender might not appreciate the positive aspects of neural and mental modification until after the change had occurred. This could weaken a refusal of the intervention by the offender. Petersen and Kragh further state, that "if the key concern is about freedom of thought, and it is possible to improve a person's freedom of thought by violating it once, it is not obvious that such violation is morally problematic" (2016, p. 32).

Still, one can take issue with their use of "violation." There may be a stronger justification for intervening in the brain if the person's thought is pathological and so cognitively and emotionally impaired that it is not free. The psychopathology undermines the person's autonomy and control of his thought. A psychopharmacological intervention would not be a violation of freedom if the thought it alters is not free in these respects. Indeed, if the intervention is safe, ameliorates a pathological state of mind, and restores some degree of autonomous agency, then it is difficult to understand in what sense it would be a violation. One can make this claim even if the intervention has to be given on a regular basis and not just on a single occasion. The intended recipient may refuse it by exercising her right to noninterference. Yet the strength of this right depends on the extent to which the offender has decisional capacity, has insight into her disorder, and understands the reasons for altering her brain. Neuromodulation as such does not undermine cognitive and emotional liberty. Whether it undermines or enables this liberty depends on whether its effects are salutary or deleterious on the recipient's thought and behavior and others who are affected by it. Nevertheless, because even the proven safety of a psychotropic drug does not rule out the possibility of adverse effects on the brain and mind, we are justified only in making the weaker claim that it may be permissible to intervene in and alter the offender's brain. We are not justified in making the stronger claim that neuromodulation should be obligatory and that violent offenders should be forced to undergo psychotropic drug treatment.

The Canadian Supreme Court case of *Starson v. Swayze* (2003) illustrates some of the contentious issues associated with freedom of thought and the legal right to refuse medication. This case involves a more complex set of issues than those that figured in *Rogers v. Okin*. Specifically, it illustrates that forced psychotropic medication does not necessarily violate cognitive liberty. Scott Starson was a Canadian engineer and computer programmer with a gift for physics. Diagnosed with bipolar depression and schizoaffective disorder with psychotic features (delusions), he was found not criminally responsible for making death threats. Starson was committed to a psychiatric hospital and detained against his will. He received various psychotropic medications to control his symptoms. Starson argued that the drugs prevented him from thinking at his full capacity and that he had the right to refuse them. A psychiatrist involved in his care (Swayze) argued that Starson lacked the mental capacity to understand the need for the medication and to know what was in his best interests. The Ontario Consent and Capacity Board confirmed Swayze's finding of incapacity. But the Ontario Court of Appeal overturned the Board's decision. In considering an appeal by Swayze to uphold the initial legal decision, the Supreme Court of Canada ruled that Starson was not incapacitated and knew what was in his best interests. The Court ruled that he was competent enough to refuse the medications.

Not long after the ruling, Starson was recommitted to a psychiatric hospital for his disorder. He was discharged on the condition that he adhere to an antipsychotic drug regimen, which reduced but did not eliminate his grandiose delusions. Although Starson repeatedly insisted that the drugs interfered with his thinking and violated his right to refuse them, his delusions indicated that he lacked insight into his condition and the degree of decisional capacity necessary to retain such a right. In these respects, he lacked freedom of thought due to a psychiatric disorder. This may be enough to claim that he did not have a right to noninterference and that there was ethical and legal justification for forced pharmacological treatment on him.

The claim that forced psychotropic treatment violated Starson's freedom of thought presupposes that he had a sufficient level and integration of the mental capacities necessary for reasoning and decision-making without the treatment. But if his mental states were severely dysfunctional because of bipolar and schizoaffective disorder, then he did not retain the freedom of thought associated with his premorbid self. This freedom could not be violated if he did not retain it to any significant degree. The issue is not whether interfering with his cognitive liberty is permissible. Rather, the issue is how this liberty could be restored when it has been lost or severely impaired by a psychiatric disorder. If psychopharmacological intervention is the only way to restore it, then forcing antipsychotic drugs on him could be justified.

There are important differences between the psychotic symptoms of someone like Starson with bipolar or schizoaffective disorder and the mental states of a criminal offender with moderately severe to severe psychopathy. In both cases, though, the disordered thought may be substantial enough to undermine cognitive liberty. Forcing safe and effective psychotropic medication on a person with severe cognitive impairment would not violate freedom of thought if the thought is not free in any plausible sense of the term. Intervening in the brain of a person with a psychiatric disorder to ameliorate its symptoms may be justified. A refusal by a person with such a disorder would not have to be respected if the person lacked a sufficient degree of decisional capacity. Indeed, healthcare providers would be obligated to force treatment on the person if his untreated condition entailed a significant risk of harm to himself or others. The strength of these claims depends on the extent of mental impairment in psychopathy. The lesser the degree of impairment, the stronger the reasons will be for upholding the right to refuse psychotropic medication. The greater the degree of impairment, the weaker the reasons will be for upholding this right.

There is no absolute right to noninterference in one's brain to change the mental capacities mediated by it. The strength of this right, and whether it can be overridden, depends on whether and to what extent the person's mental capacities are intact or impaired. It depends on whether mental impairment undermines one's reasoning and decisional capacity, and what this entails about the risk of harm to oneself and others. In cases where a person's behavior posed a significant risk of harm, there would be reasons for restricting his behavior and modifying his presumed freedom of thought. There are no decisive but at best *pro tanto* reasons for upholding cognitive liberty when cognition is impaired by psychiatric disorders in general and psychopathy in particular. These reasons may be weak when mental capacity is so impaired that the person's liberty becomes questionable. In these cases, forced intervention can be justified when it has salutary effects on the person's brain and mind. With this capacity restored, the offender may understand the therapeutic goal of the intervention and welcome it as a necessary first step in a process of rehabilitation. The upshot is that direct pharmacological intervention in the brain does not necessarily violate cognitive and emotional liberty. It can be consistent with and restore or enhance this liberty when it safely and effectively realizes its therapeutic goals.

One problem with postincarceration pharmacological intervention is that the offender may fail to adhere to the therapeutic regimen and stop taking the drug. This would disrupt the rehabilitative process and pose a risk of violent reoffending. These potential outcomes underscore the need for a supportive environment, psychiatric monitoring, and continuity of care to promote and sustain rehabilitation and prevent recidivism. It is also necessary to incorporate social and environmental factors and the relevant institutions into the treatment plan to ensure adherence. Long-term salutary changes in the offender's thought and behavior require more than psychotropic medication alone (Swanson, 2016, p. 2; Chang, Lichtenstein, Langstrom et al., 2016).

We can further elucidate the ethical and legal implications of forced psychopharmacological treatment by drawing a threefold distinction among a deontological reason against and consequentialist and nonconsequentialist reasons for this intervention in psychopathic criminal offenders. The deontological reason would be equivalent to a prohibition against brain- and mind-altering interventions. It would pertain to the right of the offender to refuse them because they would violate his dignity, intrinsic worth, and cognitive liberty (Kant, 1785/1964; Mill, 1859/1978, p. 71). The consequentialist reason would be equivalent to a permission and would pertain to the intervention as a form of deterrence to prevent harm to others (Mill, 1863/1998, Chapter 5). The nonconsequentialist reason would be equivalent to a permission and would pertain both to deterrence and the positive effects of the intervention on the offender's brain and mind. According to nonconsequentialism, the rightness or wrongness of an action or policy is not solely determined by the goodness or badness of its consequences. "Nonconsequentialism is now typically thought to include the prerogative not to maximize the good and constraints on producing the good" (Kamm, 2007, p. 14).

Regarding treatment of criminal offenders, nonconsequentialism implies that we need not always maximize potentially good outcomes, or minimize potentially bad outcomes, for society. We should duly consider the rights and interests of the offender, even if this does not promote the public good. Nonconsequentialism implies that there is more at stake in considering neurointerventions than their effects on society. Unlike deontology and consequentialism, nonconsequentialism does not construe the interests of individuals and society in disjunctive terms. It suggests that both the interests of the offender and the interests of society have to be considered in normative judgments about neurointerventions.

There are two general deontological considerations in forensic psychiatry. Punishment for violating a law resulting in harm to others is based on the deontological principle of desert or proportionality. Punishment is intended to fit the crime. Consistent with Kantian deontological ethics, an offender with the rational capacity to know what she was doing in committing a criminal act would deserve punishment (Kant, 1786/1965, Part I). This version of deontology is not relevant to what is at issue here on the assumption that the offender lacked the capacity to control his criminal behavior and be responsible for it. Moreover, safe and effective psychopharmacology could not plausibly be described as punishment. A second deontological consideration pertains to a constraint on or prohibition against interfering with the offender's thought. The freedom of thought objection to direct brain interventions could be either a deontological (Kantian) or libertarian (Millian) objection against this type of interference. It could violate the person's dignity as a rational being (Kant, 1785/1964), or it could violate the person's cognitive liberty (Mill, 1859/1978, p. 71).

Drug-induced neuromodulation would not violate the offender's dignity or liberty if it did not interfere with but restored her freedom of thought. The positive effect on the person's mental states would provide a reason against an absolute prohibition on brain-altering drugs. A nonconsequentialist justification for pharmacological intervention in the psychopath's brain could resolve conflict between the interests of society and those of the offender. By generating or improving his capacity to respond to moral reasons for or against certain actions, psychotropic drugs can be a form of deterrence. They can reduce the risk of recidivism and reoffending and thereby prevent further public harm. In addition, by improving the offender's cognitive and emotional capacities, they can enable him to have insight into his condition, restore effective reasoning and decision-making, and restore some degree of freedom of thought. Direct brain intervention could restore the offender's autonomous agency. The constraints in nonconsequentialism do not reject the importance of preventing harm but specify that social consequences should not detract from the goal of rehabilitating the offender. Nonconsequentialism in this example of forensic psychiatry focuses not only on preventing additional harm to others but also on improving the rational and moral sensitivity of the agent who would be the source of that harm.

Petersen and Kragh note that a consequentialist would argue that improving an offender's freedom of thought with direct brain interventions could be justified when comparing a positive outcome with continued incarceration (2016, p. 33). They also say, "a deontologist of a moderate kind (or a non-absolute version of deontology) could argue that if enough is at stake, the constraint against violating an offender's freedom of thought can be realized and overtrumped" (2016, p. 33). Their version of a moderate deontology could plausibly be taken as a version of nonconsequentialism. A nonconsequentialist justification would be superior to a consequentialist or deontological justification because of its deterrent effect and the direct benefit to the offender in restoring his autonomous agency. The point of the intervention would not just be to reduce recidivism and prevent additional public harm but also to improve the mental states of the offender.

Because psychopathy is a psychiatric disorder that impairs thought and results in harmful behavior, reasons for neuromodulation to restore normal thought would override reasons for noninterference in the brain and mind on the view that the offender's thought is inviolable. The impairment in psychopathy may be severe enough to preclude him from having insight into his condition and understanding the reasons for brain- and mind-modifying drugs. This would call into question any presumed right to refuse an intervention deemed safe and effective for this type of mental disorder. Claims that there is an absolute right to refuse neurointerventions and thus a deontological prohibition against them cannot be upheld because they fail to distinguish intact from impaired cognitive and emotional capacities. They also fail to appreciate that there are degrees of these capacities in mild, moderate, and severe forms of psychiatric disorders.

Nonconsequentialist reasons for direct brain interventions are consistent with the dignity and intrinsic worth of the offender insofar as they restore the capacity for rational and moral agency. Safe and effective brain interventions for a psychiatric disorder inclining one to criminal behavior would be a humane alternative to lifelong incarceration. There would be moral and legal justification for freely chosen as well as forced treatment. In light of these considerations, Patricia Churchland's comments from 2002 are still relevant:

> The movie *Clockwork Orange*, typically conjured up by the very idea of direct intervention by the criminal justice system, probably had a greater impact on our collective amygdaloid structures than it deserves to have. Certainly, some kinds of direct intervention are morally objectionable. So much is easy. But *all* kinds? Even pharmacological? Is it possible that some forms of nervous-system intervention might be more humane than lifelong incarceration or death? I do not wish to propose specific guidelines to allow or disallow any form of direct intervention. Nevertheless, given what we now understand about the role of emotion in reason, perhaps the time has come to give such guidelines a calm and thorough reconsideration. (2002, pp. 235–236)

## Preventing psychopathy

Given the pervasive social and economic cost and harm resulting from psychopathy, we should consider whether intervening in the brains of those deemed at high risk of developing the disorder could prevent it. Such preventive interventions could be given to children or adolescents whose genetic and behavioral traits strongly suggest a predisposition to psychopathy. Direct brain interventions could significantly reduce the cost and harm from the disorder by promoting prosocial behavior. This is still only a hypothesis, but one worth exploring. In Chapter 8, I will offer a more extensive discussion of interventions that might prevent psychiatric disorders in general. Here I focus exclusively on some possible ways of preventing psychopathy.

Studies conducted by Essi Viding and coauthors have shown that psychopathic traits are already present in childhood (Viding, Blair, Moffitt et al., 2005; Viding and McCrory, 2013; Viding, Price, Jaffee et al., 2013). Many children with these traits start offending at an early age and continue offending over the course of their lives. The offenses are often predatory, displaying both reactive and instrumental aggression. Viding and coauthors claim that "exhibiting high levels of callous-unemotional traits at 7 years of age, as assessed by teachers at the end of the first year of school, is under strong genetic influence" (Viding, Blair, Moffitt et al., 2005, p. 595). They further claim, "anti-social behavior for children who are high on the callous-unemotional (CU) scale is highly heritable" (2005, p. 596). Recent studies by Blair indicate that genetic and prenatal factors contribute to abnormally reduced volume in the PFC and striatum. This finding correlates with the callous–unemotional and impulsive–antisocial characteristics of psychopathy (Blair, 2013a, 2013b). Still the extent to which current genetic research can inform prediction of criminal behavior is fraught with uncertainty (Morse, 2011).

Commenting on the heritability of psychopathy, Viding and Eamon McCrory point out, "there are no *genes* for CU traits. Instead, we know that genes act in a probabilistic manner and in concert with environmental factors to make some individuals more vulnerable for developing CU traits" (2013, p. 164). These authors also state, "the legal system considers the probability of a given individual being guilty as well as the likelihood that he or she might re-offend. While they may use *population* or *group* data to inform this judgment, this is very different from behavioral genetic research. Such research focuses on the causes of *individual* differences and is concerned with determining the risk for a single individual" (2013, p. 164, emphasis added). Still, if psychopathic traits and behavior are highly heritable, and if they could be altered by psychopharmacology, then using drugs to change their brains might prevent individuals from developing the disorder and causing harm to others. Recent arguments that psychopathy should be considered a diagnostic category of a disorder in child psychiatry could support this type of intervention (Rutter, 2012).

As psychopathy correlates with abnormalities in cortical–limbic pathways, a psychotropic drug that might modulate these developing pathways in children and adolescents at risk of having the disorder could be a strategy for preventing full-blown psychopathy. Most children and many adolescents lack sufficient decisional capacity to consent to this intervention. Parents would have to give proxy consent to them on the child's behalf. The child should be able to assent to any intervention in his brain by participating in the discussion of how and by what means brain and behavior modification would occur. Because chronic use of psychotropic drugs may have unpredictable long-term effects on a child's or adolescent's developing brain, parents making decisions for and medical professionals treating them would have to weigh the potential benefits of early psychopharmacological intervention against potential adverse effects at a later time. Another factor to consider in making such a decision is that the presence of certain traits associated with psychopathy early in life would not necessarily predict future psychopathic behavior. As Morse points out, the brain of a child or adolescent deemed at risk of developing psychopathy could be altered unnecessarily based on false-positive predictions (2008, 2009). One cannot assume that any brain alteration would be beneficial. Among other processes, it could interfere with a normal degree of synaptic pruning and myelination and result in different forms of neural dysregulation and mental impairment.

Noninvasive interventions such as psychotherapy would be safer and less ethically controversial. Psychotherapy could have moderate effects on these neurodevelopmental processes and not likely result in permanent sequelae in the brain. It would be a safer intervention than pharmacotherapy. As noted, though, the efficacy of psychotherapy depends on a certain level of cognitive capacity. It is questionable how effective psychotherapy would be if the individual's frontal lobes and the cognitive capacities they mediate are not yet fully developed.

Estimating the biological risk of psychopathy in children or adolescents could potentially lead to discrimination against these individuals by labelling them as likely future criminal offenders. It could be especially harmful because it would not just apply to the individual at one stage of his life but at all stages. Prospective employers could use this information to limit a person's ability to secure and maintain employment. In this and other respects, the designation of being at risk for psychopathy could have a significant negative impact on the quality of his life. It would be unjustifiable to treat people with psychotropic drugs based solely on the probability of criminal behavior because this probability may not be actualized. Whether or not at-risk individuals display this behavior depends on a complex set of biological and social factors (Singh and Rose, 2009; Baum and Savulescu, 2013). Accordingly, legislation should be in place to ensure accurate interpretation and limit the use of biological information indicating probable criminal behavior. This is necessary to prevent misuse of this information and protect children, adolescents, and adults with certain behavioral traits from unfair discrimination.

Suppose that neuroimaging showed brain abnormalities in a child with psychopathic traits who had engaged in harmful behavior. A psychotropic drug could safely and effectively modulate these abnormalities. Suppose further that his parents refused to allow the drug to be given to him, even if it could prevent additional harmful behavior. Could the state forcibly administer the drug to the child for this purpose? The state could cite the public threat and social cost from psychopathy, the child's harmful behavior, and the safety and efficacy of the drug in preventing harmful acts to justify this action. The state could also cite the positive reason of promoting prosocial behavior in the child and enabling him to become a fully functioning member of society. These reasons would constitute a paternalistic argument for involuntary brain intervention on the basis that the child lacked the cognitive capacity to know what was in his best interests. It would also be paternalistic if the parents' rejection of the proposed treatment indicated that they were not acting in the best interests of their child. But "best interests" would have to be qualified by the probability that the changes in the brain induced by chronic use of the drug could be permanent and not salutary or benign.

Some might argue that involuntary neurointervention in a child would be categorically wrong, even if the child had a history of harmful behavior. They would argue that the child was vulnerable because he lacked decisional capacity to accept or refuse an intervention in his brain. An involuntary neurointervention would violate his intrinsic dignity and worth. Yet not intervening at an early age when he was at high risk of developing full-blown psychopathy and waiting until late adolescence or adulthood may preclude the potential for positive behavior modification. This point must be made with the caveat about the child's still-developing brain. Given the incomplete understanding of the long-term effects of brain-altering drugs, forced treatment in these cases could be justified only if the child or adolescent had already committed violent acts of aggression, there was a very high risk of further aggression, and studies indicated that the drug was safe and effective. The aggression could be a strong predictor of future violent behavior and warrant forced treatment. Any right of the child or parent to refuse the intervention could be overridden. The child's past and predictable future behavior could make public interest in avoiding harm outweigh individual interest in avoiding a direct brain intervention. This might eventually make the child more responsive to prudential and moral reasons as he lived into adolescence and adulthood. But the consequentialist argument to prevent harm to others may be sufficient to justify forced intervention in this hypothetical case.

## Conclusion

Psychopathy is a personality disorder affecting a significant percentage of the human population and resulting in significant personal harm and social cost. While there are open empirical questions about efficacy, theoretically psychotropic drugs could modify dysfunctional cortical–limbic pathways in the brains of criminal psychopaths, promote prosocial behavior, and significantly reduce the probability of violent aggression and recidivism. A drug proven to be safe and effective could be offered to a criminal psychopath to reduce a prison sentence without coercing her into accepting it. The offender could also be noncoercively offered the opportunity to participate in an experimental study testing the safety and efficacy of a drug for this particular disorder. This would assume that she gave informed consent to participate and that doing so did not expose her to unreasonable risk.

Forcibly prescribing a brain- and behavior-modifying drug would be more difficult to defend if the individual posed no risk of harm to herself or others while incarcerated. While forcing one to participate in a drug trial with significant known or unknown risks would not be defensible, forcing one to take a drug might be defensible if it was safe and more cost-effective than incarceration. It might also be defensible if, after prison release, it prevented harm to others and rehabilitated and reintegrated the person into society. In the case of children, forcibly prescribing a drug for prevention of violent aggression associated with psychopathy could be justified only if the child had already committed violent acts of aggression and was likely to commit additional aggressive acts in the future. Even if criminal psychopathic behavior could be modified by direct brain interventions, and the psychopath became more responsive to moral reasons and social norms, it is not obvious that he would be accepted within the community. The thought that a person with a history of psychopathy lived next door might not be very comforting for many people. Social reintegration of criminal offenders can be difficult to achieve.

The freedom of thought objection to direct brain interventions for criminal offenders is grounded in the idea that it violates the offender's cognitive liberty. This objection cannot be sustained in the case of the criminal psychopath if his thought is so impaired that it is not free. There would not be any violation of mental integrity if his mental states were so disordered as to indicate the absence of any such integrity. Safe and effective psychopharmacological therapy may be justified in these cases, even if the offender refuses and it has to be forced on him. It may also be justified if the public interest in avoiding additional harmful actions by the criminal psychopath outweighed his right to noninterference in his brain. The intervention could not plausibly be described as a violation of his will if his capacity for reasoning and decision-making was so impaired that he was no longer an autonomous agent in any substantive sense of the term.

It is important to emphasize that, to date, no empirical studies have shown that any brain-altering drugs could reduce or prevent psychopathic traits and criminal behavior. Changing the psychopath's thought and behavior with psychotropic drugs or neuromodulating techniques is still hypothetical. Whether these drugs or techniques would result in a positive change requires a better understanding of the neural circuits and pathways mediating cognitive-emotional processing, as well as how dysfunction in these circuits and pathways manifests in disordered thought and behavior. Many clinical trials testing the effects of drugs or techniques on the brain and mind in different cohorts would be necessary to achieve this goal. Still, modulating the neural underpinning of psychopathy is in principle possible and could have a significant impact on neurocriminology and forensic psychiatry in the future (Sadoff, 2015).

Beneficial modification of a psychopath's dysfunctional brain and behavior as a form of rehabilitation would be preferable to the current practice of prolonged adult incarceration or juvenile detention. Ultimately, whether intervening in the criminal psychopath's brain could be justified would require a careful weighing of his presumptive right to noninterference against the interests of society in avoiding harm.

# Chapter 7

# Euthanasia and assisted suicide for psychiatric disorders

A number of jurisdictions have legalized EAS for competent patients with terminal diseases. While the most common condition generating requests for EAS is cancer, an increasing number of requests have come from people with neurodegenerative diseases such as amyotrophic lateral sclerosis or severe forms of multiple sclerosis. In all of these cases, death is reasonably foreseeable. Legalization means that the act of causing or assisting in a patient's death is decriminalized and that medical professionals cannot be prosecuted for these actions. EAS is morally justified when it is consistent with a competent person's persistent wish to end her life. This is grounded in the principle of individual autonomy and the right to control the time and manner of one's death. A patient may request euthanasia when she has a desire to die and the cognitive capacity to form a plan to end her life, but lacks the physical or volitional capacity to implement that plan. A patient may request assisted suicide when she has these capacities but lacks the pharmacological or other means to do it on her own.

If EAS is morally and legally permissible for physical diseases when they are treatment-resistant and involve unbearable suffering, and if some psychiatric diseases are treatment-resistant and involve unbearable suffering, then in principle EAS should be morally and legally permissible for psychiatric diseases as well. One can make this claim even though people with severe psychiatric disorders are not imminently dying. The psychiatric disorder most often cited in this debate is treatment-resistant depression (TRD). Treatment-resistance is defined as failure to achieve remission despite adequate treatment (Holtzheimer and Mayberg, 2010, p. 1438). To permit EAS for a patient with cancer but prohibit it for a patient with severe MDD, OCD, or bipolar depression would be unfair because it would involve unequal treatment of patients with needs that were equal in all medically and morally relevant respects. This would increase the burden on people with intractable psychiatric disorders and cause additional harm to them by preventing them from ending their lives. Using this line of reasoning, Udo Schuklenk and Suzanne van de Vathorst argue that "limiting access to assisted dying to people with incurable *physical* illnesses unjustly discriminates against competent people who struggle with *psychiatric* illnesses that render their lives not worth living to them and that motivate them to request assistance in dying" (2015a, p. 577).

Some psychiatrists and ethicists have questioned the grounds for permitting EAS for psychiatric disorders. Diseases of the brain and mind are fundamentally different from diseases of the body. This difference has significant ethical implications for the permissibility or impermissibility of these practices in psychiatry. The controversy over EAS for psychiatric disorders is based on two main concerns. First, unlike physical diseases, in psychiatric diseases the desire to end one's life may be a symptom of the disorder itself. A request for EAS may be part of a pathology and a reflection of impaired cognition and emotion. A psychiatric patient may lack the mental capacity necessary to make an informed and autonomous decision about ending his life. Second, because psychiatric disorders are not terminal and can persist for years, some have questioned whether they are truly treatment-resistant. Even in cases where a patient has not responded to all available treatments, the possibility of new safe and effective therapies warrants caution in describing a psychiatric disorder as "untreatable" or "treatment-resistant" and evaluating requests for EAS from psychiatric patients on these grounds.

Having a psychiatric disorder does not necessarily undermine a person's decisional capacity. Some people with these disorders may retain a sufficient degree of capacity to make an autonomous and informed request for EAS. Disorders with psychotic or manic episodes involve cognitive impairment that can preclude the capacity to process information and make decisions based on that information. Accordingly, I exclude psychotic depression, BD with frequent manic episodes, and the positive subtype of schizophrenia from consideration of EAS. In Chapter 4, I suggested that some people with schizophrenia may have enough cognitive capacity to consent to participate in a DBS clinical trial. The stakes in EAS are much higher. It requires a higher level of cognitive and emotional capacity to appreciate the magnitude of an action that will end one's life.

The fact that psychiatric disorders are not terminal could mean that waiting for a new treatment that may, or may not, be effective would prolong suffering and increase the burden of a disorder on the patient. Bonnie Steinbock points out that "the terminal-illness requirement forces those who have an incurable illness but who are not terminally ill to suffer much longer than those who are terminally ill" (Steinbock, 2017, p. 39). This is the main point driving the argument from unfairness regarding different assessments of psychiatric and nonpsychiatric patients requesting euthanasia or assisted dying. Beyond a certain point, a person competent enough to weigh the benefits and burdens of continuing life with a mental illness against preventing further suffering by ending his life may rationally decide on the latter. Nevertheless, there is something ethically fraught and even paradoxical about the idea of a psychiatrist participating in EAS whose goal in treating patients has been to prevent them from committing suicide. It raises fundamental questions about the role of the psychiatrist in providing optimal care and the meaning of acting in a patient's best interests.

The permissibility of EAS for patients with psychiatric disorders depends on four conditions. First, the patient must be competent enough to weigh reasons for and against EAS. Second, the patient must make an informed and persistent request for it based on these reasons. Third, the suffering the patient experiences from the disorder must be unbearable and interminable. Fourth, the disorder must be resistant to all indicated treatments given to the patient over many years. A corollary to the fourth condition is that there must be a reasonable limit to the time a competent patient could be expected to wait for a new treatment that might relieve symptoms. When these conditions obtain, a request for EAS by some patients with MDD, OCD, or other conditions can be rational, and dying can be in their best interests. Psychiatrists are permitted (but not obligated) to act on the request if the conditions just described have been met.

Psychiatric research is always open to the possibility of new therapies for severe psychiatric disorders that could modulate brain dysfunction and ameliorate symptoms. But the probability of a positive response to any such therapy may be low when there has been no response to many treatments for many years. The chronicity of the disorder may result in permanent degenerative effects on neural circuits and the mental states they mediate. The pathophysiology may be too advanced to be amenable to neuromodulation. There is also the subjective aspect of how these factors influence the patient's expectation of symptom relief. The longer the disorder has been resistant to treatment, and the greater the number of treatments that have been tried and failed, the more likely it is that the patient will have a low expectation of even partial remission and symptom relief from a new treatment. This can contribute to hopelessness and increase suffering. In some cases, it may lead competent patients to desire and make a rational, deliberative request for EAS. This could be a rational judgment for *any* person with *any* unbearable and untreatable disease—physical *or* psychiatric. At least some patients who have suffered for many years from major depression may retain enough cognitive capacity to make a sufficiently informed and autonomous decision to end their life and request EAS to do this. If a patient has a psychiatric disorder that has been and is likely to remain treatment-resistant, and if EAS is the only way to relieve a patient's suffering, then EAS can be morally justified.

## Definitions, data, and criteria for euthanasia and assisted suicide for psychiatric disorders

Euthanasia or physician-assisted suicide for medical conditions is legally practiced in the Netherlands, Belgium, Luxembourg, and Columbia. Physician-assisted suicide, or assisted dying, is legal in Switzerland, Canada, and the US states of Oregon, Washington, Montana, Vermont, California, Colorado, Hawaii, and the District of Columbia. On November 29, 2017, Victoria became the first Australian state to legalize assisted dying for the terminally ill. In a review of attitudes toward and practices of euthanasia and physician-assisted suicide in Europe and North America, Ezekiel Emanuel and coauthors found that public support for them in Western Europe has increased. But it has plateaued in the United States since the Oregon Death with Dignity Act of 1997 (Emanuel, Onwuteaka-Philipsen, Urwin et al., 2016). Less than 20% of physicians in the United States report having received requests for assisted suicide, and 5% or less acted on these requests. In Oregon and Washington, less than 1% of physicians have written prescriptions for lethal doses of barbiturates or other drugs for assisted suicide each year since legalization in the first state in 1997 and the second in 2008. In the Netherlands and Belgium, approximately 50% of physicians reported having received requests for EAS, and in the Netherlands 60% complied with them. The frequency of requests for EAS in the Netherlands has increased since legalization with the Termination of Life on Request and Assisted Suicide Act of 2002.

The typical patient requesting EAS for all medical conditions is older, well educated, and white. In all jurisdictions, more than 70% of requests were from patients with terminal cancer. Most patients do not report pain as the primary motivation for ending their lives. Many patients in Oregon and Washington requesting assisted suicide and those in Belgium requesting euthanasia were enrolled in hospice or palliative care. This is a significant fact that debunks the view held by many that EAS is incompatible with palliative care (Quill and Battin, 2004a; Bernheim and Raus, 2016; Quill, Back, and Block, 2016). It refutes the belief that allowing the first undermines the second. It also refutes the belief that allowing EAS might increase the incidence of non-voluntary death in vulnerable patients whose disease impairs their decisional capacity. Emanuel and coauthors conclude, "In no jurisdiction was there evidence that vulnerable patients have been receiving euthanasia or physician-assisted suicide at rates higher than those in the general population" (Emanuel, Onwuteaka-Philipsen, Urwin et al., 2016, p. 79).

The 30% of requests for EAS from patients who did not have terminal cancer were from those with non-terminal cancer, neurodegenerative disorders such as amyotrophic lateral sclerosis or multiple sclerosis, and psychiatric disorders. "Although the numbers remain small, psychiatric EAS is becoming more frequent. In the Netherlands, a 1999 study estimated that the annual number was between 2 and 5, and in 2013 there were 42 reported cases" (Kim, DeVries and Peteet, 2016, p. 363). In 2002, Belgium became the first country in which mental suffering caused by a somatic or mental disorder could be a valid basis for euthanasia. While Belgium, the Netherlands and Luxembourg are the only countries in which EAS is legal for psychiatric disorders, Canada is reviewing the possibility of expanding medical assistance in dying to patients whose sole medical condition is mental illness. Bill C-14 was introduced in Canada in June of 2016 following a 2015 Supreme Court of Canada ruling (*Carter v. Canada,* 2015) on the legality of medical assistance in dying. At that time, the law permitting this practice extended only to mentally competent adults who were suffering unbearably from an advanced and irreversible condition, and where a natural death was reasonably foreseeable.

Part of the controversy over permitting physician-assisted suicide in Canada for people with mental illness who retain competence is that they do not meet the criterion of a reasonably foreseeable death. The federal government has asked the Council of Canadian Academies to report on how the law might be extended to adults and mature minors with mental illness, as well as to those with early-stage dementia. The case of Canadian Adam Maier-Clayton, a 27-year-old man with OCD who took his life in April of 2017 highlights the ethically and legally charged issue of medically assisted death for people with severe psychological distress due to mental illness (Franzoi, 2017). Mr. Maier-Clayton advocated for people with severe psychiatric disorders to have this more humane and easeful option over individual attempts at suicide. When they are unsuccessful, as in failed carbon monoxide poisoning, these attempts may result in a neurologically disabled state and additional suffering for the patient.

In a retrospective analysis of requests, procedures and outcomes of euthanasia for 100 Belgian patients suffering from psychiatric disorders, Lieve Thienpont and coauthors cite the Belgian Euthanasia Law (BEL) of 2002. This defines euthanasia as "the act of deliberately ending a patient's life at the latter's request" (Thienpont, Verhofstadt, Van Loon et al., 2015, p. 1). This is typically executed by administering a lethal dose of drugs such as barbiturates. Death may also result from terminal sedation inducing a permanent coma. The Law requires that the patient should be at least 18 years of age and competent at the time of the request. The request must be voluntary and well-considered. It must be clearly and repeatedly expressed over an extended period. It must not arise from coercion or any form of external pressure. The patient should be in a "medically hopeless condition of constant and unbearable physical or mental suffering, which cannot be cured and is a consequence of a severe and incurable disorder caused by accident or disease" (2015, p. 2).

To ensure that these five criteria have been met, the patient's treating psychiatrist must consult with an independent psychiatrist not involved in the patient's care. If the patient is not terminally ill and is not expected to die in the foreseeable future, then a third physician, specifically a psychiatrist or specialist in the disorder at issue, must be consulted to assess the patient's mental state. Psychiatric review should be required in evaluating all requests for EAS (McCormack and Price, 2014; McCormack and Flechais, 2012). If the treating psychiatrist refuses to assist the patient in dying or perform euthanasia on grounds of conscience or principle, then she must inform the patient as soon as possible to allow the patient to approach another psychiatrist who might be willing to do it (Naudts, Ducatelle, Kovacs et al., 2006). The patient must make the request for euthanasia in writing, and it must be documented in the patient's file. When euthanasia occurs, the case is reviewed by a federal evaluation committee. These conditions are standard in all jurisdictions allowing these practices.

Thienpont and coauthors note: "In Europe, psychological suffering stemming from either a somatic or mental disorder is acknowledged as a valid legal basis for euthanasia only in Belgium, the Netherlands and Luxembourg. In the Netherlands and Luxembourg, the term 'assisted suicide' is used when life-ending drugs are taken orally, but in Belgium the term 'euthanasia' is used when the drugs are received orally or intravenously" (Thienpont, Verhofstadt, Van Loon et al., 2015, p. 3). Depression and personality disorders are the most common diagnoses in psychiatric patients requesting euthanasia. The Belgian Euthanasia Law states that requests for euthanasia from competent adults or 'emancipated minors' (legally independent from their parents) suffering from "unbearable and untreatable" somatic and psychiatric disorders can be granted to terminally ill as well as nonterminally ill patients. In September 2016, a 17-year-old male was the first minor to receive euthanasia in Belgium for a disease causing "unbearable physical suffering" (Duncan, 2016). He died from terminal palliative sedation. In both Belgium and the Netherlands, the parent or guardian of a mature minor cannot override the patient's request; but they must consult with the physician participating in the action. An important question is whether physical suffering should be on a par with mental suffering. If both types of suffering harm patients, then in principle there is no ethically or legally significant difference between them and they should be treated equally. EAS can be justified to prevent further harm to psychiatric patients who experience unbearable and untreatable mental suffering.

"Unbearable suffering," or indeed any form of suffering, is subjective and depends on the perspective of the patient. An "untreatable" psychiatric disorder is an objective determination that fails to meet the following three requirements articulated by the Dutch Psychiatric Association in 2009. First, treatment must offer a real prospect of improvement. Second, it must be possible to administer adequate treatments within a reasonable period. Third, there must be a reasonable balance between the expected treatment results and the burden of treatment consequences for the patient (Tholen, Berghmans, Huisman et al., 2009; also cited by Thienpont, Verhofstadt, Van Loon et al., 2015, p. 2). Significantly, the second requirement implies that it would be unreasonable to expect a patient suffering from a treatment-resistant condition to wait indefinitely for a therapy that may or may not become available in the future. I will return to this issue in discussing the arguments for and against EAS.

Psychiatric diagnoses necessary for allowing and acting on requests for EAS for mental illness in the Belgian Euthanasia Law were based on the *DSM-IV* classification. Thienpont and coauthors further state that, according to the Law: "A patient is considered to be in a medically futile situation, or treatment-resistant, if the suffering is unbearable and untreatable, and there is no prospect of any improvement" (Thienpont, Verhofstadt, Van Loon et al., 2015, p. 1). Physician and patient must both come to the conclusion that there is no remaining alternative to relieve the patient's suffering. "If the psychiatrist has reason to believe that the patient could experience further benefit from treatment options, then life-ending options cannot be granted" (Thienpont, Verhofstadt, Van Loon et al., 2015, p. 2). The most significant point is the connection between "unbearable" and "untreatable." This underscores the connection between mental suffering and treatment-resistance. These determinations in turn are linked to the criterion of "adequate treatments within a reasonable period."

In a review of 66 cases of EAS for patients with psychiatric disorders in the Netherlands, Scott Kim, Raymond DeVries, and John Peteet highlight a number of factors suggesting that a significant number of requests for and completion of EAS may have failed to meet the Dutch criteria for the practice (2016). Many of the patients cited in the review had personality disorders or a history of substance abuse. Some had comorbidities with functional impairments, including PTSD, anxiety, eating disorders, and autism. These conditions may be conflated with and complicate judgments about whether depression or a different disorder is treatable or untreatable. Among physicians performing EAS on these patients, 41% were psychiatrists, and 27% of the patients received EAS from physicians with whom they did not have a continuous relationship (Kim, DeVries, and Peteet, 2016, p. 362).

Paul Appelbaum also draws attention to a number of problems in this review, raising concern that some or many of these cases failed to meet the Dutch criteria for EAS. He notes that personality disorders are "often associated with strong reactivity to environmental or interpersonal stresses" (Appelbaum, 2016, p. 325). This raises the question of the stability of a patient's request for EAS. It seems to indicate an impulsive rather than deliberative desire and request to end one's life. The fact that 38% of the Belgian patients in the review by Thienpont and coauthors who asked for physician assistance withdrew their request to die before the evaluation was completed suggests that a significant number of them did not have a stable desire to end their life. In addition, Appelbaum points out that social isolation and loneliness, which were mentioned in 56% of the cases in the review by Kim, DeVries and Peteet, could be mitigated by psychosocial interventions (2016, p. 325). Another problem with the presumed treatment-resistance motivating requests for EAS was that many patients refused at least some recommended treatments. Analyses have suggested that some physicians may be stretching the criteria to meet the perceived needs of patients, and others are uncomfortable with some of the requests (Snijdewind, van Tol, Onwuteaka-Philipsen et al., 2018; Quill, 2018).

Neither the data from Kim and coauthors' review nor the questions raised in light of it indicate that EAS is theoretically flawed and not ethically or legally justifiable. Instead, they underscore the need to distinguish psychiatric disorders from other disorders and determine which are treatable or untreatable. They also underscore the need for continuous psychiatric care. Psychiatrists must carefully assess competence and ensure that patients with these disorders meet all other ethical and legal criteria for EAS when they make a request for a physician to end or help them end their lives. A psychiatrist must strictly follow a rigorous evaluation process to justify EAS for psychiatric patients (Vandenberghe, 2018). There are some cases in which the criteria for EAS have not been met. But there are other cases in which they have been met and the practice is permissible.

## Pain and three types of suffering

We need to distinguish between pain and suffering as well as three distinct types of suffering to understand how these mental states motivate requests for euthanasia and physician-assisted dying. Although some accounts describe pain as having both physical and emotional properties, at the most basic level pain consists of nociception, or "physical responsiveness to noxious stimulation"

(Demertzi and Laureys, 2012, p. 89; Wager, Atlas, Lindquist et al., 2013; Prescott, Ma, and De Koninck, 2014). One account of suffering defines it as a "state of severe distress associated with events threatening the intactness of the person" (Cassell, 1991, pp. 35–36). Nociception may involve conscious or unconscious responses to stimuli without involving the experience of suffering. This can occur in cases where a patient has lost the capacity for self-awareness. Based on neuroimaging studies using PET and fMRI, Athena Demertzi and Steven Laureys explain that pain perception is grounded in two distinct but related neural networks mediating physical and emotional aspects of pain. There is a lateral pain system or sensory network consisting of lateral thalamic nuclei and somatosensory and parietal cortices. There is also a medial pain system or affective network consisting of the medial thalamus, anterior cingulate, and prefrontal and insular cortices (Demertzi and Laureys, 2012, p. 89).

One can experience pain without suffering, and one can suffer without experiencing pain. Unlike pain, suffering is not traceable to a neural network or connections between the CNS and peripheral nervous system. As a subjective experience, it depends on a certain degree of cortical and subcortical brain function mediating different aspects of awareness. But it also depends on how one's experiential history shapes one's psychological responses to environmental stimuli as well as to one's own bodily and mental states.

Some have described the experience of a person with an unrelenting psychiatric disorder as "psychic pain." This may be interchangeable with suffering. It may be associated with a psychiatric disorder or a psychological response to physical injury or chronic pain syndromes (Yager, 2015). Many psychiatric disorders have somatic symptoms. Patients with depression, for example, often report feeling headaches, joint and muscle pain, nausea, fatigue, and loss of appetite (*DSM-IV-TR*) (American Psychiatric Association, 2000, p. 349; Ratcliffe, Broome, Smith et al., 2014). As Kleinman has noted, there is a "predominance of somatic symptoms" in some non-western narratives of depression (1988, p. 41). While there is variability in the incidence and subtypes of these symptoms among different cultures, there are commonalities among patients with this disorder in all cultures. Symptoms can vary among cultures and reflect different responses of affected persons to their natural, cultural, and social environments. Many patients with somatic diseases such as cancer suffer in response to pain, a perceived threat to their bodily integrity, or the loss of control and dignity caused by the disease. But suffering from a psychiatric disorder has a distinctive phenomenology that sets it apart from suffering from somatic diseases. Patients with a severe psychiatric disorder report feelings of emptiness, meaninglessness, and despair with greater intensity than patients with cancer or amyotrophic lateral sclerosis report of their experiences. Although pain and loss of control from a somatic disease can cause distress and threaten the intactness of the person, mental disease can disrupt the very source of one's thought and behavior by disrupting the brain–mind relation. The difficulty in trying to describe and convey the phenomenology of mental illness to others, and the distress from the inability to convey this feeling, can exacerbate the suffering.

Kay Redfield Jamison, who has chronicled her experience of depressive episodes in bipolar disorder, attempts to describe what it is like for a person to live with the interminable and unbearable suffering they cause. "Suicidal depression involves a kind of pain and hopelessness that is impossible to describe—and I have tried . . . How can you say what it feels like to go from being someone who loves life to wishing only to die? Suicidal depression is a state of cold, agitated horror and relentless despair. The things that you most love in life leach away. Everything is an effort, all day and throughout the night. There is no hope, no point, no nothing. There is no way out and an endless road ahead. When someone is in this state, suicide can seem a bad choice but the only one" (2014, A19, cited in Schuklenk and van de Vathorst, 2015a, p. 579). William Styron wrote that his experience with unipolar depression was "close to, but indescribably different from, actual pain" (1992, p. 14). Andrew Solomon expresses his own experience with depression. "In depression, the meaninglessness of every enterprise and every emotion, the meaninglessness of life itself, becomes self-evident. The only feeling left in this loveless state is insignificance" (2001, p. 15).

One of the most significant findings in the review of Emanuel and coauthors is that patients did not report pain as the primary motivation for requesting EAS for diseases in general. Other accounts indicate that requests for EAS are motivated by loss of control of one's life, loss of dignity, and the feeling of being a burden on others (Quill, Back, and Bloch, 2015). Suffering may be a natural response to these feelings. But the phenomenology of a psychiatric disorder such as bipolar depression, as described by Jamison, points to an unrelenting mental intensity suffusing the content of the affected person's awareness. This distinguishes it from the suffering from somatic disorders. It is not so much the loss of control of one's life but the more fundamental desire for relief from unbearable and interminable suffering that drives requests for EAS for psychiatric disorders.

These considerations may explain why improved palliative care may not meet the needs of patients with severe, treatment-resistant psychiatric disorders. Nor would it likely weaken the motivation for those with these disorders to request EAS. Palliative care controls primary somatic symptoms such as pain and secondary symptoms such as anxiety and suffering in response to pain. By controlling these symptoms, palliative care can restore some degree of a patient's feeling of control of her remaining life. Because the suffering in psychiatric disorders is primary, directly related to brain–mind dysfunction and distinct from the suffering associated with physical pain, palliative care may not relieve it and change a person's attitude about living or dying. Palliative care may not be appropriate for a patient whose symptoms are resistant to all treatments, who is not imminently dying and who may continue living for years.

Gerrit Kimsma distinguishes three types of suffering driving requests for EAS in the Netherlands: physical, mental, and existential (2006, p. 1, 2012). Physical suffering involves a response to somatic diseases. It is not "physical" in the strict sense because suffering is not equivalent to the perception of pain. Suffering has emotional and volitional components as well as a cognitive one. Mental suffering from a psychiatric disorder can result from symptoms caused by the dysregulated neural circuitry of the disease and one's psychological response to them. Part of this response may be the anticipation of continued, interminable suffering— what Jamison describes as "an endless road ahead." Existential suffering consists in being "tired with life" and lacking a desire to continue living. It is typically characterized as an attitude of people who do not have a life-threatening or serious disease. They may have one or more chronic medical conditions adversely affecting their quality of life. While existential suffering may be the result of major depression, it need not be. Nor is it traceable to any type of neural circuit dysfunction implicated in MDD or other major psychiatric disorders. Specifically, it is not a form of severe anhedonia or avolition traceable to a dysfunctional NAc or other regions in the mesolimbic dopamine reward system.

Major psychiatric disorders are not just brain disorders. But varying degrees of brain dysfunction are implicated in all of them. Reports from people requesting EAS to end their existential suffering suggest that these requests are more likely symptomatic of social isolation and loneliness than brain dysfunction. Existential suffering is not a symptom of a psychiatric disease but a type of despair (Rurup, 2012; van der Lee, 2012). There is an existential aspect to the mental suffering from psychiatric disorders. Yet this suffering is more than a subjective response to one's social situation or one or more chronic somatic diseases. Mental suffering and existential suffering need to be separated in evaluating reasons for or against EAS. Because existential suffering is not the direct result of a psychiatric disorder, it does not meet the Belgian or Dutch criteria for EAS for psychiatric disorders and thus is not a valid basis for it.

Recall that, in the data reported by Kim and coauthors, 56% of requests for EAS were from patients who mentioned social isolation or loneliness as motivating factors in their requests (Kim, DeVries, and Peteet, 2016). It seems plausible to say that existential suffering triggered many of these requests. This is different from the "existential feeling" in the phenomenology of depression, as described by Matthew Ratcliffe (2015; Maiese, 2016; Ratcliffe and Stephen, 2014). This feeling pertains to the disrupted relation of the embodied self to the world (Ratcliffe, 2015, p. 10). In many cases, psychiatrists can identify symptoms associated with isolation and loneliness and separate them from symptoms directly associated with a psychiatric disorder. Psychosocial interventions can treat the second type of symptoms. These are more likely to be effective than therapies for depression because they can change the source of the isolation or loneliness. Depending on availability of and access to counseling and community support, social factors associated with existential suffering may be more amenable to treatment than neurobiological factors associated with mental suffering. This may be the case especially among the elderly, who report feeling socially isolated and lonely more often than any other age group.

Similar remarks apply to comorbidities that are often linked to depression, such as personality disorders and substance abuse. These can complicate questions about whether depression is treatment-resistant and whether the desire behind a request for EAS is impulsive rather than deliberative. Commenting on the fact that a majority of patients in the Netherlands who requested EAS reported social isolation and loneliness as the main reasons for their requests, Appelbaum states that this "evokes concern that physician-assisted death served as a substitute for psychosocial intervention and support" (2016, p. 325). These actions could mitigate mental distress and reduce the incidence of requests for EAS.

The psychosocial interventions Appelbaum mentions are particularly pertinent to requests for EAS from the elderly on grounds of existential suffering. In 2006, Kimsma cited data from interviews with 410 Dutch general practitioners who received 400 requests from people to end their lives despite not having a serious disease. Most of these people had lost a spouse or child and were single "with social problems" (Kimsma, 2006, p. 1). Distinguishing existential suffering due to psychosocial problems from mental suffering due to psychiatric disorders is critical because of the potential of interventions to resolve the first type of suffering. This distinction is also critical because it can enable psychiatrists to identify comorbidities, determine whether they can be separated from a psychiatric disorder, and focus on the neural and mental dysfunction underlying it. This can help to clarify whether depressive symptoms are associated with the disorder itself or are a response to conditions not directly related to depression. It can help to identify and prescribe potentially effective therapies and ascertain whether or to what extent the disorder is resistant to treatment.

Kimsma reported on the 1994 Dutch Supreme Court case of Dr. Boudewijn Chabot, who was acquitted from the criminal charge of assisting in the suicide of a woman who was not suffering from a terminal somatic disease. She wanted to end her life because of loneliness following a divorce and the deaths of her two sons. The Court ruled that one could experience unbearable suffering in the absence of a physical disease. There was a different ruling in the 2002 case of family physician Dr. Philip Sutorius, who ended the life of a patient who was "deeply affected by a slow physical deterioration, feelings of social isolation and existential emptiness" (Kimsma, 2006, p. 1). After weighing expert testimony regarding the medical profession's understanding of the concept of existential suffering, the Dutch Supreme Court reasoned that "a physician has no expertise to assess the un-bearable nature of a person's suffering; therefore, a physician who ends the life of such an individual cannot be exonerated" (cited by Kimsma, 2006, p. 3). Presumably, the reasons behind the ruling in the second case would have been the same if the physician had been a psychiatrist. These reasons would be consistent with the data and recommendations from the medical professional groups cited earlier in this chapter. Yet in October 2016, Health Minister Edith Schippers defended a measure before the Dutch Parliament that would allow people who are not suffering from a medical condition to seek assisted suicide if they feel that they have "completed life" (Bilefsky and Schuetze, 2016).

This measure raises some of the same issues that figured prominently in the 1994 and 2002 cases just cited. Here too one can question whether life fatigue, loneliness, or other forms of existential suffering would be sufficient rationales for requesting and receiving EAS. Again, if these experiences are amenable to psychosocial interventions, it is likely that in many cases individuals would lose the desire to end their lives and would not request EAS. Unless physicians, psychologists, and social workers could demonstrate that existential suffering could not be ameliorated by any neurobiological, psychological, or social interventions, the reasons for requesting EAS to end them would be weak. Performing EAS on these grounds would be unjustifiable.

While stating that he could not support euthanasia for existential reasons, Kimsma points out that "what complicates an assessment of unbearable suffering is that what some people find unbearable is not 'simply pain' but pain as shaped by their character and biography" (2006, p. 2, 2012). If existential suffering is not the consequence of any disease, then it seems that "pain" is being used metaphorically for social isolation and other feelings that are not symptoms of a psychopathology. Assuming that one's biography is to some extent within one's control, and one is capable of changing one's character, existential suffering is different from the mental suffering caused by brain diseases over which one has much less, if any, control. Insofar as one form of suffering is treatable and the other is treatment-resistant, existential suffering from psychosocial problems should be distinguished from mental suffering from a moderately severe to severe psychiatric disorder.

In some cases, it can be difficult to separate major depression from other psychiatric and neurological disorders that are comorbid and co-occurrent with MDD. The neural mechanisms underlying different disorders may interact and produce a similar symptomatology. Anxiety often overlaps with depression. Symptoms associated with GAD or different disorders may increase the mental distress from depression. As I explained in Chapter 1, depression may be an early prodromal symptom of PD (Gustafsson, Nordstrom, and Nordstrom, 2015). This disease may involve mood and motor disturbances at the same time. In addition, approximately 30% of stroke patients develop depression (Anderson, 2016). If the neurological and psychiatric symptoms overlap and cannot be separated, then this could make it difficult to effectively treat depression. Controlling depression and weakening a desire for EAS could be especially challenging if a treatment for MDD exacerbated symptoms of a co-occurrent neurological disorder, or if treatment for the neurological disorder exacerbated depressive symptoms. The symptoms resulting from the combination of TRD and an irreversible neurological disorder could increase a patient's psychic suffering. They could provide a stronger motivation and reason for EAS than cases in which a patient suffered from a single psychiatric disorder.

Still, justification for EAS would depend on whether or to what extent two or more neuropsychiatric disorders interfered with a person's capacity to weigh reasons for and against EAS. This would also depend on a psychiatric assessment of the patient. It seems plausible that at least in some cases, a patient with more than one disorder could retain enough cognitive and emotional capacity to make an informed and deliberated request for a physician to end, or assist him in ending, his life.

## Arguments for and against euthanasia and assisted suicide for psychiatric disorders

The argument for permitting EAS for patients with psychiatric disorders is an argument about fairness in moral assessments of suffering. If EAS is permitted for persons who suffer unbearably and interminably from physical diseases, and if persons with psychiatric diseases suffer unbearably and interminably, then EAS should be permitted for persons with psychiatric diseases. The classification of the disease type is not morally significant. What matters is the experience of persons affected by the disease. There is no moral justification for treating the two types of disease unequally in this regard. Not allowing EAS for patients with psychiatric disorders unjustly discriminates against and results in greater harm to them because it prolongs their suffering. Schuklenk and van de Vathorst spell out five conditions that should guide regulation of assisted suicide for psychiatric disorders:

(1) The patient is competent to evaluate their current situation.

(2) The patient is competent to evaluate their future prospects based on the scientific evidence available at the point in time when they request assistance in dying.

(3) The patient's decision is voluntary and informed.

(4) The patient's quality of life is such that they do not consider it worth living, and the likelihood of improvement is exceedingly small or nonexistent.

(5) The patient repeats their request over a reasonable period of time (2015a, p. 586).

Conditions (1)–(3) and (5) all pertain to competence. Condition (4) pertains to the treatment-resistant nature of the disorder. These criteria are consistent with the criteria of competence (capacity), informed and persistent request, unbearable and interminable suffering, and treatment-resistance that I specified for the justification of EAS. When these conditions obtain, a patient with a psychiatric disorder may have a low expectation of symptom relief and make a rational decision to request EAS. Because prolonged treatment-resistance and suffering motivate requests for EAS, a critical question is whether the patient has enough cognitive capacity to consider the probability of effective treatment and amelioration of symptoms in the foreseeable future. Many who object to EAS for psychiatric disorders argue that there *is* a medically and morally significant difference between physical and psychiatric diseases and base their arguments on the issue of competence. The difference is that psychiatric diseases involve dysfunction in the brain–mind relation, which is the source of cognitive and affective capacities necessary to process information and make decisions that are in one's best interests. It is questionable whether a patient with depression or any psychiatric disorder has the mental capacity necessary to make an informed and deliberated request for EAS.

Even when comorbidities such as personality disorders associated with strong reactivity to social stress can be separated from depression, some individuals with depression or other disorders may be impaired in the cognitive capacity for information processing and decision-making. This includes decisions about ending their lives. Again, though, competence is a graded property that comes in degrees. The nature and severity of different types and subtypes of psychiatric disorders can impair competence to varying degrees without completely undermining it. Many patients may retain a sufficient degree of cognitive capacity to assess their current condition and consider the possibility of a response to future therapies in weighing reasons for and against EAS. The claim that reasoning and decisional capacity obtain to different degrees is consistent with comments from authors who have addressed this issue in the context of psychiatric disorders.

In underscoring the need for stricter regulation of psychiatric EAS, Kim and coauthors state that "psychiatric disorders contribute to suicides (a major public health problem), can *sometimes* impair decision making, and are stigmatized" (Kim, DeVries, and Peteet, 2016, p. 363, emphasis added). In their commentary on the controversy of permitting euthanasia in patients with psychiatric illness, Emilie Olie and Philippe Courtet similarly state, "mental disease *may* alter a patient's judgment. Psychopathology does *not* automatically mean the patient lacks mental capacity, but is highly likely to influence decision making" (2016, p. 657, emphasis added). In addition, Appelbaum claims, "the desire to die is *often* part of the disorder" (p. 325, emphasis added). These comments support the view that not all individuals with psychiatric disorders are unable to make considered judgments about their condition and which actions should be taken in light of them. Although a sustained level of cognitive capacity may be less difficult to assess, in some cases a disorder may wax and wane between alternating periods of clear and clouded judgment. This is more likely to occur in psychiatric disorders with psychotic episodes. Whether a patient has a sufficient degree of mental capacity to understand her condition and appreciate the magnitude of requesting and receiving EAS is not generalizable. Psychiatric assessment must determine this in each particular case. Having a psychiatric disorder as such does not imply that one cannot make sufficiently informed decisions about how one should, or should not, be treated. At least some people with these disorders have this capacity and can make a reasoned and autonomous request for EAS.

Severe depression can affect a patient's capacity to make decisions about life-sustaining psychiatric treatment. But moderately severe depression does not necessarily distort or undermine this capacity in all cases. There may even be cases in which a severe form of the disorder does not distort it. Mark Sullivan and Stuart Youngner emphasize this point regarding treatment refusal: "Discriminating those cases in which depression impairs the capacity to make medical decisions from those cases in which it does not is best accomplished through a systematic approach to assessment of competence" (1994, p. 974). However, if a sufficiently competent patient with a desire to die requests ending life-sustaining treatment, then a psychiatrist must have offered appropriate treatment that failed to control her suffering before the psychiatrist could accede to her request. Sullivan and Youngner argue: "It must be assumed—unless proven otherwise—that adults are competent to evaluate their own quality of life as tolerable or intolerable . . . The burden of proof concerning competence should be on the clinician who is seeking to override a refusal of treatment. The desire to die is by itself not adequate evidence of incompetence" (1994, p. 976).

Does the right of a competent psychiatric patient to refuse life-sustaining treatment imply a right to assisted dying? Steinbock argues that it does:

> If a jurisdiction has legalized PAD [physician-assisted dying], the distinction between the right to refuse life-sustaining treatment and the right to an assisted death is no longer pertinent, since patients are entitled to both if they meet the eligibility criteria. Moreover, it is unclear why this distinction should be relevant to the evaluation of competence in patients with major depressive disorder. Given that the stakes are the same in both cases (namely, the death of the patient), it seems that the criteria for determining competence should also be the same. If patients can be competent to refuse life-sustaining treatment, then they are equally competent to request assistance in dying. Doubts about assessing competence either apply in both situations or in neither. (2017, p. 36)

Patients with treatment-resistant unipolar and bipolar depression, OCD, and the negative subtype of schizophrenia may have a desire to end their lives and the cognitive capacity to plan how it should end. Yet they may lack the volitional capacity to implement their action plan in requesting EAS. Some are so mentally impaired that they lack the cognitive capacity to even form such a plan. They may be unable to consider suicide. For example, at the lowest stage of his illness, Solomon states that "I was too dumbly lethargic even to conceptualize suicide" (2001, p. 19). In some cases, a psychiatric patient may be so cognitively and volitionally impaired as to be unable to request euthanasia or assisted dying from a physician. In other cases, he may have enough of these capacities to request euthanasia, and a psychiatrist or other medical professional then performs the action. A patient with greater cognitive and volitional capacity may be able to perform the final act with the physician's assistance. Questions about the patient's mental states are distinct from questions about the means through which physicians perform EAS. These different scenarios illustrate the spectrum of agency in patients with psychiatric disorders. They reflect differences in patients' cognitive, emotional, and volitional capacities to form and carry out an intention to end their lives. The agency in voluntary EAS also includes the ability to change one's mind and cancel the intention. A patient's control over whether his life continues or ends requires both abilities.

Suicidal ideation is often a symptom of psychiatric disorders. This ideation is often triggered by an impulsive desire associated with the psychopathology itself or from an emotional reaction to symptoms. This can be symptomatic of depression even when one excludes the strong emotional reactivity in personality disorders. In BD, the "rate of completed suicide is approximately 5% among patients who have never been hospitalized, but may be as high as 25% early in the course of the illness" (Frye, 2011, p. 51). This is the highest risk among psychiatric disorders. It may be due to the mixed manic and depressive states, the combination of "high energy and severely dysphoric mood and cognition" (Strakowski, 2014, p. 10). This is in stark contrast to those with unipolar depression characterized mainly by avolition, as expressed in Solomon's comment about being "too dumbly lethargic" to even consider suicide. The fact that the risk of suicide is higher at an early stage of the disease might suggest that it could be the result of impulsivity or emotional reactivity.

Paul McHugh and Phillip Slavney emphasize how these mental states may lead one to take one's life: "Suicide does, as many investigators have noted, involve aggression and is often impulsively carried out" (1998, p. 240). In addition to timely prescription of SSRIs for depression and lithium for BD, an effective way of suicide prevention is to increase the number of "acute psychiatric beds in general hospitals and in public mental health hospitals to provide immediate access to 24-hour care for both patient safety and stabilization" (Bastiampillai, Sharfstein, and Allison, 2016, p. 2592).

There is considerable variability among patients with psychiatric disorders regarding the risk of reactive suicide. McHugh and Slavney add, "the genetic propensity for impulsivity could explain why equally depressed individuals are not equally suicidal" (1998, p. 241). The genetics and epigenetics of unipolar and bipolar depression may explain why some individuals suffer mentally more than others or tolerate mental suffering better than others (Nestler, 2015). Not all desires to die in response to suffering from psychiatric disorders are impulsive. They are not all associated with acute disease onset or a relapse triggered by a psychological or psychosocial crisis. Nor do all of these desires imply a cognitive inability to rationally weigh the value and disvalue of continuing to live.

We need to distinguish an impulsive or temporary desire to die as a symptom of depression from a deliberative and persistent desire to die as a response to living with the disorder for an extended period. The longer one has lived with and suffered from a psychiatric disorder, the more likely a desire to end one's life will be deliberative rather than impulsive. As Schuklenk and Van de Vathorst express it, "a prolonged TRD creates a depressing reality by any stretch of the imagination" (2015a, p. 580). If the desire to die is deliberative and persists through a number of failed treatments, then it is less likely to be irrational and more likely to be rational. The patient may be competent enough to have insight into her condition and decide that ending her life would be preferable to continuing it. "Suffering from a psychiatric disease such as depression does not automatically preclude patients from being aware of what they are experiencing and of what their future prospects are" (Schuklenk and Van de Vathorst, 2015a, p. 579). Prolonged suffering can be compatible with competence when the disorder is ego-dystonic and the patient feels distressed by having experience she does not want to have. This may not be the case in psychotic depression when competence is absent or severely impaired and the patient lacks insight because the disorder is ego-syntonic.

An irrational choice is not necessarily indicative of noncompetence or incapacity (Brock and Wartman, 1990). In one form of motivated irrationality, people often display weakness of will in acting on inclinations they know are not in their best interests. They are competent enough to have this knowledge but fail to act in accord with it. Also, what may be an irrational choice for some with a particular belief and value system may be rational for others with a different system. The potential for harm in ending a person's life is significant, however, and therefore a request for EAS must be both competent and rational. Such a momentous decision must reflect the cognitive and emotional capacity to consider reasons for and against ending one's life, to consistently and coherently explain the motivation for wanting it, and to make it clear that it is in one's best interests.

Some authors have suggested that the judgment that a person with a psychiatric disorder would be better off dead may be a sign of impaired competence because it involves an incoherent comparison between being alive and being dead. The claim that a person is better or worse off at a later time than at an earlier time presupposes a comparison between two states of affairs in which the same person exists. We cannot coherently compare a person's welfare when she is living to her welfare when she is dead because she ceases to exist after she dies. Matthew Broome and Angharad de Cates cite a passage from the last section of Wittgenstein's *Tractatus Logico-Philosophicus* to underscore the presumed incoherence of such a comparison: "Death is not an event in life; we do not live to experience death" (Wittgenstein, 1961, 6.4311). Broome and de Cates claim that "the reason this idea of Wittgenstein's seems key is that for issues of competence and capacity, the decision maker has to weigh information about the outcome of their choices. Death is non-existence; epistemologically, there is no information about that prospect to be weighed alongside a continued suffering-filled existence" (2015, p. 586).

We can apply Shelly Kagan's reasoning to respond to this claim and support the coherence of requests for EAS for psychiatric disorders. If a person with such a disorder is cognitively and emotionally able to weigh the overall balance of pleasurable and painful experiences in his life, and the latter far outweigh the former, then he may conclude that he is so badly off that he would be "better off dead" (Kagan, 2012, pp. 330, 335). Despite what this conditional statement might suggest, the relevant comparison is not between the state of being alive and the state of being dead. A person cannot be "better off" in the second state because "she" does not exist in it. The relevant comparison underlying requests for EAS is not between existence and nonexistence, but between *continuing* a life filled with unbearable and interminable suffering and ending suffering by *ending* that life. The comparison is between a state of affairs in which the patient suffers and one in which the patient cannot suffer because she has ceased to exist. The fact that one cannot experience death is not what matters but that death will ensure that one can no longer experience suffering. At issue is not what occurs *after* death but what occurs *at* death. It ends a life of suffering. A patient who reasoned in this way would be making a coherent comparison between continuing and ending life. He would not be displaying impaired competence or irrationality in doing so.

A related question is whether suicide can be *morally* justified (Kagan, 2012, pp. 344–361). There are two aspects to this question applied to EAS for psychiatric disorders. The first pertains to the duty of care and professional autonomy of physicians asked to perform euthanasia or assist a patient in dying. I will address this in the next section of this chapter. The second aspect pertains to the effects that the suicide might have on others, and whether this imposes constraints on the person considering suicide when it is a rational choice for him. The *rationality* and *morality* of suicide may come apart, and this may affect the permissibility of suicide. For example, the responsibility of a father or mother to their dependent children could be a decisive reason against taking one's life because it could cause distress or other forms of harm to them. While those with an emotional relationship to the person who commits suicide or receives EAS are often harmed, in some cases they may benefit from knowing that his mental suffering has ended. Employing a consequentialist argument, Kagan spells out what he calls "a moderate conclusion" about the moral justification of suicide: "In certain circumstances suicide will be morally justified. Roughly speaking, it will be justified in those cases where you would be better off dead, and the effects on others aren't so great as to outweigh that fact" (2011, p. 352).

Mental suffering could release one from obligations to others. This may include suicide in response to this suffering, which would be the ultimate release. The patient's mental state could severely impair his ability to attend to his own affairs, much less to the affairs of family members. A person diagnosed with unipolar or bipolar depression at an early age may marry and have children. These actions entail certain responsibilities that obtain despite the disorder. They may include making appropriate financial arrangements for one's survivors during periods of remission in the event that one decided to end one's life. This could be considered as part of a responsible planning process preceding EAS. Yet many people affected by mental illness are not capable of considering the probable effects of suicide on others. If a decision to end one's life was motivated by unbearable and interminable suffering, then there would be no compelling moral reasons for prohibiting it because of potential adverse effects on others. The reasons for ending one's life would override the reasons for continuing it. In that case, the question of obligations to others and the moral justification of EAS would dissolve. The main question would still be whether a request for EAS was rational for the person making it.

Suppose that a patient had been suffering from TRD for 30 years. Despite some degree of desperation after failing to respond to multiple therapies and experience symptom relief, he was deemed sufficiently competent to participate in a DBS clinical trial for the disorder. If continuous bilateral stimulation of the dysregulated neural circuits failed to modulate them, and his symptoms were not even partly relieved, then he might rationally conclude that he had exhausted all therapeutic options. His desires and reasons for continuing to live might be exhausted as well. Without deceiving or giving him false hope, his psychiatrist may point out that an effective therapy might be developed from new clinical trials in the foreseeable future. Yet because the patient had been suffering for many years despite receiving many treatments, it would be reasonable for him to conclude that the likelihood of an effective therapy in the future would be low and the likelihood of continued unremitted suffering would be high. It may be unreasonable to expect the patient to wait until a new treatment was tested and approved. This could impose an undue burden on him by prolonging his suffering (Schuklenk and van de Vathorst, 2015a, p. 581). It would thus be reasonable for him to request EAS. If all available therapies had been attempted and failed, then it would be rational for him to conclude that his symptoms would not remit, that he would experience them for the remainder of his life, and that it would be better for him to end it.

One lingering question is whether "all" treatment options would have been attempted if the patient was a candidate for neural ablation but refused it. Unlike DBS, which is adjustable and generally reversible, electrolytic radiofrequency ablation, GKR, and HIFUS can permanently destroy targeted neural tissue. Even with high-precision targeting, ablation may have unwanted and unpredictable expanding effects on nontargeted tissue. The risk of permanent neurological and psychological damage from neural ablation, and the mixed results from ablation trials, may lead some to conclude that it should an exclusionary rather than inclusionary criterion in determining whether a psychiatric disorder is treatment-resistant. Capsulotomy (of the ventral capsule/ventral striatum) and cingulotomy (of the anterior cingulate cortex) have been the main types of ablation for severe OCD. The first of these procedures could be used for a more limited number of cases of MDD. If ablation were an established safe and effective means of controlling psychiatric symptoms, then it could influence the motivation and evaluation of requests for EAS from patients with these disorders. Yet whether ablation is a viable therapy can be shaped by the patient's perception of benefit and risk and concern about whether this procedure would improve or worsen his quality of life. A continued life of poor quality could have more disvalue than value for the affected person. These subjective factors may influence responses to the question of whether the disorder is treatment-resistant and whether a request for EAS may have included or excluded neural ablation as a treatment of last resort. Failed attempts at treating symptoms with many other interventions may be enough to justify the request.

It is also important to emphasize that certain comorbidities for some patients may exclude interventions that might be effective for others. A person with MDD or OCD who also had a seizure disorder would not be a candidate for ECT. A patient with an implanted cardiac pacemaker or defibrillator to control atrial fibrillation would not be a candidate for DBS. The impact of these comorbidities on the evaluation of treatment-resistance depends on the mechanisms and effects of these techniques and how they interact in the body and brain. These factors must be considered in evaluating a patient's condition as treatable or treatment-resistant. The impact of comorbidities of MDD and OCD on suffering and treatment options is different from those from comorbidities such as PD and stroke. If they do not significantly impair reasoning and decision-making, then these neurological disorders may not be exclusionary conditions. Nevertheless, they might increase the patient's suffering and provide a stronger reason for EAS.

Results from a recent study of Swedish patients indicate that those with OCD are ten times more likely to commit suicide than the general population (Fernandez de la Cruz, Rydell, Runeson et al., 2017). The risk is significant even in the absence of other psychiatric conditions and is higher among those who have previously attempted suicide. The authors of the study emphasize the need to closely monitor these patients and design preventive strategies against suicide. They note that the risk is less likely a measure of impulsive or reactionary behavior and more likely a measure of long-term suffering from the disorder.

It is instructive to cite responses in a treating team's interview of a patient successfully treated with DBS of the central thalamus after experiencing severe OCD for many years. Her responses suggest that a desire to end one's life may not just be an impulsive and irrational reaction as a symptom of the disorder. On the contrary, it can be a deliberative, considered response to long-term experience of obsessions and compulsions and many failed treatments.

Asked about the severity of the disorder before the electrodes were implanted and stimulated in her brain, she replied "I surely would have committed suicide if the surgery hadn't taken place." Asked whether the surgery changed her life in any way, she replied: "After surgery, there was a major change in my life. I can enjoy life again, which was impossible before. My compulsions and obsessions are greatly reduced. They do not bother me so much anymore, and I can live with them. I am neither depressed nor anxious anymore." (Merkel, Boer, Fegert et al., 2007, pp. 181–182). Her comment that she was pleased with the outcome and that her obsessions and compulsions were greatly reduced indicates that they did not completely remit. Her psychological response to the outcome indicated that she understood what a successful outcome was for DBS. She had reasonable expectations about what the technique could do in ameliorating her symptoms. They are an indication of decisional capacity that she had in consenting to undergo the procedure and which she likely would have retained if it had not been effective.

One might think that experiencing compulsions 8 hours each day, as this OCD patient did, would undermine the cognitive capacity to weigh reasons for and against suicide. A psychiatric assessment could resolve this question by determining whether she had or lacked this capacity. The psychiatric disorder itself would not necessarily undermine it. Admittedly, in discussing this case for the justification of DBS, one must be cautious in drawing inferences from a retrospective interview following a successful application of a procedure to the patient's state of mind before the procedure. Caution is warranted especially in light of the difference in symptoms before and after the procedure and the fact that the disorder involved disturbed mental content. But the reasoned responses the patient gave in the interview regarding her preoperative expectation of DBS as a therapeutic option that would not automatically result in full remission suggest that she was competent at the earlier time. Her responses suggested that she had some degree of insight into her condition. They suggested that there was incongruity between the mental states associated with OCD and the mental states she wanted to have. This caused her to experience mental distress. These considerations support a determination of a sufficient level of competence to make informed and deliberative decisions about treatment. In light of this, if the procedure failed to meet her reasonable expectations and failed to ameliorate her symptoms, and if this was the last possible treatment, then a subsequent request for EAS could have been a rational decision for her.

Broome and de Cates present an apparent dilemma about competence and illness severity required for assisted dying in cases of TRD. "Hopelessness and suicidal ideation are core symptoms of the illness such that, if the wish to die, and belief in lack of improvement, were rebadged as non-pathological in the assessment of competence, then that same individual would necessarily have a less severe illness, as based on symptom severity. Conversely, if they were deemed to remain a psychopathology, then the individual would lack competence. Hence there is a bind for decision-making in depression—those who may be competent to make decisions would necessarily have a less severe illness that then wouldn't meet the other criteria of Schuklenk and van de Vathorst" (2015, p. 587).

There are two responses to this comment. First, competence is a matter of degree, and some patients with moderate to moderately severe depression may retain enough competence to make an informed and considered request for EAS. While hopelessness and suicidal ideation are core symptoms of the disorder, they do not necessarily preclude the degree of cognitive and emotional capacity necessary to make such a request. Second, severity of symptoms in terms of impaired mental function does not necessarily align with severity of suffering. It is not so much the cognitive and emotional symptoms of the disorder but the suffering that one experiences as part of, or in response to, the symptoms that motivates and sustains a request for assisted dying. Those with a lesser degree of cognitive impairment who experience their symptoms as ego-dystonic may suffer more than those with a greater degree of impairment who experience their symptoms as ego-syntonic. Insight and the incongruity between one's actual disordered mental states and the ordered mental states one wants to have may cause more distress in patients who have this experience than in those who lack it. This is similar in some respects to dementia. Those at a less advanced stage of the disease may suffer more than those at a more advanced stage because the former retain an awareness of their deterioration that is absent in the latter.

Insight in an ego-dystonic disorder presupposes a certain degree of cognitive capacity. This may be enough for a patient to make a well-considered and autonomous request for EAS. One can remain competent while suffering from TRD and meet the conditions articulated by Schuklenk and van de Vathorst. Less severe psychiatric symptoms, specifically less severe cognitive impairment, may involve greater suffering, though this depends on the unique experience of each patient. The strength of a claim for EAS depends on the extent of suffering, not on the extent of cognitive impairment or capacity. Still, a patient must have a sufficient degree of cognitive capacity to consider and request EAS as a rational choice for him.

The soundness of these claims and arguments rests not only on the judgment that the patient has enough decisional capacity, but also on the judgment that the patient's disorder is treatment-resistant. While each of these criteria can be determined objectively by psychiatric assessment, the patient's attitudes about procedures entailing greater neurological and psychological risk and poor quality of life can influence judgments about whether the condition can be treated. My discussion of neural ablation illustrates this point. In fact, questions of competence and treatment-resistance are interconnected. A patient's judgment that, after many failed treatments, the probability of an effective therapy emerging in the future was low and that requesting and receiving EAS was in his best interests presupposes a certain degree of competence. In cases where no treatment has been effective up to the patient's current state, there is always the possibility that a new treatment will be effective, relieve symptoms, and attenuate or eliminate the patient's desire for EAS. This raises two questions. Will the mere possibility of such a treatment become a probability? How long would it be reasonable to expect a patient to wait for such a therapy while continuing to suffer?

All available therapies must have failed in order for psychiatrists to conclude that a patient's condition is treatment-resistant. These would include antidepressants (monoamine oxidase inhibitors, tricyclics, SSRIs, and SNRIs to modulate monoamines; ketamine to modulate glutamate; and aripiprazole to increase circulating levels of dopamine in late-life depression), CBT, ECT, TMS, rTMS, tDCS, FUS, DBS, and possibly neural ablation. The patient would have to be an appropriate candidate for these interventions in the brain. Some comorbidities would exclude some of these interventions as therapeutic options. One study published in 2008 estimated that 20% of patients with major depression were refractory to existing therapies (Abosch and Cosgrove, 2008). Three years later, Paul Holtzheimer and Helen Mayberg stated that "approximately 10–20% of depressed patients may show virtually no improvement despite multiple, often aggressive treatments" (2011, p. 2). Estimates of this percentage may be even higher today. The point is that a sizeable minority of patients remain treatment-resistant, despite the fact that the number of approved and experimental treatments for psychiatric disorders has increased.

Some commentators have underestimated the incidence of TRD. They have claimed that the condition is treatable but either untreated or undertreated. This may partly explain their objection to EAS. For example, McHugh and Slavney claim, "As psychiatric knowledge of suicide—a behavior driven by mental disorders and dispositions—increases, the concept of euthanasia and physician-assisted suicide becomes more suspect. The doctors supporting euthanasia emphasize the patient's medical burdens and assumptions about life and death but tend to overlook how underlying and treatable psychiatric conditions lead to these assumptions. By over-identifying with the patient's distorted and depressive attitude about the future, these doctors may well be encouraging both demoralization and aggression against the self" (1998, p. 241).

McHugh and Slavney further state, "psychiatrists . . . should teach people to realize that depression is a disease of nature, that is often associated with an irrational view of the world, that it is eminently treatable . . ." (1998, pp. 249–250).

There are two responses to this passage. First, suicide is not always or necessarily driven impulsively by a mental disorder. Depending on the degree of a patient's competence, it may be a deliberative rational response to chronic suffering from the disorder. Second, current data on the incidence of TRD belies the claim by McHugh and Slavney that major depression is "eminently treatable." While their comments may be dated, it is likely that many psychiatrists and ethicists currently take the same or a similar position.

Olie and Courtet recommend short-term use of ketamine or buprenorphine as antisuicidal treatment. This recommendation suggests that the desire and request for EAS by patients with psychiatric disorders is impulsive or only briefly considered (Olie and Courtet, 2016). If the mental suffering in these disorders is caused by chronic dysfunctional neural circuitry, then the treatment options proposed by Olie and Courtet would have at best a temporary beneficial effect. They would not ameliorate symptoms for any extended period and thus would not resolve the condition motivating the request for EAS.

Franklin Miller writes, "In making a request of a physician for aid in dying, these patients may be seeking 'permission' or endorsement by an authority figure for the decision to end their lives. Physicians should be reluctant to play this role for patients with depression, who need help in coping with rather than ending their lives" (Miller, 2015, p. 886). Like the passage from McHugh and Slavney, the first part of this passage is paternalistic in some respects. It fails to acknowledge that many patients request EAS, not because they want validation of their desire to end their life, but because of an autonomous judgment that they have suffered enough and want a physician to help them end it. Moreover, "coping" suggest that there are available strategies to manage the mental suffering in psychiatric disorders. Yet if the disorder is truly treatment-resistant and symptoms persist, then there may be no such coping strategies. Miller righty emphasizes the uncertainty surrounding treatment-resistance, and that "it is doubtful that a clinician can know that the patient has no possibility of significant therapeutic help" (2015, p. 886.). A clinician cannot know that such help would be forthcoming, either. The decreased funding by the pharmaceutical industry for research into new psychotropic drugs, as well as the limitations of TMS, DBS, and other neuromodulating techniques, raises serious questions about the potential of these modalities to overcome treatment-resistance. A patient may be offered "proper treatment" that has relieved symptoms in other patients with the same disorder (Miller and Appelbaum,

2018, p. 883). But proper treatment may not be effective treatment in all cases and may fail to relieve a patient's symptoms and suffering.

While objective measures are necessary to determine competence and treatment-resistance, the patient's own diachronic experience of living with a psychiatric disorder and its influence on his expectation about therapy should be the main factor in assessing requests for EAS. If the conditions of competence, chronic treatment-resistance, and unbearable and interminable suffering are present, and if a patient has a low expectation of effective future treatments based on these conditions, then she may rationally decide that she has suffered enough and would be better off ending her life. Solomon reports that, with depression, "you cannot remember a time when you felt better, at least clearly, and you cannot imagine a future time when you will feel better . . ." (2001, p. 55). This does not mean that a patient with major depression cannot have positive expectations about the future. He may not remember when he felt better; but he likely will remember the failed treatments. With this memory, he can form an expectation that the probability of an effective treatment in the future is low. It can be difficult to sustain hope. Contrary to what McHugh and Slavney claim, a patient's attitude about the future and its influence on a request for EAS need not be distorted and may be a clear reflection of his considered judgment and best interests. Suffering can distort one's judgment about which actions and consequences would benefit or harm one. But this is less likely to occur when one has been suffering for years and the suffering suffuses much of one's experience. Even if there were some distortion, it would not necessarily be of such a degree to make the person unable to know that ending suffering by ending his life would be preferable to continuing his life. EAS would be the lesser of two evils.

The main reason for leaving open the possibility of an effective therapy is that it could relieve depressive symptoms and remove the motivation for EAS. As Broome and de Cates point out, "TRD doesn't do a terribly good job of marking out a clinical state that is wholly 'irreversible' or 'debilitating, incurable'" (2015, p. 587). "Incurable" implies no possibility of remission. The chronicity of TRD may indicate that it probably will not remit, but it does not imply that it could never remit. More importantly, what motivates requests for EAS is suffering, and Broome and de Cates emphasize that "remission is not equivalent to response and some degree of amelioration of suffering" (p. 587). The comments by the OCD patient in the interview cited earlier suggest that a neurophysiological response involving less than complete remission can weaken or eliminate suicidal thoughts in patients with severe psychiatric disorders. Some positive response without remission may be adequate. Moreover, Broome and de Cates point out that "depression is a disorder in which feasibly new treatments may be discovered, as the recent interest in ketamine and glutaminergic targets attests" (2015, p. 587).

As I explained in Chapter 3, results of initial studies of ketamine for MDD have been promising. The monoamine hypothesis and the serotonergic and dopaminergic pathways targeted by antidepressant and antipsychotic drugs may not accurately explain the pathophysiology of depression and may account for suboptimal responses to treatment in many cases. Research into the role of glutaminergic, GABAergic, and other pathways involving other neurotransmitters may yield a better understanding of depression and result in more effective treatment. Ketamine modulates the glutaminergic receptor NMDA, dysregulation of which may have some role in the pathophysiology of depression. Through their modulating effects, drugs like ketamine may be able to ameliorate depressive symptoms more effectively than current drugs. They may result in improved cognition, mood, and motivation. Remission, interpreted as full recovery, is not necessary to relieve suffering. Since suffering is the motivation for requesting EAS, an outcome with some degree of symptom relief may be enough to relieve suffering, weaken this motivation, and reduce the incidence of these requests. Novel therapies would not have to result in complete disease remission to benefit patients in these respects.

I have questioned the claim by McHugh and Slavney that psychiatric disorders are "eminently treatable." This conflicts with the high incidence of treatment-resistance in depression and other forms of mental illness. Novel drugs and neuromodulating techniques have the potential to overcome this problem. But one cannot assume that this potential will be actualized in effective therapies. Let us suppose that researchers will develop interventions that will do more to control psychiatric disorders and relieve patients' suffering. Even if this occurs, whether these interventions had these effects would depend on the extent of structural and functional changes in the brain and associated mental states.

In some cases of chronic treatment-resistant anxiety and depression, chronic high circulating levels of cortisol from a dysregulated HPA axis and other circuits can result in reduced volumes in prefrontal regions and impaired cognition and emotion (Saplosky, 2000; Sorrells, Caso, Munhoz et al., 2009; Charney, Sklar, Buxbaum et al., 2013, Chapters 37, 43; Schmall, Hibar, Samann et al., 2017). Chronic depression can also result in reduced hippocampal volume and memory impairment. In severe cases, these neuroanatomical and psychological consequences may not be amenable to new treatments. It is not known whether adverse neural circuit changes resulting from these processes could be reversed by novel drugs. Nor is it known whether these drugs could reverse white matter deficits and reduced interhemispheric connectivity in persons with BD that has not responded to lithium or other therapies. Cognitive-emotional deficits that have developed from brain dysfunction over many years may be permanent. In unipolar and bipolar depression or OCD, new interventions might not be able to restore normal mental functions. Instead of resolving feelings of emptiness, helplessness, and despair, failed attempts at treatment could increase feelings. The possibility of new treatments alone is not enough to generate a realistic sense of hope. Even if new treatments had positive effects, differences in people's brains and responses to drugs would likely result in improved mental capacities for some patients but not others. A drug or technique that was safe and effective in modulating brain function and improving symptoms for some patients would not have the same therapeutic outcome for all patients.

If pharmacological treatments fail, then psychiatrists and neurosurgeons might identify a new neural target for DBS as a treatment for TRD. The technique might be able to modulate dysfunctional neural circuits that have not responded to other interventions. It might relieve a patient's mood disturbance in the same way that stimulating the central thalamus relieved the obsessions and compulsions of the patient with OCD. But not all patients with severe OCD respond to DBS of this brain region or the internal capsule. Nor do all patients with severe MDD respond to DBS of the subgenual cingulate, NAc, or other targets. The results of the BROADEN study are a good example of this. Dysfunctional connectivity in neural circuits in these disorders may remain too intractable for neuromodulation. Stimulating the brain at an earlier disease stage might promote neuroplasticity and neurogenesis and possibly slow or prevent further development of the disease. Yet this could mean using DBS or similar experimental techniques as first-line treatment. This would involve greater risk than pharmacotherapy and could preclude new less invasive and safer treatments that might be equally effective.

The risk of early DBS may be less acceptable in light of the fact that its neuroplastic and neurogenerative effects are hypothetical and not proven. Similar remarks apply to novel interventions such as optogenetics, TI, and delivery of trophic factors in the brain. One cannot assume that they would alter the disease process and ameliorate symptoms without any side effects. Decisions about the sequence of treatments patients should receive, as well as which treatments they should receive, are fraught with uncertainty because of uncertainty about pathophysiology. What is known is that the chronicity of the disease can cause changes in the brain that can limit the extent to which any interventions can restore neural and mental function. Many failed treatments and persistent symptoms can generate a patient's desire for EAS. After suffering from a psychiatric disorder for many years, the mere possibility of a new treatment that might alter its pathophysiology and relieve suffering is unlikely to weaken this desire.

Is it fair to expect a patient to wait indefinitely for a clinical trial that may or may not establish the safety and efficacy of a novel drug or technique? How long would it be reasonable to expect a patient to wait when she has suffered from refractory MDD, OCD, or BD for many years? It is the competent patient's decision to wait for a new treatment or decide that they have suffered enough and request EAS. Not waiting longer and making this request would not necessarily be indicative of impulsivity or irrationality.

Combined with uncertainty in psychiatric research about new treatments, Kagan's comment on the possibility of future medical treatments sheds light on a patient's motivation for requesting EAS as a response to disease. He writes: "Those who deny the rationality of suicide might insist that since you never know for sure that you won't recover, suicide never makes sense. After all, we all know that medicine is constantly making advances. Researchers are always making breakthroughs. What seems like an incurable disease one day may have some sort of cure the next. But if you kill yourself, you throw away any chance of getting that cure" (2012, p. 337). "If you can just hold on, things will eventually get better" (2012, p. 336). Kagan then makes a more critical point: "If your condition is so bad that you are better off dead, and the chance of recovery is vanishingly small, then it might well be rational to decide to kill oneself" (2012, pp. 343–344). Applying Kagan's comments to TRD, the request for EAS can be rational if a long history of failed treatments and suffering cause the patient to reasonably expect that no effective treatment and no relief of suffering will be forthcoming. The chance of these coming about is vanishingly small. In these circumstances, assisted dying in a case of TRD can be a rational choice for the patient and ethically justified.

When death is imminent, assisted dying shortens a patient's life by days, weeks, or months at most. This is typical in cases of severe brain injury and end-stage cancer. When death is not imminent, assisted dying can shorten a patient's life by years. This may seem difficult to justify given the number of life years that could be lost. But these years may be filled with unbearable and interminable suffering. This raises the questions of what the person would lose by not remaining alive and whether having more life years would make her better or worse off. There are no objective answers to these questions in psychiatry. They involve subjective judgments that only a competent person affected by a psychiatric disorder can make.

Kagan reasons further: "Even if pain and stress inevitably cloud your thinking and leave you worried and uncertain, you might nonetheless still find the odds in favor of suicide sufficiently strong so as to eventually make it reasonable to trust your judgment on the matter. In principle, then, suicide can be a rational choice." (2012, p. 344). There will be cases in which cognitive and emotional impairment associated with a disorder may cloud a patient's judgment. Prolonged suffering may have the same effect. But there will be other cases in which the patient will retain enough cognitive and emotional capacity to critically reflect on and weigh the reasons for continuing or ending her life. This will depend on the duration and severity of the illness. Assuming that a patient has a sufficient degree of this capacity, beyond a certain point it may not be reasonable to expect her to "hold on" any longer. Not holding on would not necessarily be indicative of noncompetence or irrationality but more indicative of having reached the limits of tolerable suffering.

EAS should not be permitted for adolescents and, arguably, young adults with psychiatric disorders. This claim is not based on noncompetence. Many individuals under 18 may be mature minors and thus capable of making informed decisions about medical care. Rather, they should be excluded because they do not meet the chronicity condition. The exclusion would be based on the fact that they have had the disorder for a relatively short period and might not have suffered as long or to the same extent as older adults. It would also be based on the likelihood that not all available treatments would have been offered to them. A psychiatrist caring for an adolescent or young adult patient whose condition had been treatment-resistant would not be able to determine that the disorder would remain treatment-resistant. There would be too much uncertainty about the possibility of effective therapies to support a request for EAS and any action by the psychiatrist that would lead to the patient's death. In these cases, the default positon would be to err on the side of caution and not allow the practice.

## Rights, obligations, and the noncompetent psychiatric patient

A right is a claim by a person on others to act or refrain from acting in ways that affect that person. As claims, rights entail certain obligations for those to whom they are directed. Although there is considerable debate about the content and scope of rights, a negative right is generally interpreted as a claim on others *against* unwanted interference in one's body or brain. A positive right is generally interpreted as a claim on others *for* assistance in promoting or realizing a certain goal. Any right to end one's life through direct action or assistance from others is a positive right. It is a claim by a patient on a healthcare provider to facilitate the realization of a patient's intention to die. This applies to EAS for both physical and mental diseases. In the latter, the positive right would be a claim by the patient on a psychiatrist from whom he had received continuous care to bring about his death.

In medicine, negative rights include the right of a competent patient to refuse life-sustaining medical interventions and a corresponding perfect, or absolute, obligation for a physician to respect this refusal. The principle of respect for patient autonomy grounds this right and obligation. Positive rights do not entail the same strong sense of individual autonomy and sovereignty as negative rights. They have less moral and legal force and entail at most an imperfect, non-absolute, obligation for others to act on a patient's claim (Kant, 1785/1964; Thomson, 1990, Chapters 2, 9, 11; Kamm, 2007, Section II). An imperfect obligation allows some latitude in how a physician discharges her duty of care in responding to patient requests. Because imperfect obligations do not require an agent to perform particular actions, they are permissions. As an imperfect obligation, a physician is not required to accede to any request for a medical intervention. This is typically grounded in the physician's professional judgment that the intervention may not be in the patient's best interests and not consistent with best medical practices. In cases where these issues are unclear, the physician has the prerogative to offer a requested treatment, consistent with her professional autonomy and medical judgment.

Requests for EAS are significantly different from patient requests for questionable medical treatment. If physicians have at most an imperfect obligation to assist in or directly cause a patient's death, then they are not required to act on a request for EAS and may refuse to act on it. A psychiatrist or indeed any health professional would at most be permitted to act on a patient's request to end his life. The physician could refuse to participate in or perform the final act if it conflicted with her professional integrity and understanding of her duty of care to patients on principled grounds. Acting on the patient's request may conflict with her goal of preventing suicide in the patients she treats in her clinical practice. She would be exercising the latitude her professional autonomy allows her in discharging this duty. "Conscience clauses" in jurisdictions where EAS is legal allow the professional the right to opt out of the practice.

Conscientious objection to certain treatments and procedures is a vexed issue (Giubilini and Savulescu, 2017; Sulmasy, 2017; Wicclair, 2017). There is considerable debate about whether a medical professional can choose to opt out of a service on grounds of conscience. Yet if a psychiatrist has an imperfect duty to act on a request for EAS from a psychiatric patient, then refusing to act on this request may be consistent with her general duty of care. Refusing to perform euthanasia or assist in a patient's death would not necessarily reflect a paternalistic view that the patient did not know what was in his best interests. But it may generate a conflict between the physician and the patient if the patient has a broader interpretation of medical care and his interests are not just medical. The physician's refusal may interfere with the patient's considered interest in dying. It could preclude realization of the patient's wish to die if the physician is not obligated and chooses not to act on it. It is one thing to argue that a psychiatric patient's request for EAS is justified and that EAS would be in his best interests. It is quite another to argue that a psychiatrist has an absolute obligation to accede to the request by prescribing or administering a lethal dose of drugs to the patient. Nevertheless, consistent with her professional duty and the law, the psychiatrist would be obligated to refer the patient to another psychiatrist or other physician who would be capable and willing to perform the desired action (Cowley, 2017).

This type of situation could be problematic if a significant number of physicians refused to participate in EAS. It could restrict the positive right of patients who choose to die. It could make the exercise of this right unduly burdensome if patients had to make many requests and undergo many psychiatric assessments for EAS. This could increase the suffering these patients already have endured and could cause additional harm to them. Timothy Quill provides guidance for physicians who are uncomfortable with requests for EAS from their patients: "Physicians must know the limits permitted by law but also must continue to respect their own personal boundaries. The challenge is always to respond as thoughtfully and compassionately to the patient's clinical situation and preferences without violating fundamental personal principles and with full knowledge of the boundaries set out by the law in one's own setting." (2018, p. 2).

As in assisted dying or euthanasia for physical diseases, some might believe that, in psychiatric diseases, there is a morally significant difference between providing the means for a patient to take her own life and directly causing her death. Because the physician performs only an intermediate facilitating act, and the patient performs the final act, it seems that assisted dying is more morally defensible than euthanasia for psychiatric disorders. Which of these actions is performed will depend largely on the volitional capacity of the patient and the extent of his ability to form and carry out a plan to die. Regarding the agency of the physician, euthanasia and assisted dying are not fundamentally medically or morally different because in each case the physician has causal control—physical and cognitive—over the sequence of events that results in the patient's death. In euthanasia, the physician controls the sequence of events by infusing the drug or drugs that kill the patient. In assisted dying, the physician controls the sequence of events by providing the patient with the drug or drugs and knowing that it will result in her death. The physician has control over the patient's demise because of what he does and what he knows, or foresees, will be the consequence of what he does. Thus, in asking whether a physician is permitted to participate in a patient's death, the answer does not depend on whether the act is euthanasia or assisted suicide. Because the physician has the same control over the causal sequence of events resulting in death in both cases, there is no fundamental normative difference between them.

In a response to the review by Emanuel and coauthors, Daniel Sulmasy, E. Wesley Ely, and Charles Spring argue that "the distinction between euthanasia and PAS [physician-assisted suicide] cannot hold based on 5 reasons" (2016, p. 1600). Three of these reasons are especially pertinent to EAS for psychiatric disorders. First, "PAS does not give physicians moral distance from the act. Some assert that PAS is different from euthanasia because it puts the ultimate decision in the hands of patients and therefore distances the physician from the act. This claim is spurious. A physician who writes any prescription is morally and legally implicated in its use, although the patient decides on its use" (Sulmasy, Ely, and Spring, 2016, p. 1600). Second, "permitting PAS without euthanasia is discriminatory. If PAS is justified for some patients, it is discriminatory not to provide equivalent access to death for patients with paralysis, dementia, or other neuropsychological conditions" (Sulmasy, Ely, and Spring, 2016, p. 1600). This point reinforces the argument by Schuklenk and Van de Vathorst (2015a, 2015b) and others that is unfair to those suffering from mental illness to permit EAS for physical diseases but not permit it for psychiatric diseases. Third, "from a practical perspective, euthanasia is more efficient. Some patients cannot afford barbiturates. Others are unable to consume all the pills, prone to vomit them, or are under-dosed and require active assistance" (Sulmasy, Ely, and Spring, 2016, p. 1600).

Although Sulmasy and coauthors do not explicitly mention them under "other neuropsychological conditions," major depression and other psychiatric disorders could be included in this category. In these disorders, euthanasia by terminal sedation may be the most effective means and involve the least amount of suffering for the patient. In this second respect, it may be the most humane form of EAS. The more general upshot is that the permissibility of EAS does not depend on medical differences between these two life-ending actions. Nor does an answer to the question of whether a psychiatrist has an imperfect obligation to act on a request for EAS or a right to refuse to act on it depend on these differences. These issues depend on the suffering of the patient and a judgment of what would be the most appropriate and effective means of ending it.

If a certain degree of decisional capacity is a necessary condition for requesting and receiving euthanasia, then what are the implications for those with severe and unrelenting psychiatric disorders who completely lack this capacity? If they lack the cognitive and volitional capacity to form and carry out a plan of taking a lethal dose of a drug, then assisted suicide would not be an option. If they lack the cognitive capacity to make an informed request for a physician to end their life, then voluntary euthanasia would not be an option either. Proxy consent to discontinue life-sustaining treatment from noncompetent patients is permissible when the condition is irreversible and continued treatment is clearly not what the patient would have wanted. This could be expressed by the patient in an advance directive when he or she was competent. But proxy consent for euthanasia is not permitted for EAS for physical or psychiatric diseases. The stakes are too high for allowing families or caregivers to consent to non-voluntary or involuntary euthanasia for a patient who could not clearly and consistently express his wishes about continuing or ending his life. Among other factors, the burden of caring for a person with a severe psychiatric disorder could cause a caregiver to mistakenly judge that continued life had no value for the person and that he would be better off dead. This may not be what the affected person would have wanted, even if it ended his suffering.

But preventing these vulnerable patients from ending their lives without their consent could make their lives worse for them. They may not suffer at the same level of intensity as competent patients experiencing their symptoms as ego-dystonic. Nevertheless, excluding them from EAS because they were not competent could cause them to suffer longer. They would lack the capacity to form a plan to end their lives. It seems unfair to deny euthanasia to these patients on this basis. Suffering is the motivation and justification for euthanasia, and suffering is not measured by competence. These patients would be denied access to euthanasia to end their suffering because they were not competent.

The phenomenology of suffering cannot be reduced to the cognitive and volitional capacities to manipulate information about a condition and choose between treatment options for it. A well-considered, voluntary request for euthanasia from a competent patient is necessary for a medical professional to act on the request. But amelioration or prevention of suffering is in *any* person's best interests, independently of the extent to which he is competent and has decisional capacity. Patients whose depression or obsessions and compulsions severely impair or undermine the capacity to make an informed, sustained, and voluntary request for euthanasia may suffer interminably without any recourse.

Solomon's comment about being "too dumbly lethargic even to conceptualize suicide" (2001, p. 19) suggests the situation I am describing. The patient lacks the cognitive and volitional capacity to end his suffering. These situations may include patients who have lost the capacity to reason because of severe mood disturbance or psychosis. Psychotic states involving delusions need to be distinguished from psychotic states with hallucinations for the issue at hand. Despite having impaired agency, individuals with delusions may not experience any incongruity or distress in their mental states and may not suffer in what would be an ego-syntonic state. Those with auditory hallucinations symptomatic of schizophrenia may feel tortured by what they experience as alien voices. They may suffer from this experience even though it may not be accurate to describe their condition as either ego-syntonic or ego-dystonic. Some of these individuals take their own lives. Depression is the strongest risk factor for suicide in people with schizophrenia (Castle and Buckley, 2015, p. 20). Suicidal desire is typically not attributed to the flat affect, anhedonia and avolition in the negative subtype of schizophrenia. Instead, "the typical situation for suicide in schizophrenia is a young man who has been recently diagnosed and has become depressed by the way schizophrenia has changed his life" (Castle and Buckley, 2015, p. 20). Like many cases of suicidal desire in TRD, the desire for suicide in schizophrenia is not necessarily an impulsive or reactive mental event. It may develop gradually and be reinforced by its chronicity and the individual's expectation that it will be a life-long burden. In fact, it is not suicide but the adverse cardiovascular and metabolic effects of antipsychotic drugs that account for the premature death of many people with schizophrenia (Castle and Buckley, 2015, p. 23).

Jukka Varelius claims that "restricting psychiatric assisted dying to autonomous, or rational, psychiatric patients would not be compatible with endorsing certain end-of-life practices commonly accepted in current medical ethics and law, practices often referred to as 'passive euthanasia'" (2016, p. 227, 2013). This is a stronger claim than the claim that sufficiently competent and autonomous individuals with psychiatric diseases should have the same access to EAS as those with physical diseases. Waiving the autonomy requirement might remove the main obstacle to relieving the suffering of noncompetent psychiatric patients. Still, the risk of harm from waiving it may be significant enough to outweigh the potential benefit.

"Passive euthanasia" has been interpreted by some as equivalent to "letting die" (Rachels, 1975). Varelius seems to be using the term in the sense of nonvoluntary euthanasia. This is based on the assumption that only autonomous decisions and actions can be voluntary. If a patient was not competent to make a sufficiently informed request for EAS, then any request he made would not be voluntary. It can be rational for a person who has suffered for many years from a treatment-resistant psychiatric disorder to want to die. This is a subjective assessment of the person's own life. The patient must clearly and consistently express this assessment to those who would be asked to assist in or cause his death. This expression requires a certain degree of competence and autonomy. Without a clear, autonomous and persistent request for euthanasia, it may not be known whether a patient would want to die or continue living.

Even if it is obvious that he is suffering, it may not be obvious that euthanasia is what he would want. Varelius states, "it would seem that the suffering experienced by psychiatric patients who lack autonomy can be as bad as the distress that autonomous, or rational patients undergo, if not worse" (2016, p. 227). This would require a comparison between the two groups measuring the intensity and duration of the suffering they experience. Although this may be difficult to measure, not removing the autonomy requirement would allow a noncompetent patient to continue suffering. Still, if the wishes of noncompetent and nonautonomous psychiatric patients are not known, then the potential for abuse and harm to them may be too great to justify removing the requirement. Protecting these patients in these respects may be necessary despite failing to resolve the problem of their mental suffering. Laws designed to protect patients from dying against their wishes could exclude EAS as an option for them and cause them to suffer more.

## Conclusion

EAS may be morally and legally permissible in some cases of patients with intractable psychiatric disorders. EAS is permissible when a patient is competent enough to weigh reasons for and against it, make an informed and persistent request for it, experiences unbearable and interminable suffering, and the disorder has been resistant to all available treatments over many years. It would be unreasonable to expect a patient who meets these conditions to wait indefinitely for a new treatment that may or may not relieve her symptoms. When these conditions have been met, a patient can make a rational request to a psychiatrist or other physician to end or assist in ending her life. The physician's action can be morally justified in being consistent with the goals of medicine and in the patient's best interests. As in cases of patients with physical diseases, a psychiatric patient's right to EAS is a positive right. This right does not entail an absolute or perfect obligation but at most an imperfect obligation for a psychiatrist to accede to a patient's request for EAS. Insofar as imperfect obligations imply a certain latitude in how one discharges them, a psychiatrist receiving such a request from a patient is permitted to assist in or bring about the patient's death. But she is not required to perform these actions. This is consistent with the physician's professional autonomy and right to refuse to cause or contribute to the patient's death on principled or "conscientious" grounds. However, this imperfect obligation includes a professional duty to refer a patient requesting EAS to another physician who may be willing to perform it.

The main motivation and justification for EAS for psychiatric disorders is unbearable and interminable mental suffering. "Interminable" implies that the disorder is treatment-resistant. The argument for EAS for psychiatric diseases compared with physical diseases is an argument about fairness. If patients with physical diseases are permitted to receive EAS because of unbearable and interminable suffering, and if patients with severe, treatment-resistant psychiatric disorders also suffer unbearably and interminably, then psychiatric patients should also be permitted to receive EAS. Not permitting it would be unfair to them.

The fact that a psychiatric patient is not imminently dying is not a morally or legally decisive reason against allowing EAS for that patient. Severity of cognitive, emotional, and volitional symptoms may not align with severity of suffering. A patient with less severe cognitive impairment who retains insight into her condition may suffer more than a patient with more severe cognitive impairment and little or no insight. The internal conflict and distress she experiences in the incongruity between the mental states she has and the mental states she wants to have may cause her to suffer more than those who experience their disorder without any such conflict. Suffering could be measured in terms of intensity and duration, and each of these measures may have its own scale of severity that may not map directly onto the other. Although noncompetent psychiatric patients may not suffer at the same level of intensity as competent psychiatric patients, the first group may suffer longer than the second group because they would not meet the first condition for the ethical justification of EAS.

The moral and legal permissibility of a psychiatrist to assist in or directly cause the death of a psychiatric patient seems paradoxical when one of the goals of psychiatric care is to prevent patients from committing suicide. This care rests on the assumption that treatment will eventually control or ameliorate the symptoms associated with suicidal desire. Brendan Kelly and Declan McLoughlin claim that "the shift of therapeutic role from alleviating psychic despair to facilitating suicide would be anathema to many psychiatrists" (2002, p. 278). But in some cases, treatment may increase rather than decrease the risk of suicide. The case of the patient who committed suicide in reaction to akathisia from the SSRI paroxetine, cited in Chapter 3, is one example. In other cases, the condition is resistant to all attempted treatments, and symptoms cannot be relieved. The only way of relieving suffering may be to end it by ending the patient's life. These cases may be relatively rare. But EAS can be morally permissible in them for the reasons I have discussed. Policies and laws need to be in place to protect vulnerable patients from interventions they do not want. Ultimately, though, whether euthanasia or assisted dying for TRD or other psychiatric disorders can be justified depends on the particular condition and how it affects the particular patient.

The most effective way of resolving the problem of mental suffering in treatment-resistant psychiatric disorders and avoid resorting to EAS is to prevent them. This requires a better understanding of the genetic, epigenetic, environmental, psychological, and neurobiological factors in the etiology and pathophysiology of these disorders. This is necessary at both population and individual levels. Given the causal complexity of these factors and differences in symptoms, severity, and responses to therapies, achieving this understanding is a challenging process. The RDoC's goal of explaining the causes of neural circuit dysfunction could contribute to this understanding. It could lead to new therapies and preventive interventions for psychiatric disorders. McHugh and Slavney's comment on unveiling the genetic propensity for the suicidal impulse and the variability among individuals in having this propensity alludes to the importance of research confirming the genetic mechanisms in these disorders. These mechanisms could help to explain why some individuals are more likely to develop depression. They may also help to explain why some people with depression commit suicide or develop treatment-resistance that motivates them to request EAS.

Recent studies have identified genome-wide methylation changes associated with dysfunction in the hippocampi of impulsive suicide completers (Labonte, Suderman, Maussion et al., 2013; Turecki, 2014). There are neurophysiological and molecular differences between psychiatric disorders. These differences might be part of an account of why BD has such a high suicide rate (Strakowski, 2014, p. 9). Common molecular genetic changes in the brain might also explain why severe forms of major psychiatric disorders are refractory to all forms of psychopharmacology and neuromodulation. With the goal of reducing both impulsive suicide and requests to end patients' lives, identifying these changes and other biomarkers at an early symptomatic or presymptomatic stage might provide a clearer sense of which individuals were at risk of developing psychiatric disorders. This could lead to interventions that could prevent the disorders that generate requests for EAS when they become treatment-resistant. I discuss these predictive and preventive measures in the last chapter.

# Chapter 8

# Prediction and prevention

In the Introduction, I cited reports stating that mental illness constitutes the greatest global burden of disease and that depression would be the leading cause of this burden by 2030. I also noted that schizophrenia affects approximately 24 million people worldwide. Commenting on schizophrenia, Owen, Sawa, and Mortenson state: "More than 50% of individuals who receive a diagnosis have intermittent but long-term psychiatric problems, and around 20% have chronic symptoms and disability. Unemployment is staggeringly high at 80–90%, and life expectancy is reduced by 10–20 years. In England, schizophrenia costs 11.8 billion pounds per year, with around a third of this figure accounted for by direct expenditure on health and social care, provided both in hospitals and in the community" (2016, p. 86). The long-term outlook for schizophrenia has not improved significantly since 1988. In that year, at the height of the AIDS epidemic, the editor of *Nature* commented, "schizophrenia is arguably the worst disease affecting mankind, even AIDS not excepted" (cited by Insel, 2010, p. 191).

According to a recent report of the WHO, 322 million people—4.4% of the world's population—are living with depression (World Health Organization, 2016). This makes this psychiatric disorder the leading cause of disability, defined in terms of functional impairment, inability to work, lost income, and poor quality of life. The number of people with depression increased by 18.4% between 2005 and 2015. Anxiety disorders affect 4.3 million working adults in the United States (Jacob, 2015) and more than 260 million people globally. This constitutes 3.6% of the world's population (Friedrich, 2017a). Many people experience depressive and anxiety disorders simultaneously. The two most populous nations in the world, China and India, account for 32% of the total burden of mental illness, which is higher than all Western countries combined. Yet less than 10% of people in these countries with a mental disorder receive treatment (Charlson, Baxter, Cheng et al., 2016; Cheng, Shidhaye, Charlson et al., 2016). There has been an increase in the burden of mental illness, particularly depression and anxiety, in Eastern Mediterranean regions (Friedrich, 2017b). Much of this is attributable to ethnic, religious, and military conflict. This is one example of the harmful effects of environmental stressors on the brain and mind. Other forms of environmental stressors and biological processes occurring early in life are also implicated in these disorders. Clearly, the most desirable course of action is not just to reduce the incidence of mental illness but prevent it from developing.

Preventing psychiatric disorders is challenging because of their complex etiology and pathophysiology. Therapeutic interventions aim to modulate abnormal neurotransmission and dysfunctional neural circuits and thereby ameliorate symptoms. Yet the psychomotor, cognitive, emotional, and volitional symptoms of these disorders often result from dysfunction in distributed neural networks rather than discrete, localized nodes within circuits. Interactions between genetic, immune, endocrine, and environmental factors and the brain can influence neural function or dysfunction. Focusing on the brain alone may lose sight of the multifactorial nature of psychiatric disorders and the therapeutic potential of interventions that can affect these interactions. Moreover, treatments that are effective in relieving symptoms for some patients may not be effective for others because of neuroanatomical and neurophysiological differences between them. These differences may reflect causal pathways involving factors inside and outside of the brain that are unique to each patient.

Even when treatments are effective in controlling symptoms and disease progression, they cannot reverse the underlying pathophysiology. In Chapter 3, I described a four-dimensional approach to treating schizophrenia based on a biopsychosocial model. The combination of antipsychotic medication, psychotherapy, family and social support, and work can be effective when initiated shortly after a first episode of psychosis. When psychosis occurs, however, deleterious changes may have already occurred in the brain and may be irreversible. Similar changes may have occurred in the brains of people diagnosed with unipolar or bipolar depression. This raises the question of whether intervention during the prodromal phase could prevent the disease process from progressing to full-blown schizophrenia, major depression, or BD. It also raises the question of whether earlier intervention in people at risk of having these or other psychiatric disorders could reduce or eliminate this risk.

Many psychiatric disorders have been linked to genetic polymorphisms resulting in abnormal neural circuitry and neural transmission. Thus is especially the case in schizophrenia, where genome-wide association studies and large-scale sequencing have shown this to be a highly polygenic disorder. It involves alleles on more than 100 distinct genetic loci (Owen, Sawa, and Mortensen, 2016, p. 87). There is a significant genetic component in depression as well. One study found 17 genetic variations linked to depression at 15 genome locations in people of European ancestry. These variations influence the regulation of gene expression and the generation of new neurons in the developing brain (Hyde, Nagle, Chao et al., 2016). The heritability of BD is 80– 85%, which is higher than that of any other psychiatric disorder (Strakowski, 2014, p. 48). The fact that many genes and epigenetic processes are involved in the etiology and pathogenesis of these disorders rules out the possibility of any form of "editing" or "correcting" psychiatric disease-causing genes. Gene–environment interactions influence how genes are expressed during neural development. Differences in these interactions among people may explain why some people are more susceptible than others in developing schizophrenia, depression, BD, or other mental illnesses. These differences can make it difficult to design therapies to prevent the expression of alleles associated with a particular disease. Nevertheless, genetic analysis can clarify which individuals are at risk of developing psychiatric disorders. It can guide monitoring of behavior from an early age and inform decisions about whether or when to initiate treatment.

Neuroimmune interactions may also have a causal role in psychiatric disorders. Studies have indicated correlations between abnormal synaptic pruning in adolescent and young adult brains and schizophrenia. One hypothesis is that an overactive immune response by microglia to infection in the brain causes synaptic overpruning (Paus, Keshavan, and Giedd, 2008; Talbot, Foster, and Woolf, 2016). Release of inflammatory cytokines in response to infection may influence gene–brain–environment interactions and contribute to the development of depression or exacerbate depressive symptoms. Abnormal microglial and cytokine activity may be traceable to prenatal events, where stress or infection in the womb can disrupt gene expression regulating subsequent neurotransmission and synaptic connectivity. Neuroendocrine processes may also be significant in the pathogenesis of psychiatric disorders. Chronically elevated glucocorticoid signaling from prenatal or psychosocial stress in childhood and adolescence may alter normal brain processes and impair neural development. The sex hormones estrogen, progesterone, and testosterone play a critical role in myelination, which, together with synaptic pruning, is necessary for brain maturation (Arain, Haque, Johal et al., 2013). Hormonal changes during adolescence and early adulthood may interfere with myelination. Depending on how changes in the endocrine system influence brain development, they may promote or disrupt neural functions and the cognitive and emotional functions they mediate.

Psychiatric disorders are neurodevelopmental disorders. They may become neurodegenerative disorders when they are treatment-resistant and result in long-term structural and functional changes in the brain. Reduced gray matter volume, enlarged ventricles, and chronic dysfunctional frontal–temporal–parietal connectivity are examples of neurodegeneration in schizophrenia. These features correspond to increasing cognitive and emotional impairment over the course of an affected person's life. Reduced prefrontal and hippocampal volumes and chronic dysfunctional frontal–limbic connectivity are examples of neurodegeneration in major depression. These features also correspond to increasing cognitive and emotional impairment as an affected person ages. Failing to intervene in the brain when symptoms first appear, or before they appear, could harm a person by failing to prevent what could become an entrenched disease with significant functional limitations and poor quality of life. Yet using psychotropic drugs to alter the brain of an adolescent who would not subsequently have a disease could unnecessarily disrupt normal neural development.

More accurate prediction and diagnosis and early treatment may prevent psychiatric disorders from developing beyond an initial stage. Actions taken shortly after or before birth may prevent them from developing at all. In this chapter, I first discuss reasons for and against interventions during the prodromal phase, when subtle signs of disease begin to appear. Then I discuss the predictive value of biomarkers in psychiatry, highlighting uncertainty about what they can predict, and consider some of the ethical implications of this uncertainty. I explain how neuroimmune and neuroendocrine interactions can shape brain development throughout a person's life. In addition, I discuss gene–environment interactions and genetic and epigenetic analysis to identify individuals susceptible to psychosocial stress resulting in anxiety and depression. This analysis could lead to pharmacological or noninvasive environmental interventions that could mitigate stress and reduce or eliminate the risk of having the disease. Addressing the hypothesis that inflammatory immune responses have a causal role in schizophrenia and depression, I explore the use of immune-modulating drugs that could weaken or prevent these responses.

More speculatively, I explore the possibility of infusing growth factors in the brains of people with advanced psychiatric disorders to prevent further neurodegeneration. It is possible that these factors could stimulate neuroplasticity and induce neurogenesis that could stop or even reverse the disease process. In the last section, I consider the influence of prenatal processes on brain development. In light of the fact that medical interventions do not always control psychiatric disorders, conceiving at certain times rather than others, not conceiving, or terminating a pregnancy when risk factors are present, may be effective means of preventing them.

## Intervening in the prodromal phase

The prodrome is the phase when nonspecific changes in thought and behavior precede characteristic overt symptoms of a psychiatric disorder. Pointing to changes in subjective experience for people later diagnosed with the disorder, Josef Parnas claims that "disturbances of presence seem to be the earliest type of prodromal experience in schizophrenia" (2003, p. 224). In this disorder, there are early, subtle changes in the phenomenology of presence. Instead of feeling embodied and embedded in the environment, the person feels detached from his body and disconnected from the world. This feature of schizophrenia classifies it as a disorder of consciousness. Other more commonly mentioned prodromal features of schizophrenia include impaired sensory gating, attention, and working memory (Castle and Buckley, 2015, p. 42). These early signs may initiate a transition to psychosis and warrant preventive treatments at this time. Insofar as the cognitive and experiential aspects of this disorder are traceable to underlying neurobiological abnormalities, drug therapy would seem an effective means of prevention. Dopamine dysregulation is one characteristic of schizophrenia. If prodromal symptoms correlate with this dysregulation, then a drug that modulated baseline synaptic dopamine levels and dopamine release would be one way of preventing it from progressing to a severe disorder (Howes, McCutcheon, Owen et al., 2017). Whether prepsychotic symptoms lead to psychotic episodes and schizophrenia is uncertain, however, as is the benefit of early pharmacological intervention.

In Chapter 3, I pointed out that antipsychotic drugs could have significant metabolic and cardiovascular side effects. These have to be weighed against the ability of these drugs to control cognitive symptoms in the positive subtype of schizophrenia. There are sound reasons for administering these drugs in the prodromal phase as potentially preventive treatment. But the likelihood of adverse effects of drugs used before a definitive diagnosis has been made should raise questions about this practice. One study of patients in the prodromal phase prior to clinical psychosis showed that "medications appeared to be associated with greater impairment in attention and working memory" (Reichenberg and Mollon, 2016, p. 1249; Seidman, Shapiro, Stone et al., 2016). Rather than improving cognitive functions, the drugs made them worse. While the authors of and commentators on the study point out that "the results are complex and should be interpreted with caution" (Reichenberg and Mollon, 2016, p. 1249), this is an example of how early intervention does not always benefit individuals at risk of having a psychiatric disorder. Abraham Reichenberg and Josephine Mollon mention heterogeneity of cognitive functions among individuals at risk of schizophrenia as a confounding factor in estimating outcomes of preventive interventions. "There is . . . considerable heterogeneity within clinical high-risk samples because studies have consistently observed that most high-risk individuals do not go on to develop clinical psychosis, and a substantial minority may even recover symptomatically and functionally. Future research should focus on understanding the neurocognitive and psychosocial factors that characterize non-converters, as well as those who recover" (Reichenberg and Mollon, 2016, pp. 1249–1250).

These comments underscore the need to interpret cognitive symptoms within the context of biological, psychological, and social factors, as well as how the combination of these factors influences symptoms and underlying disease mechanisms. This broader approach may be one way of addressing the problem of false positives in identifying individuals who are at high risk for but do not develop psychosis (Wehler and Preskorn, 2016). False positives may be more likely to arise from studies focusing on genetics and neuroimaging data from populations rather than individuals. The 50% concordance rate of homozygous twins is a reminder that genetics cannot predict all forms of risk for schizophrenia (Insel, 2010, p. 190). Other biological and psychosocial influences on different people's brains might explain variability in neurocognitive functions. Without a better understanding of these complex causal relationships, and their connection to disease, many people who would not develop schizophrenia or other psychiatric disorders would take psychotropic drugs with no therapeutic benefit and only harm from adverse effects on the body and brain. The changes induced by psychoactive substances could be especially harmful if they were given during adolescence, when the brain is still developing. The reasons for intervening during this period are understandable, since the onset of most psychiatric disorders typically occurs during adolescence. Yet these reasons must be weighed against the potential harm in attempting to prevent a disease that might not develop.

Longitudinal studies have provided evidence for prodromal symptoms in depression. These include anxiety, irritability, and sleep and mood disturbances as early signs of the disorder. The fact that these are among the symptoms included in a diagnosis of major depression suggests that the differences between earlier and later symptoms of the disorder are of degree rather than kind and are all part of its pathogenesis (Belmaker and Agam, 2008). A similar prodromal pattern has been observed in studies of bipolar depression, where individuals later diagnosed with the disorder had earlier isolated hypomanic and depressive episodes (Frye, 2011; Strakowski, 2014). In addition, studies conducted over many years confirm that many patients with OCD report at last one prodromal symptom, such as somatic anxiety, irritability, or indecision before a definitive diagnosis of the disorder has been established (Hirschtritt, Bloch, and Mathews, 2017).

Nevertheless, symptoms described as prodromal do not necessarily convert to disease. Although these symptoms may indicate a moderately high or high probability of developing a psychiatric disorder, the appearance of symptoms alone does not imply that a person will go on to have schizophrenia, MDD, BD, or OCD. Even an individual at risk of developing schizophrenia based on having a first-degree relative with the disorder may have schizophreniform disorder for 1 month but not continue to have symptoms for the 6-month period necessary for a diagnosis of schizophrenia. This is significant when considering that all psychotropic drugs prescribed for these disorders have side effects, some more serious than others. While these drugs can relieve symptoms, they can also have neurological, psychological, and somatic sequelae. The heterogeneity of the effects of biological, psychological, and environmental influences on the brain should influence decisions about psychopharmacological intervention when an individual presents with prodromal symptoms. In many cases, the intervention could mitigate the disease process and clearly benefit the individual. In other cases, the intervention may be unnecessary and could cause more harm than benefit. This is one of the challenges of probabilistic risk assessment in making decisions about whether to treat psychiatric disorders, and which treatments to use.

Endophenotypes may help to clarify the probability of early changes in thought and behavior progressing to psychopathology. These traits are phenotypic abnormalities with a clear genetic connection to a disorder. They appear before overt symptoms and indicate susceptibility to disease (Gottesman and Gould, 2003). Some may appear well before diagnosis. For example, "preschizophrenic phenotypic abnormalities are traceable to the neonatal period and to early childhood" (Parnas, 2003, p. 236). The ability of researchers to use endophenotypes to confirm the connection between genes and psychiatric disorders distinguishes them from biomarkers, or makes them a unique type of biomarker. They are often included in explanations of the pathogenesis of heritable conditions such as schizophrenia and BD. Impaired sensory gating and working memory could be endophenotypes in schizophrenia. Impaired face-emotion labelling and first-episode hypomania could be endophenotypes in BD. Sleep disturbances in MDD and somatic anxiety and irritability in OCD are additional examples. Whether these features should be categorized as endophenotypes or prodromal features may depend on the extent of the role of genetics in these disorders (Misiak, Frydecka, and Rybakowski, 2016). For disorders that have a clear genetic component and are highly heritable, identifying behavioral changes as endophenotypes may indicate a high probability that disease risk will be realized in overt symptoms. This identification could provide stronger reasons for intervening in the prodromal phase.

Still, while the probability of these changes converting to psychiatric disease may be higher than the probability associated with more ambiguous changes, this does not mean that they will necessarily manifest in disease. Nor does it alter the fact that not all psychotropic drugs can control the underlying path-ophysiology or symptoms, or that some of these drugs may initiate a different pathophysiology. In the absence of a disease, there would be no benefit to offset or compensate for the adverse effects of antipsychotic, antidepressant, anxio-lytic, or other psychotropic drugs.

## Biomarkers for psychiatric disorders: genetics and neuroimaging

A biomarker is a biological feature that can detect or measure the presence or progression of a disease and predict or confirm responses to treatment. Biomarkers can also clarify risk and predict disease in people who are asympto-matic. As I explained in Chapter 1, these signatures may be mutations detected through genetic testing and screening. They may also be abnormal proteins discovered in bodily fluids, or structural and functional changes in the brain detected by neuroimaging. For example, abnormal alpha-synuclein and tau proteins in the cerebrospinal fluid have been identified as biomarkers for neu-rodegenerative diseases such as Alzheimer's (Doecke, Laws, Faux et al., 2012). Biomarkers associated with psychiatric disorders may be detected earlier than endophenotypes. They may have more predictive value for these disorders by indicating a high risk of people developing them. In these respects, they may provide indications for earlier preventive interventions. Biomarkers could be especially significant in the field of child and adolescent psychiatry. They could be used to predict which asymptomatic or early symptomatic individuals would likely develop a disorder.

There is uncertainty about the predictive value of biomarkers. Nonspecific symptoms may or may not develop into the set of symptoms that characterize psychopathologies. This depends on how epigenetic, environmental, and psychosocial events and processes influence these early symptoms (Rothen-berger, Rhode, and Rothenberger, 2015). Identifying specific causal disease mechanisms is problematic because of the complexity of interactions between these events and processes. In Chapter 3, I described a study of neurophysio-logical biomarkers identified by PET to predict treatment responses to the SSRI escitalopram and CBT for subjects with depression. I also mentioned an im-aging study identifying a biomarker associated with first-episode schizophrenia that could guide antipsychotic treatment, and a different study distinguishing brain biomarkers for bipolar and unipolar depression.

Biomarkers could identify early signs of brain pathology to justify initiating therapy. "More refined use of biomarkers might be beneficial, for example, if a biomarker could predict the presence of an early disorder that is not yet clinically evident but would show improved outcome with early treatment" (Boksa, 2013, p. 75). Identifying these biological signatures might lead to interventions that would not just slow the progression of a disease but prevent it from developing (Strawbridge, Young, and Cleare, 2017). Intervening in the brain with psychotropic drugs carries its own risks. By clarifying disease risk, biomarkers may indicate when pharmacological intervention is or is not appropriate. Commenting on actual cases where psychotic-like symptoms appear in individuals as young as 11 or 12 years of age, Michael Rutter writes, "Clearly this presents the possibility of early intervention in late childhood. However, only some individuals with psychotic-like experiences go on to develop schizophrenia, and this highlights the need to develop effective biomarkers to identify those individuals at risk who will actually show schizophrenia" (2013, p. 201).

There is considerable debate about whether there are "effective biomarkers" for specific psychiatric disorders. Presumably, these would be individual biological signatures with a clear role in the etiology and pathogenesis of the disorder. There are questions about just how refined biomarkers could be and whether they could initiate or be part of a new era of personalized psychiatry. These questions are not only about accuracy in predicting responses to treatments but also about accuracy in predicting who will develop psychiatric disorders and whether early intervention can prevent or mitigate them. In the remainder of this section, I consider genetic biomarkers and biomarkers detected by structural and functional brain imaging. Then I explore some of the ethical and social implications of these two types of biomarkers for psychiatry.

The Cross-Disorder Group of the Psychiatric Genomics Consortium states, "Most psychiatric disorders are moderately to highly heritable" (Lee, Ripke, Neale et al., 2013, p. 984). According to Patrick Sullivan, 60–65% of the risk for schizophrenia is attributable to genes. In contrast, 30–40% of the risk for major depression is heritable, with the remaining risk attributable to environmental factors (cited by Abbasi, 2017a, p. 14). Depression is a disorder with many gene variants producing subtle effects in the brain. Due to its heterogeneity, researchers need to collect data from large cohorts of people with depression to gain a better understanding of the genetics of this disorder. The Group further states, "the degree to which genetic variation is unique to individual disorders or shared across disorders is unclear" (Lee, Ripke, Neale et al., 2013, p. 984). Even more unclear is whether a particular person with a genetic susceptibility to a particular disorder will develop it. "Big Data" and genome-wide association studies cannot answer this question. Statistical analysis alone cannot explain why a disorder affects some people at risk but not others. Having a first-degree relative with schizophrenia may entail a high probability of developing the disorder, but it does not determine that one will in fact develop it.

The link between genes and behavior is probabilistic rather than deterministic. It might seem that identifying loci of genetic variations in the DNA of people with schizophrenia could lead to a better understanding of why they develop it. But more than 100 such variations have been discovered thus far, and it is not known which of these variations have a causal role in what is a complex polygenic disease (Ripke, Neale, Corvin et al., 2014). Part of this epistemological problem is that genetic variation by itself cannot account for gene–environment interactions and their effects on neural circuits and neurotransmitters. Disease risk for individuals cannot be assessed independently of these interactions. Kenneth Kendler points out that molecular genetic findings may be informative in revealing pathophysiological mechanisms underlying psychiatric disorders. But it is not likely that they will be diagnostically informative in their own right (Kendler, 2006; Rutter, 2013).

Endophenotypes may be more diagnostically informative. They could confirm risk if they were early symptoms of a disorder. This would provide a sound basis for pharmacological intervention. Still, it is not clear whether starting pharmacotherapy when phenotypic traits appear would stop or slow further development of a disorder and mitigate its effects on the patient. Ideally, interventions should prevent the earliest events in the pathogenesis of a psychiatric disorder. Yet by the time endophenotypes have been identified, prevention may no longer be possible.

Despite challenges in assessing an individual's risk for developing a psychiatric disorder, the combination of genetic analysis and epigenetic analysis may lead to interventions that could mitigate its symptoms or prevent it. Epigenetics refers to changes in gene expression that occur without changes in the DNA sequence. These changes may occur in the body and brain from methylation or interactions between a person's genes and her environment. One study of methylation in people with schizophrenia has identified blood biomarkers of environmental insults in peripheral tissue in some subjects (Aberg, McClay, Nerella et al., 2014). The authors conclude that this information about disease mechanisms may be one component in improved disease management. A more desirable goal of epigenetics in psychiatric research is not just to manage but prevent mental illness.

Eric Nestler notes how "growing evidence supports the hypothesis that epigenetics is a key mechanism through which environmental exposures interact with an individual's genetic constitution and influence gene expression to determine risk for depression throughout life" (2014, p. 454). He adds that "according to this hypothesis, severe stress triggers changes—in vulnerable individuals—in chromatin structure at particular genomic loci in the brain's limbic regions, which drive sustained changes in gene expression that contribute to episodes of depression" (2014, p. 454). Limbic abnormalities partly account for the disrupted emotional processing in depression. Related studies have shown that a high anxiety trait is a vulnerability phenotype for depression associated with stress (Weger and Sandi, 2018). An additional critical feature of the epigenetic hypothesis is that "such stress-induced epigenetic modifications also occur early in life and help determine an individual's lifetime vulnerability or resistance to subsequent stressful events" (Nestler, 2014, p. 454). "Vulnerable" individuals in this context are those with a genetic risk of depression based on heritability.

There is a significant correlation between the timing of many epigenetic modifications and the onset of depression and other psychiatric disorders. Both tend to occur in adolescence or early adulthood. Environmental stimuli perceived as stressors can disrupt synaptic transmission and neural signaling, especially in limbic and frontal–limbic circuits regulating emotion. Although it is still an imperfect science, epigenetics might indicate whether an individual would perceive stimuli and social situations as stressful or threatening or as events to respond to in an emotionally neutral way. Gene–environment interactions can influence negative or positive perceptions of stimuli, which are critical to vulnerability or resilience. In cases where epigenetics suggested vulnerability, avoiding stressful living or working situations and seeking and securing salutary alternatives in a stable and supportive social environment could be part of a preventive strategy. This would depend on how much control an adolescent or young adult and his family had over factors such as income, housing, and access to healthcare. These environmental interventions would not be as direct as pharmaceutical interventions in their effects on the brain. But they could mitigate psychosocial stress as a causal factor in depression.

Biomarkers detected by neuroimaging could be integrated with genetic and epigenetic analysis as part of a more general preventive strategy in psychiatry. Imaging studies could complement findings on the effects of gene–environment interactions on brain function, or clarify these effects when the connection between these interactions and brain function is ambiguous. Combining structural and functional neuroimaging could confirm decisions about which form of treatment—pharmacological, psychological, or a combination of the two—would be most effective in an individual case (Rutter, 2013, p. 201). Vince Calhoun and Muhammad Arbabshirani claim, "There are several biological markers (so-called biomarkers) that can be extracted from each of these complementary imaging techniques" (2013, p. 207). These techniques may include MRI, PET, fMRI, and other imaging modalities. Imaging-detected biomarkers "have the potential to explain effects of psychiatric disorders on the brain" (Calhoun and Arbabshirani, 2013, p. 207). The authors point out that functional imaging showing abnormalities in the default mode network is a neurophysiological biomarker for schizophrenia. They also note that structural imaging showing "reductions in gray matter volume and increased ventricular cerebrospinal fluid are neuroanatomical biomarkers for the disorder" (Calhoun and Arbabshirani, 2013, p. 210). In addition, volumetric MRI, VBM, and DTI have revealed gray matter reductions and reduced connectivity in cortico–cortical and cortical–limbic pathways in individuals with schizophrenia that have not been evident in the brains of healthy controls (Bluhm, Raczek, Broome et al., 2015). These abnormalities may be detectable early in the pathogenesis of the disorder.

Other imaging techniques can detect biomarkers for other disorders. In one study, investigators used arterial spin labelling, which, like fMRI, measures blood flow in the brain, to differentiate early changes in the anterior cingulate cortex associated with bipolar depression from changes associated with unipolar depression (Almeida and Phillips, 2013). This is one respect in which arterial spin labelling can help to establish a definitive diagnosis of BD. It is significant because only one in five patients with this disorder is accurately diagnosed when a healthcare professional first evaluates them. In addition to helping psychiatrists avoid prescribing drugs that could precipitate hypomania, this and other hemodynamic biomarkers may be able to predict future bipolar behavior in younger adults or adolescents who are asymptomatic. These biomarkers may indicate earlier and possibly more effective interventions.

Psychiatric biomarkers need not be genetic, neuroanatomical, or neurophysiological. Hypertension and cardiac arrhythmia may be symptoms of a hyperactive response of the autonomic nervous system to psychosocial stress. In some cases, these cardiovascular changes may be early precursors of anxiety and depression. Increases in heart rate and blood pressure may increase circulating levels of glucocorticoids such as cortisol and catecholamines such as norepinephrine, which can be risk factors for these disorders. Abnormal levels of thyroid hormone in the blood may also be a precursor of depression (Joffe, 2011). It is important to emphasize, however, that many people with these cardiovascular and endocrine symptoms do not develop anxiety or depression. Because psychiatric disorders have a multifactorial etiology, there is no single and direct causal connection between a biomarker and a disorder.

Some psychiatrists and social scientists are skeptical about identifiable biomarkers for psychiatric disorders. For example, Owen, Sawa, and Mortensen write, "no diagnostic test or biomarkers are available" for schizophrenia, "which is made clinically on the basis of history and by examination of the mental state" (2016, p. 86). Even among psychiatrists who acknowledge the presence of these biological signatures, they are circumspect about their ability to predict whether an individual with them will have a disorder. Neuroimaging is the most common means of detecting psychiatric biomarkers. Yet there is uncertainty about the predictive value of the data generated by imaging for psychiatric disorders. Neuroimaging data can be ambiguous and not sufficient to confirm the presence of a particular disorder independently of other features.

Biomarkers detected though neuroimaging can provide a higher level of precision about brain structure and function than genetic analysis. Early signs of abnormal functional connectivity in frontal–temporal–parietal connectivity, imbalance between GABAergic and glutaminergic signaling, or reduced gray matter volume detected by imaging could be early signs of schizophrenia. These findings could warrant preemptive intervention. Still, detection of a biomarker associated with a disorder by neuroimaging at an early stage does not mean that an individual with that biomarker will develop it. Functional imaging measuring levels of neural connectivity may be more useful in this regard than structural imaging. But the information derived from fMRI scans, for example, is more pertinent to groups than individuals. It is thus unclear what the diagnostic and predictive value of functional neuroimaging would be in particular cases.

The predictive or diagnostic value of functional neuroimaging for psychiatric disorders is also unclear because of the inferential gap between the data and brain activity and problems in interpreting this data. In Chapter 1, I cited a meta-analysis showing a false-positive rate of up to 70% among researchers interpreting data from fMRI studies (Eklund, Nichols, and Knutsson, 2016). I also cited a different meta-analysis of fMRI and PET studies to assess the neurobiological basis of cognitive and emotional processing in unipolar depression. In this study, researchers found inconsistencies across individual experiments investigating aberrant brain activity (Muller, Cieslik, Serbanescu et al., 2017). Both meta-analyses illustrate the limitations in identifying the neurobiological underpinning of depression or other mental illnesses at earlier and even later stages of the disease process. Some forms of neuroimaging can provide more accurate information than others regarding early changes in the brain as possible first indications of psychopathology. VBM or DTI might not have the same limitations as fMRI in providing information about these changes. Nevertheless, questions remain about the predictive value of biomarkers detected by all forms of imaging. These in turn raise questions about the justification for intervening in and altering the brains of individuals with these features at a presymptomatic or early symptomatic stage.

Even as researchers identify an increasing number of biomarkers for psychiatric disorders, they will likely have limited predictive value on their own. This is because of the multifactorial etiology of depression and other psychiatric disorders and because of the heterogeneity in the expression of their symptoms.

It is unlikely that a single biomarker will have a significant impact on diagnosis and treatment in psychiatry (Boksa, 2013, p. 76). Although detection of more psychiatric biomarkers through genetic analysis and neuroimaging will contribute to a better understanding of psychiatric disorders, it will not offer a complete explanation of why some people develop these disorders. Nor will it explain why some disorders are more severe than others, or why some patients respond and others fail to respond to therapy. Biomarkers will not replace but supplement other investigative methods for predicting disease onset, severity, responses to treatment, and possible prevention.

Psychiatric biomarkers generate ethical and social concerns. Ideally, information about brain biomarkers would enable individuals with known risk factors for psychiatric disorders, or parents of children at risk, to make rational decisions about potentially preventive interventions. This is hypothetical regarding psychopharmacology, since there are no known drugs that could prevent schizophrenia, depression, or other mental illnesses before the first signs of psychopathology. When illness is present, identifying a particular neuroanatomical or neurophysiological feature could inform psychiatrists of which treatment would be more likely to control or ameliorate their symptoms. The study by McCabe and coinvestigators cited earlier is one example. Detecting the biomarker could benefit patients as part of a process that eventually could reduce the severity of their illness. Except for a relatively small number of cases, though, the current state of biomarker research does not have the requisite level of accuracy to do this on a broad scale. Information about a biomarker when one was asymptomatic or had what appeared to be prodromal symptoms could cause more harm than benefit in at least two respects. First, it could lead to drug treatment for a disease that might not have developed and cause serious side effects without any compensatory benefit. Second, it could generate anxiety over whether one would have a psychiatric disorder and whether available treatments could control it. The anxiety from the uncertainty about developing such a disorder might not be of the same degree as the anxiety generated by the knowledge that one had the *APOEe4* allele associated with late-onset sporadic Alzheimer's disease. There are effective therapies for schizophrenia and depression, but not for Alzheimer's. Nevertheless, the mere possibility of developing mental illness in the near or even remote future could cause a person to experience considerable distress.

If biomarker testing became widely available, then some individuals deemed at risk might refuse to undergo it to avoid the possibility of psychological harm. For those who consented to be tested, healthcare providers would have an obligation to emphasize the uncertainty surrounding biomarkers when discussing this information with them. They would be asymptomatic, or mildly symptomatic, and would not have been given a diagnosis. For these reasons, disclosing information about biomarkers would require balancing the value of this information to the person against the potential of it to cause distress and harm. Communication between psychiatric researchers, primary care physicians, practicing psychiatrists, patients, and their families would be critical for ensuring that those who wanted to know about brain biomarkers received accurate information about them. This may not eliminate the anxiety or fear of developing a mental illness for those who know they are at risk. But it could minimize the potential for psychological harm by clarifying what is currently known—and not known—about biomarkers for psychiatric disorders.

These considerations warrant caution in interpreting the earlier claim that biomarkers could be an important component of precision medicine and a more personalized approach to psychiatric diagnosis and treatment. Much of the uncertainty surrounding biomarkers in assessing the risk of developing a psychiatric disorder is associated with the fact that genetic analysis and neuroimaging research involve group studies. Biomarkers would be clinically relevant only if they had strong predictive value for specific individuals. Researchers cannot draw direct inferences from information about populations or groups to information about individuals within these groups. Risk assessment is probabilistic rather than deterministic. It could not be known whether an individual with a biomarker for depression, for example, would in fact develop the disorder. If one already had the disorder, then a single biomarker would not provide psychiatrists with knowledge of whether or how one would respond to different therapies. Biomarkers would have questionable reliability in particular cases.

Michael Rutter comments that, to be beneficial for patients, "inferences based on biomarkers must be shown to be robust and valuable at the individual level" (2013, p. 189). His comment underscores the limitations of genome-wide studies and neuroimaging in identifying biomarkers and estimating their diagnostic and prognostic potential. Again, this information is only statistically significant for groups. Rutter's comment also underscores the obligation for researchers and practitioners to explain to patients and research subjects the uncertainty in probabilistic risk assessment using biomarkers in psychiatry. This would include emphasizing the fact that psychiatric disorders arise from a complex set of factors and that biomarkers are just one of these factors. Whether an individual will develop a psychiatric disorder, how severe it will be, and whether it will respond to treatment, cannot be predicted based on biomarker information alone.

The tendency to overgeneralize and oversimplify biomarker findings could have broader social implications. Ilina Singh and Nikolas Rose point out that, in cases involving children, "biomarker information might reshape the beliefs, practices and decision-making of the people in a child's environment, including parents, teachers and health providers" (2009, p. 204). This could unduly influence how they interpret the child's behavior and their interactions with the child. The idea that a child was predisposed to mental illness could lead others to limit opportunities for him and the development of his autonomous agency. Biomarkers could also contribute to or exacerbate the stigma associated with psychiatric disorders. Phenotypically normal people could be stigmatized or discriminated against because they have a biomarker without any demonstrable disease state (Sadler, 2009). Discrimination is a major concern. Third parties such as insurance companies could gain unauthorized access to medical information that included biomarkers questionably associated with mental illness. They could use this information to unfairly deny medical insurance to individuals they considered at risk of having a costly mental illness. Companies could deny employment to individuals with biomarkers for similar reasons. More disturbing is the possible use of biomarkers to construct profiles of future antisocial or criminal behavior in children. As I pointed out in my discussion of psychopathic traits in youth in Chapter 6, this could lead to psychopharmacological intervention at an age when the brain was undergoing critical maturation of myelin and synapses. Taking psychotropic drugs at an early age could result in permanent deleterious effects on brain structure and function. Even if these drugs were safe, it is questionable whether this intervention could achieve a preventive goal and be medically and ethical justified, given that behavior is a function of neurobiological, psychological, and environmental factors. Medications with their own significant risks and toxicities could be given to children who would not subsequently engage in any criminal behavior. If the detection of brain biomarkers supported early intervention in children's brains to prevent harmful behavior, then the children could not consent to take psychotropic medication. Their parents would have to give proxy consent for drug therapy on the children's behalf. The ambiguous connection between biomarkers and future behavior makes it unclear whether this would be in a child's best interests.

Biomarkers will be an increasingly important component in more accurate diagnosis and effective treatment of psychiatric disorders. But their predictive value for mental disorders and behavior in general is uncertain because they are based on the uncertain enterprise of probabilistic risk assessment (Baum and Savulescu, 2013; Baum, 2016, Chapter 2). This should temper claims that identifying biomarkers will lead to early interventions that will prevent disease. More longitudinal studies are needed to clarify their explanatory significance in psychiatry. They are only one component among other biological, psychological, and environmental components in the onset and progression of diseases of the brain and mind. Singh and Rose emphasize, "Prospective research on these issues is needed to inform policies and practices that will maximize the positive potential of biomarker information and protect individuals and families from harm" (2009, p. 204).

## Neuroimmune and neuroendocrine interactions

Central nervous, endocrine, and immune systems interact to promote adaptability to and survival of human organisms in the natural environment. The brain processes information from the external world and the body to enable the organism to recognize and respond to external and internal threats. The combined action of the innate and adaptive components of the immune system eliminates pathogenic threats to the body and brain by responding appropriately to infection. The action of the endocrine system in releasing stress hormones in the body and brain enables the organism to fight or flee from threatening environmental circumstances. In these and other respects, neuroimmune and neuroendocrine communication maintains homeostasis (Talbot, Foster, and Woolf, 2016). In some cases, however, overactive immune and endocrine responses can trigger or aggravate inflammation and other processes in the brain, disturb homeostasis, and cause neural and mental dysfunction.

A chronic hyperactive stress response to stimuli can release chronic high circulating levels of cortisol and norepinephrine. This can result in dysfunctional prefrontal–limbic connectivity and cognitive-emotional processing characteristic of anxiety and depression. Prolonged neural and mental dysfunction can result in prefrontal and hippocampal atrophy in people with these disorders. This is an example of how adverse neuroendocrine interaction can cause both neurodevelopmental abnormalities and neurodegeneration (Sapolsky, 2000; Sorrells, Caso, Munhoz et al., 2009). Elevated activation of microglia, the brain's immune cells, is one hypothesis for the excessive synaptic pruning associated with schizophrenia. A different hypothesis is that high circulating levels of proinflammatory cytokines can cause neural circuit disturbances associated with depression or increase them in people who already have this disorder. In both schizophrenia and depression, inflammation in the brain appears to cause dysregulation in neurotransmitters and neural circuits underlying cognitive and emotional processing. Whereas the inflammation and dysregulation in the brain triggered by elevated microglia activation appears to be in response to infection or other physiological processes, the inflammation and dysregulation triggered by cytokines may be in response not only to infection but also to psychosocial stressors (Miller and Raison, 2016).

Could pharmacological or other interventions modulate inflammatory immune and endocrine responses in the brain and eliminate what could be causal factors in psychiatric disorders? Could immune- and endocrine-modulating or other drugs prevent these disorders at the earliest detectable sign of neural dysfunction? Abnormal neuroimmune interaction could be an early sign of a psychiatric disorder. Identifying this abnormality could be the first step in preventing a disorder from developing further.

Many psychiatric disorders emerge during adolescence when the brain is still developing. Adolescence is an active period of the neurobiological processes of myelination and synaptic pruning (Paus, Keshavan, and Giedd, 2008; Keshavan, Giedd, Lau et al., 2014). Myelination refers to the production of the myelin sheath around axons constituting white matter in the brain. Synaptic pruning is the natural process of eliminating excess neuronal synapses that develop in the first years of life (Boksa, 2012). Because psychiatric disorders involve dysfunction in synaptic connectivity and emerge at a time when synaptic pruning is in progress, researchers have drawn correlations between these disorders, particularly schizophrenia, and abnormal synaptic pruning. Schizophrenia could result from a defect of synaptic elimination during adolescence. This defect may be due to an overactive microglial response to infection or other insult to the brain. When functioning normally, microglia eliminate unnecessary synapses in the same way they remove pathogens and damaged cells through phagocytosis.

Approximately 40% of the total number of synapses in the brain are eliminated during adolescence. This elimination process is necessary not only for functional connectivity between neural circuits but also for the maturation of the frontal lobes, which are critical for cognitive and emotional processing. If microglial mechanisms become hyperactive, then their protective response may become a pathological response in pruning too many synapses. Overpruning may also result from a surge in sex hormones during adolescence (Hoekzema, Barba-Muller, Pozzobon et al., 2017). A similar endocrine process may have a causal role in the reduction of the volume of gray matter in the brains of new mothers. Normal neuroimmune and neuroendocrine communication becomes miscommunication, resulting in the pruning of too many synapses. This impairs connectivity in frontal–temporal–parietal and frontal–limbic pathways mediating the cognitive and emotional capacity necessary for normal thought and behavior. Abnormal immune activation can adversely affect myelination and axonal activity and result in reduction of white as well as gray matter volume in the brain (Paus, Keshavan, and Giedd, 2008; Keshavan, Giedd, Lau et al., 2014). Neural dysfunction caused by hyperactive immune and endocrine responses can result in subsequent psychomotor, cognitive. and emotional impairment. The type of neuroimmune interaction in psychiatric disorders is distinct from the neuroimmune interaction in anti-NMDA receptor encephalitis. Although this neurological disorder involves psychosis, the underlying pathogenesis is more acute and involves different mechanisms than those in the positive subtype of schizophrenia or bipolar depression (Dalmau, Gleichman, Hughes et al., 2008).

When the overpruning process has been active for an extended period, it may be too late for any intervention to stop or reverse it. But structural and functional neuroimaging may be able to detect the earliest indications of overpruning by comparing the brains of those at risk of schizophrenia with normal controls who are not at risk. In one study, PET brain imaging was able to detect increased microglial activity in subjects at high risk of psychosis (Bloomfield, Selvaraj, Veronese et al., 2016). If synaptic overpruning is the result of a hyperactive immune response to infection in the brain, then even those without a first-generation relative with schizophrenia could develop the disease. Genetic susceptibility to the disorder may make synaptic overpruning more likely. But not having the alleles associated with schizophrenia would not necessarily preclude it in people with abnormal neuroimmune interaction. Those without the typical risk factors would not be likely candidates for imaging studies. This could overlook other early signs of psychopathology.

Assuming that there is a causal connection between elevated microglia activation and excessive synaptic pruning, immune-modulating drugs capable of downregulating this activation could be administered at the first detectable sign of abnormal pruning. This would occur before disease onset and might stop the pathophysiology. Crucially, any such drug would have to be immunomodulating without being immunosuppressive. It would have to avoid disruption of protective innate and adaptive immune functions in the brain. Blocking elevated microglial activation should leave other neuroimmune interactions intact. If a drug suppressed innate and adaptive immune functions in the brain, then it could leave subjects vulnerable to infectious agents that could damage healthy brain cells and tissue. Because this is hypothetical, one can only speculate on how this intervention would affect not just neuroimmune interaction but brain functions in general. This is a promising area of research with the potential to yield a better understanding of neuroimmune interaction. It could lead to preventive interventions for some major psychiatric disorders.

The connections between microglial activation, synaptic pruning, and schizophrenia are still unclear. Clinical trials are underway to investigate how interfering with hyperactive microglial activation could reduce symptoms and possibly prevent this disorder (Howes and McCutcheon, 2015). Researchers would introduce the blocking mechanism in subjects in whom there was a correlation between immune hyperactivation and early symptoms. Yet this raises the same issues that arise regarding initiating treatment based on early detection of biomarkers and prodromal symptoms. Some individuals considered to be at high risk based on genetics and abnormal synaptic pruning may develop full-blown symptoms of schizophrenia. Others may have more synaptic pruning than normal but not develop the disorder. Still others with similar risk factors may have a normal rate of synaptic pruning and not develop it either.

The combination of genetic analysis and imaging could indicate the probability of a person having schizophrenia. Like information about biomarkers, though, information about synaptic pruning alone could not predict that a person would actually develop the disorder. This is significant because any drug infused into the brain could have adverse effects. Specifically, intravenous immunoglobulin to modulate microglial function may cause hematologic toxicities in the brain (Baxley and Akhtari, 2011). A subject who had some neuroimmune dysfunction but did not develop schizophrenia could be exposed to these toxicities. In that case, there would be harm without any compensatory benefit. In addition, there would be uncertainty about the timing of the intervention and how intervening too early could interfere with normal developmental processes in a maturing brain.

To be ethically justified, clinical trials designed to test the safety of this intervention would depend on investigators judging that the risk of microglial hyperactivity, excessive synaptic pruning, and mental illness for certain individuals was greater than any risk of adverse effects of drugs designed to weaken or block these processes. If the goal of the research was to test whether early drug intervention could prevent disease onset, then only asymptomatic or early symptomatic individuals deemed at *high* risk of schizophrenia should be allowed to participate as subjects in the active experimental arm of a controlled study. This would be the only way of answering the research question.

The study on the connection between hyperactive microglia and schizophrenia refers to the research subjects as "people at *ultra high risk* of psychosis" (Bloomfield, Selvaraj, Veronese et al., 2016, p. 44, emphasis added). A small number of these subjects in phase I trials would be necessary to establish the safety of the drug before later phase II and phase III trials could establish its efficacy. Healthy subjects are allowed to participate in phase I trials for other experimental drugs without any probable benefit and with some risk. The difference between these subjects and those at risk of schizophrenia who are asymptomatic or with prodromal symptoms but no diagnosis of disease may not seem ethically significant. Nevertheless, the potential for adverse effects in the brain and body from drugs altering immune and neural functions suggests that a higher standard of protection of research subjects should be in place before initiating the trials. The additive risk of harm from altering both central nervous and immune systems could be significantly higher than the risk from altering one of these systems alone.

There is also the question of whether an adolescent whose brain has undergone excessive synaptic pruning would have enough cognitive capacity to give informed consent to participate in research testing neuroimmune modulating drugs as a form of psychiatric prophylaxis. Ordinarily, an 18-year-old would be of consenting age, as would a younger mature minor. But it is unclear whether this neuropathology would impair her capacity to process information and make a reasoned decision about treatment or participation in research. This would be in addition to the fact that the frontal lobes mediating this capacity are naturally immature during adolescence. Imaging showing structural and functional brain changes confirming overpruning might suggest impaired mental capacity. Nevertheless, a determination of capacity would be based on the individual's behavior, specifically how she responded to questions from researchers conducting a clinical trial. In the case of an adolescent at high risk who did not meet criteria of capacity because he was not a mature minor, a parent could give proxy consent to enroll him in a trial. This could be justified if the same protections were in place that would be in place if the subject were capable of consenting on his own. This would follow earlier proxy consent to allow the adolescent to undergo brain imaging to clarify risk.

Two separate acts of informed or proxy consent would be necessary, one regarding brain imaging, and the other regarding neuroimmune modulation. The first act would be required for the second, but consenting to the first would not entail an obligation to consent to the second. Given the risk of a drug altering neuroimmune function, a parent giving proxy consent would have to demonstrate a higher level of understanding of the purpose and potential effects of the drug infusion than what would be required for imaging. This risk would also entail a stronger obligation of the researchers conducting the trial to explain the biochemical mechanism of the drug and the reasons for testing it.

Another challenge for delivering such a drug into the brain would be the blood-brain barrier. If the drugs consisted of large molecules, then they might not be able to cross the BBB. One way of overcoming this problem would be to use FUS, which can open the BBB and allow drugs to enter the brain that otherwise would be blocked from entering it. Still, delivering a drug into the brain is one thing; controlling any immunosuppressive of immunogenic effects of the drug in the brain is quite another. Solving the delivery problem would not resolve questions about potential positive and negative effects of psychoactive drugs on brain structure and function. Only a sufficient number of phase

I and phase II trials with a sufficient number of subjects could answer these questions.

Abnormal neuroimmune interactions may also influence the pathophysiology of a subgroup of patients with depression (Miller, Meletic, and Raison, 2009; Raison and Miller, 2011; Felger and Lotrich, 2013; Miller and Raison, 2016). Perceived or actual environmental threats to the subject can trigger a hyperactive stress response and a cascade of neurophysiological events. This can cause an adverse biochemical environment in the brain and disturb neural mechanisms mediating normal mental functions. In addition to cortisol and norepinephrine, psychosocial stress can cause the release of high circulating levels of inflammatory cytokines such as tumor necrosis factor 1, and interleukins 1 and 6. These can also cause or contribute to brain inflammation. This neurophysiological process can disrupt the innate capacity of the organism to regulate internal functions and maintain equilibrium in the body and brain by counteracting adverse influences from the environment.

Andrew Miller and Charles Raison claim that "the greater the inflammatory response [in the brain] to a psychosocial stressor, the more probable the subject is to develop depression over the ensuing months" (2016, p. 22). They add, "As the field [of neuro-immunology] has matured, it has become increasingly apparent that inflammatory markers are elevated not only in subgroups of patients with depression but also in patients with other neuropsychiatric disorders including anxiety disorders and schizophrenia" (2016, p. 25). Miller and Raison state that psychosocial stress can also lead to the activation of microglia (2016, p. 26). This is significant because it suggests that different inflammatory responses may be involved in depression and other psychiatric disorders. It also suggests that something other than pathogens and tissue injury may be the source of these responses. Equally significant, "inflammation has been associated with antidepressant non-responsiveness" (Miller and Raison, 2016, p. 25). Chronic inflammation in the brain resulting in monoamine dysregulation may be part of an explanation for treatment-resistant major depression.

Although inflammatory cytokines are relatively large molecules, they can influence brain function by crossing through "leaky" sections of the BBB (Miller and Raison, 2016, p. 27). The main pathophysiological consequence of inflammatory cytokines in depression is a reduction of synaptic availability of monoamines such as serotonin and dopamine (Miller and Raison, 2016, p. 27). Cytokines can also disrupt glutamate and neuropeptide signaling pathways (Felger and Lotrich, 2013). This dysfunction of neurotransmitters can cause dysfunction in frontal–limbic circuits—including the PFC, dorsal anterior cingulate cortex, insula, and amygdala—and contribute to anhedonia, avolition, and impaired cognition from abnormal fear responses to stimuli (Miller and

Raison, 2016, p. 29). Miller and Raison note, "fMRI studies have demonstrated that increased inflammation is also associated with increased activation of threat-and anxiety-related neurocircuitry" in these regions (2016, p. 29). Some people with depression linked to inflammation experience somatic symptoms in the form of nonspecific pain and disturbance of the phenomenology of the subject's relation to his body. Not all depressed patients have these symptoms and this experience (Ratcliffe, Broome, Smith et al., 2014, pp. 177–180). More generally, the role of psychosocial stressors in this account of depression supports a biopsychosocial model for explaining depression. It does not result from biological factors alone.

Similar to research into neuroimmune interaction in schizophrenia, anti-inflammatory drugs could be an intervention in depression when there is a correlation between inflammation and the mental and behavioral features of this disorder. Clinical trials have used this class of drugs to block overactive immune responses in depressed patients (Miller and Raison, 2016, pp. 31–32). Reducing inflammation in the body and brain could relieve depressive symptoms in some affected persons. High levels of inflammatory biomarkers such as C-reactive protein in the blood might indicate intervening with drugs that could reduce inflammation before the onset of symptoms, or when they first appear. Interventions could be therapeutic or preventive. However, there are good reasons for caution regarding pharmacological attempts to prevent depression by targeting inflammatory mechanisms. Even when there are correlations between inflammation and depression, this does not mean that the first causes the second. It is difficult to justify using psychotropic drugs with potentially adverse effects in the body and brain in the absence of a known causal relation between them. It is especially difficult to justify this action when a person is asymptomatic, or mildly symptomatic, and may not fully develop major depression.

Within the subgroups of depressed patients with corresponding high levels of inflammation, the hypothesis of immune dysregulation as a causal factor in this disorder is inconclusive (Ratcliffe, Broome, Smith et al., p. 177). Miller and Raison acknowledge the need for the "balanced perspective that anti-inflammatory therapies are unlikely to be all-purpose antidepressants" (2016, p. 31). The presence of one or more reliable inflammatory biomarkers in the brain does not imply that a person with them will develop depression. An anti-inflammatory drug could modulate neuroimmune interaction and some of the mechanisms underlying this disorder. On the other hand, it might disrupt innate and adaptive immune functions and make individuals susceptible to infection in the brain. An intervention designed to prevent depression could result in preventable harm.

Identifying patients with both depression and brain inflammation and confirming a correlation between them would be critical for determining whether neuroimmune modulating drugs could benefit them. At an early stage of research, knowing whether these drugs could cause adverse changes in the brain would be more difficult. Miller and Raison mention other potentially harmful aspects of pharmacological intervention in the brain: "Anti-inflammatory drugs may harm patients without increased inflammation. Inflammatory cytokines and the innate immune response have pivotal roles in synaptic plasticity, neurogenesis, long-term potentiation (which is a fundamental process in learning and memory) and possible antidepressant response" (2016, p. 31). This suggests that the potential for adverse consequences of altering neuroimmune functions goes beyond increased susceptibility to infection. It underscores the need for additional studies to clarify whether or in which cases brain inflammation causes depression. It also underscores the need to determine which interventions could safely and effectively modulate or reduce inflammation and reduce the severity of or prevent the disorder. This would depend on an optimal dose of the drug and the timing of infusion so that it coincided with the critical processes in the brain.

Those who already have a psychiatric disorder are beyond the possibility of preventing its onset. Some may control symptoms and disease progression with pharmacotherapy. A substantial number of others do not respond to any therapies, and their brains undergo a gradual process of neurodegeneration. In these cases, a neurodevelopmental disorder becomes a neurodegenerative disorder. This does not foreclose all possibilities of slowing or even reversing neural degeneration, however. It is instructive to consider a particular intervention that might have these effects.

Focused ultrasound can increase the permeability of the BBB to promote drug delivery into the brain. This could overcome the problem of drugs consisting of large molecules that cannot penetrate this barrier. It could be one form of early treatment of diseases of the CNS (Baseri, Choi, Deffieux et al., 2012; Burgess and Hynynen, 2014). These are typically characterized as degenerative neurological diseases such as PD or Alzheimer's disease. But chronic psychiatric disorders may result in similar patterns of neurodegeneration. Although it is experimental, the use of FUS of a certain intensity could open the BBB and allow delivery of exogenous brain-derived neurotrophic factor (BDNF) and other neurotrophic factors into the brain. It is possible that this could prevent further progression of schizophrenia after the disease already had developed.

Studies have shown reduced BDNF protein and mRNA levels in patients with schizophrenia (Balu and Coyle, 2011; Boksa, 2012, p. 76). The levels of this protein correlate positively with spine density in the PFC. Reduced levels of BDNF protein and mRNA correlate with reduced prefrontal volume. Theoretically, infusion of BDNF into the brains of patients with schizophrenia could stop progression of the disease by restoring normal synaptic connectivity. Infusion of these factors at a later disease stage might induce or enhance neuroplasticity and neurogenesis in psychiatric disorders with neurodegeneration from chronic treatment-resistance. Researchers could deliver these growth factors into brains with substantially reduced gray and white matter volumes, reduced prefrontal volume, and impaired functional connectivity in neural circuits disrupted in schizophrenia, depression, and BD. These may be cases of advanced disease resulting from brain inflammation and chronic and extensive synaptic overpruning. Neuroanatomical and neurophysiological degeneration may be from other causes as well. The aim of the intervention would not just be to prevent further development of disease but to reverse it. In cases of extensive neurodegeneration, attempts to regenerate neurons and synaptic connectivity may fail. In cases of moderate degeneration, there may be potential for neurogenesis.

Still, investigators would have to weigh this potential against the potential for excitotoxicity and uncontrolled proliferation of growth factors that could damage healthy cells and tissue in the brain. These processes could defeat the purpose of the intervention and leave research subjects worse off than they were with the mental illness. Depending on the extent to which neurodegeneration impaired their cognitive capacity, questions about their capacity for informed consent to participate in these experiments would arise here too. Given the risk of deleterious proliferative effects of trophic factors in the brain, only subjects with a sufficient level of cognitive capacity and clear imaging-based signs of neurodegeneration should be allowed to participate in these studies. The lack of knowledge about the possible effects of delivering exogenous growth factors into the brain may lead some to question whether even competent individuals could give informed consent to participate in proof-of principle phase I trials testing the safety of the technique. Some might cite studies I mentioned in Chapter 4 suggesting the possibility of increased neuroplasticity from the use of DBS in patients with early-stage PD. Thy might argue that, like early DBS, delivering growth factors in the brain when a psychiatric disorder was less advanced could induce endogenous regenerative processes and prevent further abnormal neurodevelopment and subsequent neurodegeneration. Early intervention would be more likely to achieve both a preventive and therapeutic goal.

At least two qualifications are in order, however. First, inducing neurogenesis through exogenous neural growth factors is still an unproven hypothesis. One cannot assume that this intervention would stop the underlying pathophysiology in psychiatric disorders. Second, researchers do not know whether any unintended proliferative effects of growth factors in the brain would be reversible. The magnitude of any harm to patients and research subjects from factors gone awry in the brain could be substantial. Nevertheless, these trials would be necessary to generate knowledge about the potential benefits and risks of the technique and answer questions about its therapeutic potential. Consistent with the first stage of any ethically justified clinical trial, a series of phase I trials testing toxicity levels of growth factors incrementally could provide adequate protection of research subjects. They would be a critical first step in addressing all of the medically and ethically relevant issues regarding the use of these factors to treat diseases of the brain.

In the last part of Chapter 4, I mentioned a study indicating that some patients with PD would prefer to wait until an advanced disease stage before undergoing DBS. Their attitudes about the risks associated with the procedure outweighed their attitudes about the therapeutic potential of earlier use of the technique. In the issue at hand, only patients with treatment-resistant schizophrenia or depression and early signs of neurodegeneration would be candidates for the experimental infusion of neural growth factors to slow or reverse this pathology. It is not known whether psychiatric patients with these features, given the opportunity, would want to participate in this research earlier or later in the disease process. Specifically, it is not known how the risks associated with the procedure would influence their attitudes about whether or when to participate in the research. If the risks associated with infusing growth factors in the brain were the same regardless of the stage of disease when the drug was infused, and if the neurogenerative potential of the procedure were greater if administered at an earlier stage, then many patients would probably decide to participate in the research at an earlier rather than later time. These decisions would also depend on the judgment of psychiatrists, neurologists, and neurosurgeons about the optimal timing and dose of the infusion. This judgment would also depend on the extent of neurodegeneration.

As noted, there are noninvasive ways of preventing anxiety and depression linked to psychosocial stressors. Epigenetic analysis of the type proposed by Nestler could identify which individuals with certain risk factors would be susceptible or resilient to these stressors and these disorders. For those identified as being susceptible, altering the natural and social environment could preempt or weaken a hyperactive emotional reaction to fear-inducing stimuli. In addition, techniques such as CBT could enable them to reframe their beliefs and modulate their responses to stimuli so that they did not perceive them as threats. Psychotherapeutic interventions alone, or in combination with psychopharmacology, have been effective in controlling and relieving symptoms of anxiety and depression. It is uncertain whether psychotherapeutic treatments, combined with environmental changes, could prevent these disorders if they were initiated at a presymptomatic or early symptomatic stage. Epigenetic analysis could clarify this question by identifying at-risk individuals who may be more likely to respond to these interventions.

The idea of preventing anxiety and depression by avoiding or neutralizing psychosocial triggers of hyperactive neuroendocrine and neuroimmune responses linked to these disorders is at least intuitively plausible. If this early identification and intervention were successful, then it could obviate the need for psychotropic drugs or exogenous neurotrophic factors. It could avoid the side effects of drugs and result in a much more favorable ratio of benefit to harm.

## Prenatal interventions

Many studies have indicated an association between certain events in the fetal environment and the development of some psychiatric disorders (Brander, Perez-Vigil, Larsson et al., 2016; Fernandez and Leckman, 2016). These events are associated with neuroimmune and neuroendocrine interactions in the fetus and the biological mother. Insel writes, "Environmental factors identified so far have also [in addition to genetics] implicated prenatal or perinatal events Maternal malnutrition during famine, infections in the second trimester, perinatal injury and cytokine exposures have all been associated with subsequent increased risk for schizophrenia. Most of these effects are modest (less than a twofold increase in risk) and none seem specific for schizophrenia, but in aggregate they demonstrate that early adverse experiences, including mid-gestational insults, are a risk factor for psychosis occurring two decades later" (2010, p. 188). Insel further notes, "The model that emerges from this neurodevelopmental perspective is that of an early insult, a latent period through much of neural development, and the emergence of psychosis in late adolescence or early adulthood" (2010, p. 189). These adverse experiences include epigenetic factors that influence gene expression in the brain and how genes regulate neural and mental functions. An example is a link between prenatal nutritional deficiency and extremely low gestational weight and subsequent nonaffective psychosis in offspring (Mackay, Dalman, Karlsson et al., 2017).

Prenatal risk factors are particularly significant in the etiology of depression, OCD, and schizophrenia. Preventing these events and processes at an early stage of human life could prevent these disorders. Yet researchers have not identified a single event or process as the sole cause of any of these disorders. Biological and environmental factors inside and outside of the womb and fetal brain may all have a causal role in their pathogenesis. Moreover, the long-term effects of interactions between these factors may be unpredictable. This can make it difficult to control how processes in preconceptual, prenatal, and perinatal periods influence the emergence of psychiatric disorders. Nevertheless, researchers have established associations between these earlier and later processes. Mental illness may have its origin in fetal development. It may even be traceable to events occurring before conception. These considerations raise several related questions. Could prospective biological parents prevent an adverse prenatal environment and harmful effects on brain development linked to subsequent psychiatric disorders? Could a male or female parent modify their behavior to reduce the risk of prenatal processes later manifesting in psychopathology? Which actions could they, with the aid of health professionals, take to avoid having a child who would later experience the burden of mental illness?

Although there is no conclusive evidence establishing a causal connection between viral infection during pregnancy and schizophrenia in offspring, inflammatory biomarkers associated with early-life infection can increase the risk of this disorder (Patterson, 2011, pp. 64 ff.; Hartwig, Borges, Horta et al., 2017). Whether it is due to inflammatory or other processes, abnormal brain development may begin during embryogenesis. Not all children born to mothers with viral infections during pregnancy develop schizophrenia. Yet the type, severity, and timing of infection may influence a child's mental health. The infection and the immune response to it can disturb the activity of transcription factors in the brain. There is evidence linking paternal age with an increased risk of schizophrenia. Epigenetic changes in human sperm may contribute to abnormalities in neural and synaptic development. This can increase the risk of offspring developing this disorder in the second or third decade of life. The mechanisms of these changes may be related to parental age, diet, weight, and alcohol consumption, or a combination of some or all of these factors. They can contribute to a range of adverse health outcomes, including cardiovascular disease, obesity, diabetes, behavioral problems, and disorders such as schizophrenia and depression (Abbasi, 2017b, p. 2049).

One of the conclusions of the Newborn Epigenetics Study at Duke University conducted between 2013 and 2015 was that "a man's lifestyle may be imprinted on his child's epigenome" (Abbasi, 2017b, p. 2050). There are prenatal and perinatal risk factors for OCD as well. These include "maternal smoking of 10 or more cigarettes per day during pregnancy, caesarian section delivery, preterm birth, low birth weight, large for gestational age, breach presentation at labor, and low Apgar scores at 5 minutes after delivery" (Fernandez and Leckman, 2016, p. 1117). Prenatal stress may influence inflammatory mechanisms in offspring and result in chronic elevated glucocorticoid signaling associated with adolescent-onset anxiety and depression (Cottrell and Secki, 2009).

Biological and environmental changes inside and outside of a woman's body can influence fetal brain development and the mental health of a person years after birth.

Many events occurring during fetal gestation that adversely affect fetal, childhood, and adolescent brain development are beyond the control of parents, obstetricians, and perinatologists. They are not preventable. This does not mean that all events occurring prenatally are beyond human control. Actions that one or both prospective biological parents take during the prenatal period or earlier may decrease or eliminate the known risk of a psychiatric disorder affecting their children. These actions can affect fetal development. They may include not conceiving, terminating a pregnancy during a viral epidemic, or conceiving at a different time. They may also include limiting alcohol consumption, smoking cessation, and adequate prenatal nutrition. These behaviors can affect the identities and well-being of the people biological parents bring into existence.

Suppose that stress in the prenatal environment, viral infection during pregnancy, prenatal nutritional deficiency, or epigenetic changes in sperm linked to male behaviors cause abnormalities in fetal brain development. These abnormalities interfere with neural and synaptic maturation and subsequently manifest in a psychiatric disorder in a person when he is in his late teens or early twenties. Assuming that certain actions could have prevented this outcome, we can compare two life trajectories of the person who comes into existence. In one trajectory, the person develops normally through adolescence and early adulthood and has a life without mental illness. In the other trajectory, the person develops normally until the age of disease onset. It then diverges and becomes a significantly different life from the life the person would have had without the disorder. There are two *distinct lives* with different levels of well-being of the *same person* existing after birth. This is one way of describing the effects of moderate to moderately severe psychiatric disorders on individuals affected by them. They involve significant changes in one's mental states, but not to the extent that they alter identity.

The biological and psychological properties that constitute a person are not equivalent to the biological, psychological, and biographical properties that constitute a person's life. The same person can have a better or worse life depending on his state of health or disease, how he experiences these states, and the extent to which he has opportunities to form and complete action plans. Persons and lives are separable ontological categories. In severe psychiatric disorders there may be a substantial disruption in mental content, psychological connectedness, and continuity and thus a change in identity. There may be a substantial change from one's premorbid self. In these cases, there would be two *distinct lives* of two *distinct people* with distinct levels of well-being before and after the onset of symptoms (Parfit, 1984, Part III; McMahan, 2002, Part IV).

A woman who knew of the risk of viral infection during fetal gestation for a psychiatric disorder in her offspring may wait to conceive, or terminate a pregnancy, during a viral epidemic. If she later began a different pregnancy and brought it to term, then the person who existed at the later time would be different from the person who would have existed at the earlier time. If the risk of the disorder from the viral infection was high, then her decision could mean the difference between a person who would have the disorder and a person who would not have it. This would also be the case if there were a different biological father who did not have the genetic mutations in sperm identified as one of the causes of schizophrenia. The identities of the people who existed at the two times would be distinct because of the presence or absence of the viral infection and genetic mutations and their effects on the brain. They would also be distinct because of differences in the timing of conception, fetal gestation, and birth and the different biological and psychological properties that would result from these factors. These issues are particularly important for psychiatry because psychopathology may not only cause a person to experience psychic pain and suffering. It may also disrupt the psychological connectedness and continuity in terms of which a person experiences herself persisting through time.

The harm in severe psychiatric disorders would be greater than the harm in moderate or moderately severe disorders because of the symptoms and degree of functional impairment. It would also be greater because affected individuals may become different persons. Assuming that an affected individual would have wanted to retain the mental states and psychological relations he had before the onset of symptoms, the change in identity is a harm because it defeats the person's interest in remaining the same individual. Even without identity change, the different life can be harmful. It can limit the person's capacity for functional independence and opportunities to achieve a decent minimum level of well-being. A research model clarifying the role of genetic, epigenetic, endocrine, immune, and environmental factors in the etiology of psychiatric disorders is critical for preventive actions during perinatal, prenatal, and preconceptual periods.

Disability in psychiatric disorders beginning in adolescence or early adulthood is significantly different from disability that develops immediately after birth regarding the effects on identity. Because the onset of psychiatric disorders can occur many years after birth, there is a disruption of psychological connectedness and continuity in the first part of an affected person's life. In contrast, many children born with disabilities may grow into them. At this early stage of life, there is no substantial change in identity because there is not yet a unified set of psychological relations that could be disrupted. The disability is an essential aspect of how they develop as persons after birth. Regardless of whether they benefit from having lives that are worth living or are harmed by the disability, identity change is not part of any harm they could experience.

These issues bring to mind prenatal genetic testing for mutations associated with Mendelian diseases and decisions to terminate or bring a fetus to term in light of this information. Even when a disease of this type is late onset and does not affect a person until the age of 40 or 50, the suffering in the last 10 or 15 years of the person's life may give it a net disvalue. The presence of the mutation at the embryonic or fetal stage may incline a parent to prevent the disease by terminating embryonic or fetal development. This would prevent the existence of the person who would have had the disease. Genome editing in the form of CRISPR (clustered regularly interspersed short palindromic repeats) may enable parents to eliminate or correct disease-causing alleles and have children without disease (Cyranoski, 2016; Doudna and Sternberg, 2017).

However, there are important differences between Mendelian and psychiatric disorders regarding genetic processes during the prenatal period. The number of alleles implicated in the second type of disorder is so extensive that it would be an oversimplification to think that identifying and editing or deleting certain alleles would prevent it. A decision to terminate a pregnancy because of the risk of a psychiatric disorder could not be based on a single allele. The causal factors in psychiatric disorders are much more numerous and complex. They involve more than genetic mutations alone. For parents informed of prenatal risk factors for psychiatric disorders, their deliberation and decision about whether or when to have children may be even more difficult than it is for Mendelian disorders. Because the collective harm that may result from what prospective biological parents do, or fail to do, prenatally is greater in psychiatric than Mendelian disorders, the ethical magnitude of these actions or omissions is greater in the first type than it is in the second.

The main medical and ethical question is whether actions before birth could prevent psychiatric disorders and the burden on people who experience them. Not all psychiatric disorders emerge during adolescence or early adulthood. Others, such as MDD or OCD, may not emerge until later in life. Even in later-onset disorders, the functional limitations they impose on a person and the suffering they may entail in the last 20 or more years of their life could make later negative experiences outweigh earlier positive experiences. This may be the case if we have asymmetrical attitudes about the past and future and care more about avoiding bad experiences in the future than recalling good experiences in the past (Parfit, 1984, Part II). If so, then a severe later-onset psychiatric disorder could significantly reduce an affected person's lifetime well-being.

The point here is not to determine whether a biological parent or parents would be morally blameworthy for failing to take steps that could reduce or eliminate the risk for psychiatric disorders in their offspring. It is not helpful to ask whether they would be negligent and liable for wrongful life for conceiving or not terminating a pregnancy when risk factors were present and the child developed a disorder. In any case, it would be difficult to assign responsibility or blame when the link between prenatal and perinatal events and subsequent psychiatric disorders was probabilistic rather than deterministic and many causal factors could influence whether a person would be affected. Instead, the point should be the more constructive one of focusing on actions by all relevant parties—prospective parents, geneticists, psychiatrists, and obstetricians—before birth that could reduce or eliminate the risk. The focus should be on interventions that could prevent the burden of mental illness that people may experience for the balance of their lives.

Preventing psychiatric disorders by preventing the existence of people who would have them may seem an extreme position. It may not be extreme if potential parents can prevent a psychiatric disorder and harm to a person who would develop it by making certain reproductive choices. Yet despite the causal role of genetic mutations in psychiatric disorders and schizophrenia in particular, no single allele has been isolated as having a particularly deleterious effect on transcription and other factors influencing brain maturation.

Suppose that, in the near future, researchers identified high-penetrance genetic mutations in a man's sperm entailing a high risk of his future children developing schizophrenia. If genetic analysis enabled researchers to predict that the disorder would be severe, and the potential father knew of this risk, then there would be a decisive reason for him not to conceive. The reason would be to prevent harm by preventing a possible person from existing. This could override any reason to conceive. Alternatively, if potential parents were aware of the genetic risk and had the financial means, they could conceive through in vitro fertilization. They could create several embryos and use preimplantation genetic diagnosis to determine which embryos had the mutations. With this information, they could selectively terminate affected embryos, implant a mutation-free embryo, and allow it to develop to a live birth. In a different hypothetical scenario, suppose that a woman knew that contracting a flu during fetal gestation entailed a high risk of schizophrenia, BD, or a different type of mental illness in the child who would come into existence. Terminating the pregnancy would eliminate the risk by preventing the birth of the child. She could conceive later and have a different child who would not be exposed to this risk.

Despite the suffering experienced by people with major psychiatric disorders, it would be controversial to claim that their lives were not worth living. Assuming that they are worth living, any reasons for preventing their existence would seem weak. This situation is similar in some respects to what Derek Parfit calls the nonidentity problem (Parfit, 1984, pp. 351 ff.; Boonin, 2014). If a person would exist with a disease or disability, then one should bring a different person into existence who would not have it. Choosing the first person rather than the second would appear to cause preventable harm and thus be the wrong choice. Yet if the first person had a life that was worth living, then the parents' decision to bring her into existence would not be morally wrong. There would be no identifiable person who was harmed or wronged.

In severe psychiatric disorders, it may seem wrong to cause a person to exist with a disease or disability who would be worse off than a physically and mentally healthy person. Given the choice between having a child with a high probability of developing a psychiatric disorder and a child who would not have the disorder, the prospective parent should make the second choice (Kamm, 2002; McMahan, 2002, Part IV; Wasserman, 2005; Glover, 2006, Part II). While both people would have lives worth living, the second person would be better off than the first. This involves a shift in focus from a person-affecting principle to an impersonal comparative principle (Parift, 1984, pp. 351 ff.). The second principle involves a comparison between two distinct lives of two distinct people. It does not suggest that the first person's life would be less valuable to her subjectively than the second person's life would be to him. Objectively, though, the first life would be preferable because of the absence of a disorder and the absence of functional limitations. Some might argue that this type of choice could reinforce the stigma associated with mental illness. This does not follow. Rather, it suggests making a choice that would prevent harm to people who would exist with a psychiatric disorder. It does not promote discrimination against existing people who have these disorders but aims to prevent additional functional impairment, disrupted thought, and mental suffering that additional people would experience by developing a disorder. Besides, better education and increased understanding of the biological, psychological, and social dimensions of mental illness may be the most effective way of reducing the stigma associated with it. In addition, it would be an expression of parents' reproductive autonomy to make choices about whether to cause people to exist and, to a certain extent, the sorts of lives their children would have (Glover, 1984).

Not causing people to exist who would have a severe psychiatric disorder, or indeed not bringing any person into existence, would not harm anyone (Parfit, 1984, pp. 351 ff.). Only actual people, not possible people, can be harmed. Harm consists in making a person worse off than she was or would have been. This claim presupposes that the same person exists in two different states of affairs at earlier and later times. Before birth, there is no person who could be affected by any action at that time. One cannot coherently compare existence with non-existence in making value judgments about people and their lives. Still, causing a person to exist who would subsequently have a disorder could harm her by defeating her interest in not living with disease or disability. Once she exists, the disease could make her worse off than she would have been without it.

Therapies that could control these disorders and ameliorate symptoms could change these assessments. A parent knowing of the risk of having a child with a psychiatric disorder would not be harming or wronging the child if a drug or other intervention could treat it safely and effectively. This cannot be known before birth. What *is* known is that major psychiatric disorders involve significant functional impairment and that the incidence of treatment-resistance among them is relatively high. These facts and the risk factors for a psychiatric disorder could inform decisions about birth during the prenatal period. They could support a reason for preventing the disorder by intervening before birth. Predicting psychiatric disorders based on events occurring before conception, during fetal gestation, and in the perinatal period is still an inexact science.

In the current state of reproductive medicine and psychiatry, potential parents do not have the information to know whether a future child would develop a disorder, or how severe it would be. Nor do they have the information to know whether new therapies would become available to treat severe disorders. All of this could change if research determined that events occurring before birth would result in neural and psychological dysfunction after birth and throughout a person's life. It could also change if new therapies resulted in a higher incidence of positive responses in psychiatric patients. These considerations show how questions in psychiatric neuroethics are inextricably linked to questions in reproductive ethics.

## Conclusion

Research into preventing psychiatric disorders is still at an early stage. Advances in this area of psychiatry require a better understanding of genetic risk factors, reliable biomarkers, and neurobiological mechanisms underlying the first signs of pathogenesis and psychopathology. Progress in disease prevention also depends on knowledge of how epigenetic processes influence gene expression in the brain and how this shapes thought and behavior. Prevention also requires knowledge of how environmental influences such as psychosocial stress can disrupt neurotransmitter signaling and functional connectivity in neural circuits. It requires an understanding of psychiatric disorders as neurodevelopmental disorders extending from embryogenesis and fetal gestation through childhood, adolescence, and adulthood. The fact that many neurodevelopmental disorders become neurodegenerative disorders can also contribute to preventing psychiatric disorders by elucidating disease mechanisms that are active over the course of an affected person's life.

One of the challenges with preventive interventions is that the neurobiological and behavioral changes that would indicate them are of limited predictive value. Prodromal symptoms may indicate early treatment that could block further development of a psychiatric disorder. Treatment could at least reduce its severity. Yet these symptoms would not necessarily result in a disorder. In these cases, people deemed at risk may be exposed to adverse effects of psychotropic drugs without any benefit. Endophenotypes could clarify the connection between genetic risk factors and the phenotypic traits of a disorder. Here too, though, these biological signatures would not determine that an individual would go on to have a major mental illness. The same concern about weighing potential benefit and harm from pharmacological intervention would apply.

Biomarkers may improve prediction of responses to drugs and other treatments. Yet these signatures alone do not determine mental health outcomes. In some cases, identifying biomarkers for psychiatric disorders may be more harmful than beneficial. Third parties could take this information to calculate risk assessments that could lead to various forms of discrimination against certain individuals seeking employment or applying for health insurance. Like the potential adverse psychological effects of presymptomatic genetic testing, knowing that one had a biomarker associated with mental illness could generate chronic anxiety and distress in asymptomatic individuals. This may occur even when any predictive value of a biomarker is probabilistic rather than deterministic. Simply knowing that there was a chance of developing a psychiatric disorder could be enough to harm a person. Biological parents could take some actions and avoid others during fetal gestation to reduce the risk of abnormal fetal brain development resulting in a neurodevelopmental disorder later in life.

There are many causal factors in the pathogenesis of these disorders. Eliminating or mitigating some of these factors may reduce this risk but will not eliminate it. Behavioral changes by biological parents, modulation of neuroimmune interactions during fetal gestation, childhood, or adolescence, and modification of the external environment are necessary components of any preventive strategy. The etiology of psychopathy is more difficult to ascertain, and this may present greater challenges in preventing this disorder than the other psychiatric disorders I have discussed. Although some studies indicate that psychopathy is heritable, there is no conclusive evidence that early pharmacological, psychological, or environmental intervention could prevent it.

Despite the challenges and limitations I have outlined, the importance of prevention cannot be understated. Due largely to the high incidence of treatment-resistance, the magnitude of harm from schizophrenia, MDD, OCD, BD, and other psychiatric disorders is considerable. One preventive strategy for depression would be to screen adolescents at risk for this disorder in primary care settings (Hirschtritt and Kroenke, 2017). Patients with early depressive symptoms could be prescribed antidepressant medication and/or CBT to prevent the disease from developing further. Yet the success of this strategy would depend on continuity of care for younger patients. This may be difficult for those whose disease is linked to the stress of extenuating social situations. In addition, some adolescents might have to be nudged to adhere to treatment. In spite of these problems, Pam Cuijpers, Aartan Beekman, and Charles Reynolds note progress in preventing depression: "More than 30 randomized trials have demonstrated that preventive interventions can reduce the incidence of new episodes of major depressive disorder by about 25% and by as much as 50% when preventive interventions are offered in stepped-care format. Methods with proven effectiveness involve educational, psychotherapeutic, pharmacological, lifestyle and nutritional interventions" (2012, p. 1033).

More effective disease prevention is clearly the most effective way of reducing its global burden. Whether the incidence of schizophrenia, major depression, and other psychiatric disorders increases or decreases depends on the extent to which psychiatry researchers and practitioners, other health professionals, prospective parents, families, and patients themselves can control the biological, psychological, and social factors that cause them. Complete control of disease mechanisms and prevention is unlikely. Nevertheless, changes in people's behavior and further research into these mechanisms can at least approximate these goals.

# Epilogue: Psychiatry, neuroscience, philosophy

Advances in neuroscience in the last 30 years have shown that major psychiatric disorders are disorders of the brain. Biological psychiatry provides the theoretical framework for the RDoC, which complements the *DSM-5* in accounting for the etiology, pathophysiology, and symptomatology of these disorders. According to biological psychiatry, sensorimotor, cognitive, emotional, and volitional impairments in psychiatric disorders are associated with dysfunctional neural circuits and neurotransmitters. Genetic and epigenetic analyses have also contributed to a better understanding of these disorders by elucidating how genes are expressed in brain structure and function. Neuroimaging has confirmed the underlying abnormal neurobiology and helped to monitor their progression. These techniques have contributed to more accurate diagnosis and prognosis and to safer and more effective responses to psychopharmacological, psychological, and neurosurgical interventions.

Psychiatric disorders are not *just* disorders of the brain. They are also disorders of the mind and the affected person's relation to other persons and the world. Neuroscience alone cannot explain how these disorders develop and progress. Neuroimaging can reveal the neurobiological correlates of mental illness, but correlation is not causation. We should therefore be circumspect in claiming that neural circuit or neurotransmitter dysfunction causes mental illness. Imaging is limited in explaining diseases of the brain and mind not only because of inferential distance between data from brain scans and real-time brain activity but also because of inferential distance between neural dysfunction and mental dysfunction. Detecting abnormalities at the brain-systems level is necessary but not sufficient for explaining abnormalities at the mental-systems level. Neural dysfunction can only partly account for disordered mental states. Focusing on neural mechanisms alone cannot entirely explain the psychopathology in schizophrenia, depression, or other forms of mental illness. Ordered and disordered mental states have neural representations, but they are more than just products of brain function or dysfunction. The phenomenology of impaired mental capacities and distorted mental content is associated with but is not identical to structural and functional brain abnormalities.

In the positive subtype of schizophrenia, for example, MRI and VBM may reveal reductions in cortical gray matter and PET and fMRI may reveal dysfunctional connectivity in frontal–temporal–parietal pathways associated with auditory hallucinations. Yet imaging revealing these brain abnormalities cannot reproduce what it is like for a subject to have these cognitive symptoms because neither the voices nor the person's experience of them are located in the brain. Nor can imaging revealing dysfunctional connectivity in frontal–limbic pathways associated with mood disturbances capture the darkness of severe depression. This experience is not located in the brain either. Imaging cannot "read" the disordered content of the person's mind. The psychopathology of psychiatric disorders emerges from but involves more than dysfunctional neural circuits and neurotransmitters. This view rejects ontological and explanatory reductionism and supports nonreductive materialism as an explanatory model of the neural and mental processes underlying psychiatric disorders.

These remarks do not suggest a substance dualist model in which brain and mind are separate and independent systems. Rather, brain and mind are interdependent systems that interact and influence each other in a circular causal process involving a series of bottom-up and top-down re-entrant loops. Ordinarily, interacting and mutually influencing neural and mental processes maintain homeostasis by enabling the organism to balance internal functions of the brain and body with information from the external world. This balance promotes flexible thought, behavior, and the subject's capacity to adapt to the demands of the environment. In major psychiatric disorders, dysfunctional neural and mental processes can cause the loss of homeostasis and result in psychopathology that impairs or undermines this adaptive capacity. Dysfunction at the neural level corresponds to dysfunction at the mental level, and vice versa. According to the biopsychosocial model of mental health and mental illness, genetic, epigenetic, immune, endocrine, psychological, and environmental factors influence brain–mind interaction.

Although the onset of psychiatric disorders typically occurs in adolescence or early adulthood, pathogenesis may begin before birth. The underlying mechanisms of these disorders may involve adverse events and processes during fetal gestation. They may be traceable to epigenetic changes in human sperm and eggs prior to conception. This requires a broader temporal perspective than the time of onset of symptoms in gaining a better understanding of psychiatric disorders. Such a perspective may lead to earlier interventions that could control or prevent them.

Commonalities between neurology and psychiatry support relaxing the categorical distinction between these disciplines that has predominated in clinical neuroscience for the last century. Many psychiatric and neurological disorders involve dysfunction in interconnected neural networks associated with motor and mental symptoms. These symptoms may be present at the same time or at different times and different disease stages. The extent of overlap between traditional neurological and psychiatric disorders warrants broadening diagnostic categories and treatment modalities for people with diseases of the brain and mind. It also warrants closer monitoring of patients' mental and neural health, not just at one period of life, but over their lifespan.

Despite this overlap and the fact that both types of disorder have a common neurobiological underpinning, psychological and social factors play a greater role in psychiatric than neurological disorders. This has important philosophical implications. Biological, psychological and social factors associated with mental illness have a critical role in enabling or disabling free will and autonomous agency. These factors also have a role in maintaining or disrupting the psychological relations necessary for personal identity. In addition, they are critical for explaining the respects in which mental illness harms people and how interventions to treat it can benefit them. Psychiatry is more germane to these philosophical concepts than neurology. There are also differences in the phenomenology of psychiatric and neurological disorders in that the first type more directly alters an affected person's subjective experience than the second type. While there are sound medical and philosophical reasons for relaxing a strict distinction between neurology and psychiatry, there are equally sound reasons for not collapsing them into one category of neuropsychiatry.

Cognitive neuroscientists have been developing computational and mechanistic models of the brain that go beyond the current state of biological psychiatry. DBS is an artificial form of neuromodulation enabling shared control of thought and behavior between the device and the subject in whose brain it is implanted. Some might be concerned that more advanced neural prosthetics could threaten the conviction that persons are autonomous agents who can have an impact on events in the world. This is what makes the capacity for agency meaningful for us. Presumably, devices alone could ensure the right balance of neural inputs and outputs in the brain for the organism to adapt to the demands of the environment. Instead of restoring the subject's control of her thought and behavior, these devices would eliminate it. Replacing natural neural circuits and networks with an increasing number of implanted devices could alter our conception of the brain–mind relation and human agency. It could also alter our conception of mental health and mental illness.

Yet even if an artificial device performed the same functions as natural neural networks, it would not completely replace the human brain and explain away the mental capacities it mediates. Like DBS, newer implantable devices could be designed to modulate dysfunctional neural circuits and compensate for neural functions impaired by diseases of the brain. Neural prosthetics would supplement rather than supplant natural neural functions. These devices would not undermine control of thought and behavior but would restore varying degrees of this control through their enabling effects.

Although complete replacement of a natural brain with an artificial one consisting of implants and engineered tissue is not likely in the near future, it is a theoretical possibility. The Human Brain Project began in 2013 as a 10-year European collaborative endeavor in cognitive neuroscience. Its original goal was to achieve a multilevel, integrated simulation of the entire brain to increase "understanding of brain function and its effects on society" (Markram, Meier, Lippert et al., 2011, p. 39; Kandel, Markram, Matthews et al., 2013). In the wake of organizational problems and criticism that its approach was too narrow to account for the brain's role in thought and behavior, the Project now has the more modest goal of developing platforms for neurocomputing and neurorobotics research and development (Fregnac and Laurent, 2014). In addition, the Human Connectome Project aims to create a comprehensive network map of brain circuitry and connectivity through different imaging modalities (Sporns, 2012; Fornito, Zalesky, and Breakspear, 2015). Because psychiatric disorders are disorders of neural circuits and neural connectivity, this and other initiatives in brain simulation and reconstruction could advance research into them.

But it is questionable whether an artificially constructed brain could replicate all the dimensions of the brain–mind relation. One can be skeptical of the idea that a mechanistic model could reproduce the complex interactions between the central nervous, immune, and endocrine systems, genes, and epigenetic processes and how these interactions shape, and are shaped by, the subject's interaction with the environment. One may also be skeptical of the idea that an artificially constructed brain could generate the intentionality and phenomenology of our mental states, or the ordered and disordered mental content that emerges from these interactions. Nor should we assume that an artificially constructed brain would function as well as a natural brain. Initiatives aimed at simulating neural networks may at best make a limited contribution to achieving a better understanding of mental illness and developing safer and more effective treatments for it. Mental health and illness are organic functions of natural, dynamic processes rather than artificial ones.

Persons are constituted by their brains but are not identical to them. The content of our healthy and diseased mental states is the product not only of the brain but also of the other biological systems in which we are embodied and the natural and social environment in which we are embedded. A biopsychosocial model of mental illness should be integrated into psychiatric research, teaching, and clinical practice (Arbuckle, Travis, and Ross, 2017; Gask, 2018). Factors both inside and outside of the brain influence the pathogenesis and psychopathology of psychiatric disorders. These factors should inform philosophical questions about how psychiatric disorders affect free will, personal identity, and the respects in which they harm people. These questions in turn should inform current and future neuroscience research aimed at gaining a better understanding of differences between healthy and diseased brains and minds. They should also inform the development of therapies and preventive strategies that will minimize harm, maximize benefit, and improve the quality of life of the millions of people who suffer from psychiatric disorders.

The debilitating effects of major psychiatric disorders can impede functional independence. Although the symptoms are often more covert than overt, people with mental illness can be as functionally impaired and suffer as much as people with cancer, neuromuscular diseases, and spinal cord injuries. Diseases of the brain and mind can disable thought and behavior to the same extent as diseases of the body. Indeed, psychiatric disorders constitute a larger percentage of the global burden of disease than physical disorders. Mental illness is undertreated or untreated in many countries. Even when treatments are available, many psychiatric disorders are treatment-resistant and do not result in positive responses in the people who have them. For these reasons, funding for research into major psychiatric disorders should have priority over funding for other medical conditions. This is a matter of justice and fairness in meeting a stronger claim of need from a larger population. It is especially important in light of the reduction in the development of new psychotropic drugs by the pharmaceutical industry. With the global incidence of mental illness increasing exponentially, there is a critical need for a better understanding of its biological, psychological, and social causes. Adequate funding should be given to research that will generate this understanding and result in safer and more effective treatment and prevention. This is necessary to enable people who have or would have psychiatric disorders to be functionally independent with productive and fulfilling lives.

# References

Abbasi, J. (2017a). 23andMe, Big Data, and the Genetics of Depression. *Journal of the American Medical Association* **317**: 14–16.

Abbasi, J. (2017b). The Paternal Epigenome Makes its Mark. *Journal of the American Medical Association* **317**: 2049–2051.

Abbate-Daga, G., Amianto, F., Delsedime, N., De-Bacco, C. and Fassino, S. (2014). Resistance to Treatment and Change in Anorexia Nervosa: A Clinical Review. *BMC Psychiatry* **14**: 62. doi: 10.1186/1471-244x-14-62.

Abbott, A. (2005). Deep in Thought. *Nature* **436**: 18–19.

Aberg, L., McClay, J., Nerella, S., Clark, S., Kumar, G., Chen, W. *et al.* (2014). Methylome-Wide Association Study of Schizophrenia. *JAMA Psychiatry* **71**: 255–264.

Abi-Dargham, A. (2015). Imaging the "GABA Shift" in Schizophrenia. *American Journal of Psychiatry* **172**: 1062–1063.

Abosch, A. and Cosgrove, G.R. (2008). Biological Basis for the Surgical Treatment of Depression. *Neurosurgery Focus* **25**: e2. doi: 10.3171/FOC/2008/25/7/E2.

Abramowicz, M., Zuccotti, G. and Pflomm, J-M. (2014). Deep Brain Stimulation for Parkinson's Disease with Early Motor Complications. *Journal of the American Medical Association* **311**: 1686–1687.

Achey, R., Yamamoto, E., Sexton, D., Hammer, C., Lee, B., Butler, R. *et al.* (2018). Prediction of Depression and Anxiety via Patient-Assessed Tremor Severity, not Physician-Reported Motor- Symptom Severity, in Patients with Parkinson's Disease or Essential Tremor Who Have Undergone Deep Brain Stimulation. *Journal of Neurosurgery* **126**. doi: 10.3171/2017.8. JNS1733.

Agnesi, F., Johnson, M. and Vitek, J. (2013). Deep Brain Stimulation: How Does it Work? *Handbook of Clinical Neurology* **116**: 39–54.

Agren, T., Engman, J., Frick, A., Bjorkstrand, J., Larsson, E.M., Furmark, T. *et al.* (2012). Disruption of Reconsolidation Erases a Fear Memory Trace in the Human Amygdala. *Science* **337**: 1550–1552.

Aharoni, E., Vincent, G., Harenski, C., Calhoun, V., Sinnott-Armstrong, W., Gazzaniga, M. *et al.* (2013). Neuroprediction of Future Re-Arrest. *Proceedings of the National Academy of Sciences* **41**: 6223–6228.

Almeida, J. and Phillips, M. (2013). Distinguishing Between Unipolar Depression and Bipolar Depression: Current and Future Clinical and Neuroimaging Perspectives. *Biological Psychiatry* **73**: 111–118.

Alonso, J., Chatterji, S. and He, Y. (eds.) (2013). *The Burden of Mental Disorders: Global Perspective from the WHO World Mental Health Surveys*. Cambridge: Cambridge University Press.

Alphs, L., Benedetti, F., Fleischhacker, W. and Kane, J. (2012). Placebo-Related Effects in Clinical Trials in Schizophrenia: What is Driving this Phenomenon and What Can Be Done to Minimize It? *International Journal of Neuropsychopharmacology* **15**: 1003–1014.

**American Psychiatric Association**. (2000). *Diagnostic and Statistical Manual of Mental Disorders*. Fourth Edition, Text Revision (DSM-IV-TR). Washington, DC: American Psychiatric Association.

**American Psychiatric Association**. (2013). *Diagnostic and Statistical Manual of Mental Disorders*. Fifth Edition (DSM-5). Washington, DC: American Psychiatric Association.

**Anderson, G.** (2016). Depression after Stroke—Frequency, Risk Factors, and Mortality Outcomes. *JAMA Psychiatry* **73**: 1013–1014.

**Annas, G.** (2004). Forcible Medication for Courtroom Competence—The Case of Charles Sell. *New England Journal of Medicine* **350**: 2297–2301.

**Appelbaum, P.** (2007). Assessment of Patients' Competence to Consent to Treatment. *New England Journal of Medicine* **357**: 1834–1840.

**Appelbaum, P.** (2016). Physician-Assisted Death for Patients with Mental Disorders—Reasons for Concern. *JAMA Psychiatry* **73**: 325–326.

**Appelbaum, P.** and **Grisso. T.** (1988). Assessing Patients' Capacities to Consent to Treatment in Psychiatric Research. *International Journal of Law and Psychiatry* **5**: 319–329.

**Appelbaum, P., Grisso, T., Frank, E., O'Donnell, S.** and **Kupfer, D.** (1999). Competence of Depressed Patients for Consent to Research. *American Journal of Psychiatry* **156**: 1380–1384.

**Appelbaum, P., Roth, L.** and **Lidz, C.** (1982). The Therapeutic Misconception: Informed Consent in Psychiatric Research. *International Journal of Law and Psychiatry* **5**: 319–329.

**Arain, M., Haque, M., Johal, L., Mathur, P., Nel, W., Rais, A.** *et al.* (2013). Maturation of the Adolescent Brain. *Neuropsychiatric Disease and Treatment* **9**: 449–461.

**Arbuckle, M., Travis, M.** and **Ross, D.** (2017). Integrating a Neuroscience Perspective into Clinical Psychiatry Today. *JAMA Psychiatry* **74**: 313–314.

**Aristotle** (1984). *The Complete Works of Aristotle*. Trans. and ed. J. Barnes. Princeton, NJ: Princeton University Press.

**Ashok, A., Marques, T., Jauhar, S., Nour, M., Goodwin, G., Young, A.** *et al.* (2017). The Dopamine Hypothesis of Bipolar Affective Disorder: The State of the Art and Implications. *Molecular Psychiatry* **22**: 666–679.

**Atmanspacher, H.** and **Rotter, S.** (2012). On Determinacy or its Absence in the Brain. In Swinburne, 84–101.

**Baker, J., Holmes, A., Masters, G., Yeo, T., Krienen, F., Buckner, R.** *et al.* (2014). Disruption of Cortical Association Networks in Schizophrenia and Psychotic Bipolar Disorder. *JAMA Psychiatry* **71**: 109–118.

**Baker, L.R.** (2000). *Persons and Bodies: A Constitution View*. New York: Cambridge University Press.

**Baker, L.R.** (2009). Non-Reductive Materialism. In McLaughlin and Beckerman, 109–120.

**Baker, L.R.** (2013). *Naturalism and the First-Person Perspective*. Oxford: Oxford University Press.

**Bakhshayesh, A. Hansch, S., Wynchkon, A., Rezai, M.** and **Esser, G.** (2011). Neurofeedback in ADHD: A Single-Blind Randomized Controlled Trial. *European Child and Adolescent Psychiatry* **20**: 481–491.

**Ballantine, H.T., Bouckoms, A., Thomas, E.** and **Giriunas, I.** (1967). Treatment of Psychiatric Illness by Stereotactic Cingulotomy. *Biological Psychiatry* **22**: 807–819.

Balu, D. and **Coyle, J.** (2011). Neuroplasticity Signaling Pathways Linked to the Pathophysiology of Schizophrenia. *Neuroscience and Biobehavioral Reviews* **35**: 848–870.

Bargh, J. and **Morsella, E.** (2008). The Unconscious Mind. *Perspectives on Psychological Science* **3**: 73–79.

Barrett, K. (2017). Psychiatric Neurosurgery in the 21st Century: Overview and Growth of Deep Brain Stimulation. *British Journal of Psychiatry Bulletin* **41**: 281–289.

Bartels, A. (2012). Oxytocin and the Social Brain: Beware the Complexity. *Neuropsychopharmacology* **37**: 1795–1796.

Bartz, J. (2016). Oxytocin and the Pharmacological Dissection of Affiliation. *Current Directions in Psychological Science* **25**: 104–110.

Baseri, B., **Choi, D., Deffieux, T., Samiotaki, G., Tung, Y., Olumolade, O.** *et al.* (2012). Activation of Signaling Pathways Following Localized Delivery of Systemically Administered Neurotrophic Factors Across the Blood-Brain Barrier Using Focused Ultrasound and Microbubbles. *Physics in Medicine and Biology* **57**: N65–81.

Bastiampillai, T., **Sharfstein, S.** and **Allison, S.** (2016). Increase in US Suicide Rates and the Critical Decline in Psychiatric Beds. *Journal of the American Medical Association* **316**: 2591–2592.

Bauer, C., **Diaz, J., Concha, L.** and **Barrios, F.** (2014). Sustained Attention to Spontaneous Thumb Sensation Activates Brain Somatosensory and Other Proprioceptive Areas. *Brain and Cognition* **187**: 86–96.

Baum, M. (2016). *The Neuroethics of Biomarkers: What the Development of Bioprediction Means for Moral Responsibility, Justice and the Nature of Mental Disorder.* Oxford: Oxford University Press.

Baum, M. and **Savulescu, J.** (2013). Behavioral Biomarkers: What Are They Good For? Toward the Ethical Use of Biomarkers. In Singh, Sinnott-Armstrong and Savulescu, 12–41.

Baxley, A. and **Akhtari, M.** (2011). Hematologic Toxicities Associated with Intravenous Immunoglobin Therapy. *International Immunopharmacology* **11**: 2663–1667.

Baylis, F. (2014). Neuroethics and Identity. In Levy and Clausen, 367–372.

Bayne, T. and **Hohwy, J.** (2014). Global Disorders of Consciousness. *WIREs Cognitive Science* **5**: 129–139.

Beauchamp, T. and **Childress, J.** (2012). *Principles of Biomedical Ethics.* Seventh Edition. New York: Oxford University Press.

Beauregard, M. (2007). Mind Really Does Matter: Evidence from Neuroimaging Studies of Emotional Self-Regulation, Psychotherapy and Placebo Effect. *Progress in Neurobiology* **81**: 218–236.

Bechara, A., **Damasio, H.** and **Damasio, A.** (2000). Emotion, Decision Making and the Orbitofrontal Cortex. *Cerebral Cortex* **10**: 295–307.

Bechtel, W. (2008). *Mental Mechanisms: Philosophical Perspectives on Cognitive Neuroscience.* New York: Taylor and Francis.

Becker, A. and **Kleinman, A.** (2013). Mental Health and the Global Agenda. *New England Journal of Medicine* **369**: 66–73.

Bell, E. and **Racine, E.** (2009). Enthusiasm for fMRI Often Overlooks its Dependence on Task Selection and Performance. *American Journal of Bioethics* **9**: 3–13.

Bell, R., Racine, E., Chiasson, P., Dufourcq-Brana, M., Dunn, L., Fins, J. *et al.* (2014). Beyond Consent in Research: Revisiting Vulnerability in Deep Brain Stimulation for Psychiatric Disorders. *Cambridge Quarterly of Healthcare Ethics* 23: 361–368.

Belmaker, R. and Agam, G. (2008). Major Depressive Disorder. *New England Journal of Medicine* 358: 55–68.

Belmont Report (1978). *Ethical Principle and Guidelines for the Protection of Human Subjects of Research.* Report of the National Commission for the Protection of Human Subjects of Biomedical and Behavioral Research. Washington, DC: Department of Health, Education and Welfare.

Benabid, A-L., Pollak, P., Louveau, A., Henry, S. and de Rougement, K. (1987). Combined (Thalamotomy and Stimulatiom) Stereotactic Surgery of the VIM Thalamic Nucleus for Bilateral Parkinson Disease. *Applied Neurophysiology* 50: 344–346.

Benedetti, F. (2009). *Placebo Effects: Understanding the Mechanisms in Health and Disease.* New York: Oxford University Press.

Benedetti, F. (2011). *The Patient's Brain: The Neuroscience Behind the Doctor-Patient Relationship.* New York: Oxford University Press.

Benedetti, F., Carlino, E. and Pollo, A. (2011). How Placebos Change the Patient's Brain. *Neuropsychopharmacology* 36: 339–354.

Bennett, M. and Hacker, P. (2003). *Philosophical Foundations of Neuroscience.* Malden, MA: Blackwell.

Berlin School of Mind and Brain (2016). Research Topic 5: Brain Disorders and Mental Dysfunction. Available at: http://www.mind-and-brain.de/research/topic-5-brain-disorders-and-mental-dysfunction/8/31/2016.html

Bernat, J. (2010). The Natural History of Chronic Disorders of Consciousness. *Neurology* 75: 206–207.

Bernheim, J. and Raus, K. (2017). Euthanasia Embedded in Palliative Care: Responses to Essentialistic Criticisms of the Belgian Model of Integral End-Of-Life Care. *Journal of Medical Ethics* 43: 489–444.

Bilefsky, D. and Schuetze, C. (2016). Dutch Law Would Allow Assisted Suicide for Healthy Older People. *New York Times,* October 13. http://www.nytimes.com/2016/10/14/world.eurpope/dutch-law-would-allow-euthanasia-for-healthy-older-people.html

Blair, R.J.R. (2003). Neurobiological Basis of Psychopathy. *British Journal of Psychiatry* 182: 5–7.

Blair, R.J.R. (2007a). The Amygdala and Ventromedial Prefrontal Cortex in Morality and Psychopathy. *Trends in Cognitive Sciences* 11: 387–392.

Blair, R.J.R. (2007b). Aggression, Psychopathy and Free Will From a Cognitive Neuroscience Perspective. *Behavioral Sciences and the Law* 25: 321–331.

Blair, R.J.R. (2008). The Cognitive Neuroscience of Psychopathy and Implications for Judgments of Responsibility. *Neuroethics* 1: 149–157.

Blair, R.J.R. (2013a). Psychopathy: Cognitive and Neural Dysfunction. *Dialogues in Clinical Neuroscience* 15: 181–190.

Blair, R.J.R. (2013b). The Neurobiology of Psychopathic Traits in Youths. *Nature Reviews Neuroscience* 14: 786–799.

Blair, R.J.R., Mitchell, D. and Blair, K. (2005). *The Psychopath: Emotion and the Brain.* Malden, MA: Blackwell.

Blakemore, S., Wolpert, D. and Frith, C. (2002). Abnormalities in the Awareness of Action. *Trends in Cognitive Sciences* **6**: 237–242.

Blanke, O. (2012). Multisensory Brain Mechanisms of Bodily Self-Consciousness. *Nature Reviews Neuroscience* **13**: 556–571.

Bleuler, E. (1911/1950). *Dementia Praecox or the Group of Schizophrenias*, trans. J. Zinkin. New York: International Universities Press.

Block, N. (1995). On a Confusion about a Function of Consciousness. *Behavioral and Brain Sciences* **18**: 227–287.

Block, N. (2007). Consciousness, Accessibility and the Mesh between Psychology and Neuroscience. *Behavioral and Brain Sciences* **30**: 481–499.

Bloomfield, P., Selvaraj, S., Veronese, M., Rizzo, G., Bertoldo, A., Owen, D. *et al.* (2016). Microglial Activity in People at Ultra High Risk of Psychosis and in Schizophrenia: An [(11) C] PBR 28 PET Brain Imaging Study. *American Journal of Psychiatry* **173**: 44–52.

Bluhm, R., Raczek, M., Broome, M. and Wall, M. (2015). Ethical Issues in Brain Imaging in Psychiatry. In Sadler, Van Staden and Fulford, Volume 1, 1109–1125.

Blumer, D. (2002). The Illness of Vincent Van Gogh. *American Journal of Psychiatry* **159**: 519–526.

Boksa, P. (2012). Abnormal Synaptic Pruning in Schizophrenia: Urban Myth or Reality? *Journal of Psychiatry and Neuroscience* **37**: 75–77.

Boksa, P. (2013). A Way Forward for Research on Biomarkers for Psychiatric Disorders. *Journal of Psychiatry and Neuroscience* **38**: 75–77.

Boly, M., Phillips, C., Tshibanda, L., Vanhaudenhuyse, A., Schabus, M., Dang-Vu, T. *et al.* (2008). Intrinsic Brain Activity in Altered States of Consciousness. *Annals of the New York Academy of Sciences* **1129**: 119–129.

Bomann-Larsen, L. (2013). Voluntary Rehabilitation? On Neurotechnological Behavioral Treatment, Valid Consent and (In)appropriate Offers. *Neuroethics* **6**: 65–77.

Boonin, D. (2014). *The Non-Identity Problem and the Ethics of Future People*. Oxford: Oxford University Press.

Bortolotti, L. (2009). *Delusions and Other Irrational Beliefs*. Oxford: Oxford University Press.

Bostick, N., Sade, R., Levine, M. and Stewart, D. (2008). Placebo Use in Clinical Practice: Report of the American Medical Association Council on Ethics and Judicial Affairs. *Journal of Clinical Ethics* **19**: 59–61.

Boyer, E. and Shannon, M. (2005). The Serotonin Syndrome. *New England Journal of Medicine* **352**: 1112–1120.

Brander, G., Perez-Vigil, A., Larsson, H. and Mataix-Cols, D. (2016). Systematic Review of Environmental Risk Factors for Obsessive-Compulsive Disorder: A Proposed Roadmap from Association to Causation. *Neuroscience and Biobehavioral Reviews* **65**: 36–62.

Broca, P. (1861). Remarks on the Seat of the Faculty of Articulate Language, Following an Observation of Aphemia (Loss of Speech). *Bulletin de la Societe Anatomique* **186**: 330.

Brock, D. and Wartman, S. (1990). When Competent Patients Make Irrational Choices. *New England Journal of Medicine* **322**: 1595–1599.

Brody, H. (1982). The Lie that Heals: The Ethics of Giving Placebos. *Annals of Internal Medicine* **97**: 112–118.

Broome, M. and de Cates. A. (2015). Choosing Death in Depression: A Commentary on "Treatment-Resistant Major Depressive Disorder and Assisted Dying." *Journal of Medical Ethics* **41**: 586–587.

Brown, W. (1994). Placebo as Treatment for Depression. *Neuropsychopharmacology* **10**: 265–269.

Brown, W. (2012). *The Placebo Effect in Clinical Practice*. New York: Oxford University Press.

Browne, T. (2018). *Depression and the Self: Meaning, Control and Authenticity*. Cambridge: Cambridge University Press.

Brunoni, A., Boggio., P., Ferrucci, R., Priori, A. and Fregni, F. (2013). Transcranial Direct Current Stimulation: Challenges, Opportunities and Impact on Psychiatry and Neurorehabilitation. *Frontiers in Psychiatry* **4**: 19. doi: 10.3389/fpsyt.2013.00019.

Brunoni, A., Moffa, A., Sampaio-Junior, B., Borrione, L., Moreno, M., Fernandes, R. *et al.* (2017). Trial of Electrical Direct-Current Therapy versus Escitalopram for Depression. *New England Journal of Medicine* **376**: 2523–2533.

Bu, X-L., Xiang, Y., Jin, W., Wang, J., Shen, L. Huang, Z. *et al.* (2017). Blood-Derived Amyloid-B Protein Induces Alzheimer's Disease Pathologies. *Molecular Psychiatry* **22**: 204. doi: 10.1038/mp.2017.204.

Bublitz, C. (2014). Freedom of Thought in the Age of Neuroscience. *Archives of Philosophy of Law and Social Philosophy* **100**: 1–25.

Bublitz, C. (2016). Moral Enhancement and Mental Freedom. *Journal of Applied Philosophy* **33**: 88–106.

Bublitz, C. and Merkel, R. (2013). Guilty Minds in Washed Brains? Manipulation Cases and the Limits of Neuroscientific Excuses in Liberal Legal Orders. In Vincent, 335–374.

Bublitz, C. and Merkel, R. (2014). Crimes Against Minds: On Mental Manipulations, Harms and a Human Right to Mental Self-Determination. *Criminal Law and Philosophy* **8**: 51–77.

Buchanan, A. and Brock, D. (1990). *Deciding for Others: The Ethics of Surrogate Decision Making*. New York: Cambridge University Press.

Buckholtz, J., Treaday, M., Cowan, R., Woodward, N., Benning, S., Li, R. *et al.* (2010). Mesolimbic Dopamine Reward System Hypersensitivity in Individuals with Psychopathic Traits. *Nature Neuroscience* **13**: 419–421.

Buckholtz, J. and Meyer-Lindenberg, A. (2012). Psychopathy and the Human Connectome: Toward a Transdiagnostic Model of Risk for Mental Illness. *Neuron* **74**: 990–1004.

Burgess, A. and Hynynen, K. (2014). Drug Delivery Across the Blood-Brain Barrier Using Focused Ultrasound. *Expert Opinion in Drug Delivery* **11**: 711–721.

Cacioppo, J. and Berntson, G. (2011). The Brain, Homeostasis and Health: Balancing Demands of the Internal and External Milieu. In H. Friedman, 121–137.

Calhoun, V. and Arbabshirani, M. (2013). Neuroinaging-Based Automatic Classification of Schizophrenia. In Singh, Sinnott-Armstrong and Savulescu, 206–230.

Cannon, W. (1932). *The Wisdom of the Body*. New York: Norton.

Canuso, C., Singh, J., Fedgchin, M., Alphs, L., Lane, R., Lim, P. *et al.* (2018). Efficacy and Safety of Intranasal Esketamine for the Rapid Reduction of Symptoms of Depression and Suicidality in Patients at Imminent Risk for Suicide: Results of a Double-Blind,

Randomized, Placebo-Controlled Study. *American Journal of Psychiatry* 175. doi: 10.1176/appi.ajp.2018.17060720.

Carhart-Harris, R., Roseman, L., Bolstridge, M., Demetrious, L., Pannekoek, J., Wall, M. *et al.* (2017). Psilocybin for Treatment-Resistant Depression: fMRI-Measured Brain Mechanisms. *Scientific Reports* 7: 13187. doi: 10.1035/srep41598-017-13282-7.

*Carter v. Canada (AG)* (2015). Supreme Court of Canada (SCC), 5.

Casey, B., Craddock, N., Cuthbert, B., Hyman, S., Lee, F. and Ressler, K. (2013). DSM-5 and RDoC: Progress in Psychiatry Research? *Nature Reviews Neuroscience* 14: 810–814.

Cassell, E. (1991). *The Nature of Suffering and the Goals of Medicine*. New York: Oxford University Press.

Castle, D. and Buckley, P. (2015) *Schizophrenia*. Oxford: Oxford University Press.

Castrioto, A. Lhommee, E. Moro, E. and Krack, P. (2014). Mood and Behavioral Effects of Subthalamic Stimulation in Parkinson's Disease. *The Lancet Neurology* 13: 287–305.

Chandler, J. (2013). Autonomy and the Unintended Legal Consequences of Emerging Neurotherapies. *Neuroethics* 6: 249–263.

Chang, Z., Lichtenstein, P. Langstrom, N., Larsson, H. and Fazel, S. (2016). Association Between Prescription of Major Psychotropic Medications and Violent Reoffending After Prison Release. *Journal of the American Medical Association* 316: 1798–1807.

Charlson, F., Baxter, A., Cheng, H., Shidhaye, R. and Whiteford, H. (2016). The Burden of Mental, Neurological and Substance Use Disorders in China and India: A Systems Analysis of Community Representative Epidemiological Studies. *The Lancet* 388: 376–389.

Charney, D., Sklar, P., Buxbaum, J. and Nestler, E. (eds.) (2013). *Neurobiology of Mental Illness*. Fourth Edition. Oxford: Oxford University Press.

Chatterjee, A. and Farah, M. (eds.) (2013). *Neuroethics in Practice*. Oxford: Oxford University Press.

Cheng, H., Shidhaye, R., Charlson, F., Deng, F., Lyngdoh, T., Chen, S. *et al.* (2016). Social Correlates of Mental, Neurological and Substance Use Disorders in China and India: A Review. *The Lancet Psychiatry* 3: 882–899.

Chekroud, A., Gueorguieva, R., Krumholz, H., Trivedi, M., Krystal, J. and McCarthy, G. (2017). Reevaluating the Efficacy and Predictability of Antidepressant Treatments: A Symptom Clustering Approach. *JAMA Psychiatry* 74: 370–378.

Cherkasova, M. and Stoessl, A.J. (2014). A Brain Network Response to Sham Surgery. *Journal of Clinical Investigation* 124: 3285–3288.

Cheung, T., Zhang, C., Rudolph, J., Alterman, R. and Tagliati, M. (2013). Sustained Relief of Generalized Dystonia Despite Prolonged Interruption of Deep Brain Stimulation. *Movement Disorders* 28: 1431–1434.

Choudhury, S. and Slaby, J. (eds.) (2012). *Critical Neuroscience: A Handbook of the Social and Cultural Contexts of Neuroscience*. London: Blackwell.

Christen, M., Bittlinger, M., Walter, H., Brugger, P and Muller, S. (2012). Dealing with Side Effects of Deep Brain Stimulation: Lessons Learned from Stimulating the STN. *American Journal of Bioethics-Neuroscience* 3: 37–43.

Christen, M. and Muller, S. (2018). The Ethics of Expanding Applications of Deep Brain Stimulation. In Rommelfanger and Johnson, 51–65.

Christopher, P., Appelbaum, P., Truong, D., Albert, K., Maranda, L. and Lidz, C. (2017). Reducing Therapeutic Misconception: A Randomized Intervention Trial in Hypothetical Clinical Trials. *PLoS One* **12**: e0184224. doi: 10.1371/journal.pone.0184224.

Churchland, P.S. (2002). *Brain-Wise: Studies in Neurophilosophy*. Cambridge, MA: MIT Press.

Churchland, P.S. (2011). *Braintrust: What Neuroscience Tells Us About Morality*. Princeton, NJ: Princeton University Press.

Churchland, P.S. (2013). *Touching A Nerve: The Self as Brain*. New York: W.W. Norton & Company

Cima, M., Tonnaer, F. and Hauser, M. (2010). Psychopaths Know Right From Wrong but Don't Care. *Social Cognitive and Affective Neuroscience* **5**: 59–67.

Cipriani, A., Furukawa, T., Salanti, G., Chaimani, A., Atkinson, L., Ogawa, Y. *et al.* (2018). Comparative Efficacy and Acceptability of 21 Antidepressant Drugs for the Acute Treatment of Adults with Major Depressive Disorder: A Systematic Review and Network Meta-Analysis. *The Lancet* **391**: 1357–1366.

Clark, W. (2008). *In Defense of Self: How the Immune System Really Works*. Oxford: Oxford University Press.

Clausen, J. (2009). Man, Machine and in Between. *Nature* **457**: 1080–1081.

Cleckley, H. (1982). *The Mask of Sanity*. Revised Edition. St Louis, MO: Mosby.

ClinicalTrials.gov (2015). Deep Brain Stimulation (DBS) for the Management of Treatment-Refractory Negative Symptoms in Schizophrenia. Centre for Addiction and Mental Health, University of Toronto. NCT017235334.

ClinicalTrials.gov (2017a). Deep Brain Stimulation in Treatment-Resistant Schizophrenia. The Johns Hopkins University Hospital. NCT02361554.

ClinicalTrials.gov (2017b). Deep Brain Stimulation in Treatment-Resistant Schizophrenia (DBS-SCHIZO). Hospital Santa Creu i Sant Pau, Barcelona. NCT01725334.

Cohen Kadosh, R., Levy, N., O'Shea, J., Shea, N. and Savulescu, J. (2012). The Neuroethics of Non-Invasive Brain Stimulation. *Current Biology* **22**: 108–111.

Coman, A., Skarderud, F., Reas, D. and Hofmann, B. (2014). The Ethics of Neuromodulation for Anorexia Nervosa: A Focus on rTMS. *Journal of Eating Disorders* **2**: 1–7.

Cooney, J. and Gazzaniga, M. (2003). Neurological Disorders and the Structure of Human Consciousness. *Trends in Cognitive Sciences* **7**: 161–165.

Cottrell, E. and Secki. J. (2009). Prenatal Stress, Glucocorticoids and the Programming of Adult Disease. *Frontiers in Behavioral Neuroscience* **3**: 19. doi: 10.3389/neuro.08.019.2009.

Cowley, C. (2017). Conscientious Objection in Healthcare and the Duty to Refer. *Journal of Medical Ethics* **43**: 207–212.

Craig, J. (2016). Incarceration, Direct Brain Interventions, and the Right to Mental Integrity—A Reply to Thomas Douglas. *Neuroethics* **9**: 107–118.

Craver, C. (2007). *Exploring the Brain: Mechanisms and the Mosaic Unity of Consciousness*. Oxford: Oxford University Press.

Crick, F. and Koch, C. (2003). A Framework for Consciousness. *Nature Neuroscience* **6**: 119–126.

**Crockett, M.** (2014). Moral Bioenhancement: A Neuroscientific Perspective. *Journal of Medical Ethics* **40**: 370–371.

**Crockett, M.** (2016). Morphing Morals: Neurochemical Modulators of Moral Judgment and Behavior. In Liao, 237–245.

**Crockett, M., Clark, L., Hauser, M.** and **Robbins, T.** (2010). Serotonin Selectively Influences Moral Judgment and Behavior through Effects on Harm Aversion. *Proceedings of the National Academy of Sciences* **40**: 17433–17438.

**Crosley, N., Scott, J., Ellison-Wright, I.** and **Mechelli, A.** (2015). Neuroimaging Distinction between Neurological and Psychiatric Disorders. *British Journal of Psychiatry* **207**: 429–434.

**Crowell, A., Garlow, S., Riva-Posse, P.** and **Mayberg, H.** (2015). Characterizing the Therapeutic Response to Deep Brain Stimulation for Treatment-Resistant Depression: A Single-Center Long-Term Perspective. *Frontiers in Integrative Neuroscience* **9**: 41. doi: 10.3389/fnint.2015.00041.

**Cuijpers, P., Beekman, A.** and **Reynolds, C.** (2012). Preventing Depression: A Global Priority. *Journal of the American Medical Association* **307**: 1033–1034.

**Cuijpers, P., Sijbrandij, M. Koole, S., Anderson, G., Beekman, A.** and **Reynolds, C.** (2013). The Efficacy of Psychotherapy and Pharmacotherapy in Treating Depressive and Anxiety Disorders: A Meta-Analysis of Direct Comparisons. *World Psychiatry* **12**: 137–149.

**Curfman, G.** and **Redberg, R.** (2011). Medical Devices—Balancing Regulation and Innovation. *New England Journal of Medicine* **365**: 975–977.

**Cuthbert, B.** and **Insel, T.** (2013). Toward the Future of Psychiatric Diagnosis: The Seven Pillars of the RDoC. *BMC Medicine* **11**: 126. doi: 10.1186/1741-7015-11-126.

**Cyranoski, D.** (2016). CRISPR Gene-Editing Tested in a Person for the First Time. *Nature* **539**, 479.

**Dalmau, J., Gleichman, A., Hughes, E., Rossi, J., Peng, X., Lai, M.** *et al.* (2008). Anti-NMDA-Receptor Encephalitis: Case Series and Analysis of the Effects of Antibodies. *The Lancet Neurology* **7**: 1091–1098.

**Damasio, A.** (2010). *Self Comes to Mind: Constructing the Conscious Brain.* New York: Vintage Books.

**Damasio, H., Grabowski, T., Frank, R., Galaburda, A.** and **Damasio, A.** (1994). The Return of Phineas Gage: Clues about the Brain from the Skull of a Famous Patient. *Science* **264**: 1102–1105.

**Daniels, N.** (1985). *Just Health Care.* New York: Cambridge University Press.

**Daniels, N.** (2008). *Just Health: Meeting Health Needs Fairly.* New York: Cambridge University Press,

**David, A.** and **Nicholson, T.** (2015). Are Neurological and Psychiatric Disorders Different? *British Journal of Psychiatry* **207**: 373–374.

**Davidson, D.** (2001a). Actions, Reasons and Causes. In Davidson, 2001c, 3–10.

**Davidson, D.** (2001b). Mental Events, In Davidson, 2001c, 207–224.

**Davidson, D.** (2001c). *Essays on Actions and Events.* Oxford: Clarendon Press.

**Davis, N.** (2014). Transcranial Stimulation of the Developing Brain: A Plea for Extreme Caution. *Frontiers in Human Neuroscience* **8**: 600. doi: 10.3389/fnhum.2014.00600.

**Davis, N.** and **van Koningsbruggen, M.** (2013). "Non-Invasive" Brain Stimulation Is not Non-Invasive. *Frontiers in Systems Neuroscience* **7**: 76. doi: 10.3389/fnsys.2013.00076.

Decety, J., Michalska, M. and Kinzler, K. (2012). The Contribution of Emotion and Cognition to Moral Sensitivity: A Neurodevelopmental Study. *Cerebral Cortex* **22**: 209–220.

Decety, J., Skelly, L. and Kiehl, K. (2013). Brain Response to Empathy-Eliciting Scenarios Involving Pain in Incarcerated Individuals with Psychopathy. *JAMA Psychiatry* **70**: 638–645.

De Charms, C., Maeda, F., Glover, G., Ludlow, D., Pauly, J., Soneji, D. *et al.* (2005). Control over Brain Activation and Pain Learned by Using Real-Time Functional MRI. *Proceedings of the National Academy of Sciences* **102**: 18226–18231.

Dehaene, S. (2014). *Consciousness and the Brain: Deciphering How the Brain Codes Our Thoughts.* New York: Penguin.

Dehaene, S. and Changeux, J-P. (2011). Experimental and Theoretical Approaches to Conscious Processing. *Neuron* **70**: 200–227.

Deisseroth, K., Etkin, A. and Malenka, R. (2015). Optogenetics and the Circuit Dynamics of Psychiatric Disease. *Journal of the American Medical Association* **313**: 2019–2020.

De la Fuente-Fernandez, R. and Stoessl, A.J. (2002). The Placebo Effect in Parkinson's Disease. *Trends in Neuroscience* **25**: 302–306.

DeLong, M. and Wichmann, T. (2012). Deep Brain Stimulation for Movement and Other Neurological Disorders. *Annals of the New York Academy of Sciences* **1265**: 1–8.

Demertzi, A. and Laureys, S. (2012). Wherein the Brain Is Pain? Evaluating Painful Experiences in Non-Communicative Patients. In Richmond, Rees and Edwards, 89–98.

Deng, Z.-D., Lisanby, S., Peterchev, A. (2013). Electric Field Depth Locality Trade Off in Transcranial Magnetic Stimulation: Simulation Comparison of 50 Coil Designs. *Brain Stimulation* **6**: 1–13.

Dennett, D. (2015). *Elbow Room: The Varieties of Free Will Worth Wanting.* New Edition. Cambridge, MA: MIT Press.

De Ridder, D., Vanneste, S., Gillett, G., Manning, P., Glue, P. and Langguth, B. (2016). Psychosurgery Reduces Uncertainty and Increases Free Will? A Review. *Neuromodulation* **19**: 239–248.

Doecke, J., Laws, S., Faux, N., Wilson, W., Burnham, S., Lam, C. *et al.* (2012). Blood-Based Protein Biomarkers for Diagnosis of Alzheimer Disease. *Archives of Neurology* **69**: 1318–1325.

Doudna, J. and Sternberg, S. (2017). *A Crack in Creation: Gene Editing and the Unthinkable Power to Control Evolution.* New York: Houghton Mifflin Harcourt.

Dougall, N., Maayan, N., Soares-Weiser, K., McDermott, L. and McIntosh, A. (2015). Transcranial Magnetic Stimulation for Schizophrenia. *Schizophrenia Bulletin* **41**: 1220–1222.

Douglas, T. (2014). Criminal Rehabilitation through Medical Intervention: Moral Liability and the Right to Bodily Integrity. *Journal of Ethics* **18**: 101–122.

Dubicka, B., Elvins, R., Roberts, C., Chicj, G., Wilkinson, P. and Goodyer, I. (2010). Combined Treatment with Cognitive-Behavioural Therapy in Adolescents with Depression: Meta-Analysis. *British Journal of Psychiatry* **197**: 433–440.

Dubljevic, V., Saigle, V. and Racine, E. (2014). The Rising Tide of tDCS in the Media and Academic Literature. *Neuron* **82**: 731–736.

Dukart, J., Regen, F., Kherif, F., Colla, M., Bajbouj, M., Heuser, I. *et al.* (2014). Electroconvulsive Therapy-Induced Brain Plasticity Determines Therapeutic Outcome in Mood Disorders. *Proceedings of the National Academy of Sciences* **111**: 1156–1161.

Duncan, J. (2016). 17-Year-Old in "Unbearable" Physical Pain Becomes First Child to Die by Euthanasia in Belgium Two Years after Law Was Passed. *Daily Mail*, September 17. http://www.dailymail.co.uk/news/article-3794054/Belgium-reports-case-euthanasia-minor.html

Dunn, L., Holtzheimer, P., Hoop, J., Mayberg, H., Roberts, I. and Appelbaum, P. (2011). Ethical Issues in Deep Brain Stimulation Research for Treatment-Resistant Depression: Focus and Risk and Consent. *American Journal of Bioethics-Neuroscience* **2**: 29–36.

Dworkin, G. (1988). *The Theory and Practice of Autonomy*. New York: Cambridge University Press.

Dyster, T., Mikell, C. and Sheth, S. (2016). The Co-Evolution of Neuroimaging and Psychiatric Neurosurgery. *Frontiers in Neuroanatomy* **10**: 68. doi: 10.3380/fnana.2016.00068.

Eklund, A., Nichols, T. and Knutsson, H. (2016). Cluster Failure: Why fMRI Inferences for Spatial Extent Have Inflated False Positive Rates. *Proceedings of the National Academy of Sciences USA* **113**: 7900–7905.

El Hady, A. (ed.) (2016). *Closed Loop Neuroscience*. Amsterdam: Elsevier.

El-Hai, J. (2005). *The Lobotomist: A Maverick Medical Genius and His Tragic Quest to Rid the World of Mental Illness*. Hoboken, NJ: John Wiley & Sons.

Elias, W., Lipsman, N., Ondo, W., Ghanouni, P., Kim, Y., Lee, W. *et al.* (2016). A Randomized Trial of Focused Thalamotomy for Essential Tremor. *New England Journal of Medicine* **375**: 730–739.

Elliott, C. (1997). Caring about Risks: Are Severely Depressed Patients Competent to Consent to Research? *Archives of General Psychiatry* **54**: 113–116.

Emanuel, E., Grady, C., Crouch, R., Lie, R., Miller, F. and Wendler, D. (eds.) (2008). *The Oxford Textbook of Clinical Research Ethics*. New York: Oxford University Press.

Emanuel, E., Onwuteaka-Philipsen, B., Urwin, J. and Cohen, J. (2016). Attitudes and Practices of Euthanasia and Physician-Assisted Suicide in the United States, Canada and Europe. *Journal of the American Medical Association* **316**: 79–90.

Engel, G. (1977). The Need for a New Medical Model: A Challenge for Biomedicine. *Science* **196**: 129–136.

European Commission (2014). *Medical Devices: Guidance Document—Classification of Medical Devices*. http://ec.europa.eu/DocsRoom/documents/10337/attachments/1/translations/en/renditions/pdf

Farah, M. and Gillihan, S. (2012). The Puzzle of Neuroimaging and Psychiatric Diagnosis: Technology and Nosology in an Evolving Discipline. *American Journal of Bioethics-Neuroscience* **3**: 34–41.

Feinberg, T. (2001). *Altered Egos: How the Brain Creates the Self*. New York: Oxford University Press.

Feinberg, T. (2009). *From Axons to Identity: Neurological Explorations of the Nature of the Self*. New York: W.W. Norton & Company.

Feinberg, T. (2011). Neuropathologies of the Self. *Consciousness and Cognition* **20**: 75–81.

Felger, J. and **Lotrich, F.** (2013). Inflammatory Cytokines in Depression: Neurobiological Mechanisms and Therapeutic Implications. *Neuroscience* **246**: 199–229.

Fenichel, O. (1946). *The Psychoanalytic Theory of Neurosis*. London: Kegan Paul.

Fernandez, T. and **Leckman, J.** (2016). The Origins of Obsessive-Compulsive Disorder: Prenatal and Perinatal Risk Factors and the Promise of Birth Cohort Studies. *JAMA Psychiatry* **73**: 1117–1118.

Fernandez de la Cruz, L., **Rydell, M., Runeson, B., D'Onofrio, B., Brander, G., Ruck, C.** *et al.* (2017). Suicide in Obsessive-Compulsive Disorder: A Population-Based Study of 36,788 Swedish Patients. *Molecular Psychiatry* **22**: 1626–1632.

Ferro, J., **Caeiro, L.** and **Figueira, M-L.** (2016). Neuropsychiatric Sequelae of Stroke. *Nature Reviews Neurology* **12**: 269–280.

Figee, M., **Luigjes, J., Smolders, R., Valencia-Alfonso, C., Van Wingen, G., de Kwaasteniet, B.** *et al.* (2013). Regaining Control: Deep Brain Stimulation Restores Frontostriatal Network Activity in Obsessive-Compulsive Disorder. *Nature Neuroscience* **16**: 366–387.

Fine, C. and **Kennett, J.** (2004). Mental Impairment, Moral Understanding and Criminal Responsibility: Psychopathy and the Purposes of Punishment. *International Journal of Law and Psychiatry* **27**: 425–443.

Fins, J. (2005). Rethinking Disorders of Consciousness; New Research and its Implications. *Hastings Center Report* **35** (2): 22–24.

Fins, J. (2015). *Rights Come to Mind: Brain Injury, Ethics and the Struggle for Consciousness*. New York: Cambridge University Press.

Fins, J. and **Schiff, N.** (2010). Conflicts of Interest in Deep Brain Stimulation Research and the Ethics of Transparency. *Journal of Clinical Ethics* **21**: 125–132.

Fins, J. and **Pohl, B.** (2016). Ethics of Neuromodulation. In Hamani, Holtzheimer, Lozano and Mayberg, 15–26.

Fins, J., **Schlaepfer, T., Nuttin, B., Kubu, C., Galert, T., Sturm, V.** *et al.* (2011). Ethical Guidance for the Management of Conflicts if Interest for Researchers, Engineers and Clinicians Engaged in the Development of Therapeutic Deep Brain Stimulation. *Journal of Neural Engineering* **8**: E033001.

Fischer, J.M. (1994). *The Metaphysics of Free Will: An Essay on Control*. Cambridge, MA: Blackwell.

Fischer, J.M. and **Ravizza, M.** (1998). *Responsibility and Control: An Essay on Moral Responsibility*. New York: Cambridge University Press.

Fitzgerald, M. (2015). Do Psychiatry and Neurology Need a Close Partnership or a Merger? *British Journal of Psychiatry Bulletin* **39**: 105–117.

Flaherty, A. (2005). Frontotemporal and Dopaminergic Control of Idea Generation and Creative Drive. *Journal of Comparative Neurology* **493**: 147–153.

Flaherty, A. (2011). Brain Illness and Creativity: Mechanisms and Treatment Risks. *Canadian Journal of Psychiatry* **56**: 132–143.

Focquaert, F., **Glenn, A.** and **Raine, A.** (2015). Psychopathy and Free Will from a Philosophical and Cognitive Neuroscience Perspective. In Glannon, 103–124.

Foltynie, T., **Brayne, C., Robbins, T.** and **Barker, R.** (2004). The Cognitive Ability of an Incident Cohort of Parkinson's Patients in the UK: The CamPaiGN Study. *Brain* **127**: 550–560.

**Foltynie, T.** and **Hariz, M.** (2010). Surgical Management of Parkinson's Disease. *Expert Reviews of Neurotherapeutics* **10**: 903–914.

**Ford, P.** (2009). Vulnerable Brains, Research Ethics and Neurosurgical Patients. *Journal of Law, Medicine and Ethics* **37**: 73–82.

**Fornito, A., Harrison, B., Goodby, E., Dean, A., Ooi, C., Nathan, P.** *et al.* (2013). Functional Dysconnectivity of Corticostriatal Circuits as a Risk Phenotype for Psychosis. *JAMA Psychiatry* **70**: 1143–1151.

**Fornito, A., Zalesky, A.** and **Breakspear, M.** (2015). The Connectomics of Brain Disorders. *Nature Reviews Neuroscience* **16**: 159–172.

**Fournier, J., DeRubeis, R., Hollon, S., Dimidjian, S., Amsterdam, J., Shelton, R.** *et al.* (2010). Antidepressant Drug Effects and Depression Severity: A Patient-Level Meta-Analysis. *Journal of the American Medical Association* **303**: 47–53.

**Fradera, A.** and **Kopelman, M.** (2009). Memory Disorders. In Squire, 751–760.

**Frank, M., Samanta, J., Moustafa, A.** and **Sherman, S.** (2007). Hold Your Horses: Impulsivity, Deep Brain Stimulation and Medication in Parkinsonism. *Science* **318**: 1309–1312.

**Franke, A., Gransmark, P., Agricola, A., Schule, K., Rommel, T., Sebastian, A.** *et al.* (2017). Methylphenidate, Modafinil, and Caffeine for Cognitive Enhancement in Chess: A Double-Blind Randomised Controlled Trial. *European Neuropsychopharmacology* **27**: 248–260.

**Frankfurt, H.** (1988a). Free Will and the Concept of a Person. In Frankfurt, 1988d, 11–25.

**Frankfurt, H.** (1988b). Coercion and Moral Responsibility. In Franfurt, 1988d, 26–46.

**Frankfurt, H.** (1988c). Identification and Externality. In Frankfurt, 1988d, 58–68.

**Frankfurt, H.** (1988d). *The Importance of What We Care About*. New York: Cambridge University Press.

**Franzoi, C.** (2017). Adam Maier-Clayton's Death Renews Debate on Assisted Dying Access for Those with Mental Illness. *The Globe and Mail*, April 16. http://www.theglobeandmail.com/news/national/adam-maier-clayton's-death-renews-debate-on-assisted-dying-access-for-those-with-mental-illness/article34718194/

**Freedman, R., Brown, A., Cannon, T., Druss, B., Earls, F., Escobar, J.** *et al.* (2018). Can a Framework be Established for the Safe Use of Ketamine? *American Journal of Psychiatry* **175**: doi: 10.1176.appi.ajp.2018.18030290.

**Freeman, M.** (ed.) (2011). *Law and Neuroscience: Current Legal Issues*, Volume **13**. Oxford: Oxford University Press.

**Freeman, W.** and **Watts, J.** (1942). Prefrontal Lobotomy: The Surgical Relief of Mental Pain. *Bulletin of the New York Academy of Medicine* **18**: 794–812.

**Fregnac, Y.** and **Laurent, G.** (2014). Neuroscience: Where Is the Brain in the Human Brain Project? *Nature* **513**: 27–29.

**Freud, S.** (1895). *Project for a Scientific Psychology*, trans. J. Strachey *et al.*, Standard Edition of the Complete Psychological Works of Sigmund Freud, Volume I. London: Hogarth Press.

**Freud, S.** (1914). *On Narcissism*, trans. J. Strachey *et al.* Standard Edition of the Complete Psychological Works of Sigmund Freud, Volume XIV. London: Hogarth Press.

**Fried, I., Katz, A., McCarthy, G., Sass, K. Williamson, P., Spencer, S.** *et al.* (1991). Functional Organization of Human Supplementary Motor Cortex Studies by Electrical Stimulation. *Journal of Neuroscience* **11**: 3656–3666.

Friedman, H. (ed.) (2011). *Oxford Handbook of Health Psychology*. Oxford: Oxford University Press.

Friedman, R. (2012). Depression Defies the Rush to Find an Evolutionary Upside. *New York Times* January 16. http://www.nytimes.com/2012/01/17/health/depression-defies-rush-to-find-evolutionary-upside/html.

Friedrich, M. (2017a). Depression is the Leading Cause of Disability Around the World. *Journal of the American Medical Association* 317: 1517.

Friedrich, M. (2017b). Mental Health Burden Increasing in Eastern Mediterranean Region. *Journal of the American Medical Association* 318: 1431.

Frith, C. (1996). The Role of the Prefrontal Cortex in Self-Consciousness: The Case of Auditory Hallucinations. *Philosophical Transactions of the Royal Society of London B* 351: 1505–1512.

Frye, M. (2011). Bipolar Disorder—A Focus on Depression. *New England Journal of Medicine* 364: 51–59.

Fuchs, T. (2011). The Psychopathology of Hyperreflexivity. *Journal of Speculative Philosophy* 24: 239–255.

Fuchs, T. (2012). Are Mental Illnesses Diseases of the Brain? In Choudhury and Slaby, 331–344.

Fuchs, T., Breyer, T. and Mundt, C. (eds.) (2014). *Karl Jaspers' Philosophy and Psychopathology*. Berlin and Heidelberg: Springer.

Fuster, J. (2013). *The Neuroscience of Freedom and Creativity: Our Predictive Brain*. New York: Cambridge University Press.

Gallagher, S. (2005). *How the Body Shapes the Mind*. Oxford: Clarendon Press.

Gallagher, S. (2006). Where's the action? Epiphenomenalism and the problem of free will. In Pocket, Banks and Gallagher, 109–124.

Galpern, W., Corrigan-Curay, J., Lang, A., Kahn, J., Tagle, D., Barker, R. *et al.* (2012). Sham Neurosurgical Procedures in Clinical Trials for Neurodegenerative Diseases: Scientific and Ethical Considerations. *The Lancet Neurology* 7: 643–650.

Gask, L. (2018). In Defense of the Biopsychosocial Model. *The Lancet Psychiatry* 5: 548–549.

Gerrans, P. (2014). *The Measure of Madness: Philosophy of Mind, Cognitive Neuroscience and Delusional Thought*. Cambridge, MA: MIT Press.

Geschwind, M. and Picard, F. (2016). Ecstatic Epileptic Seizures: A Glimpse into the Multiple Roles of the Insula. *Frontiers in Behavioral Neuroscience* 10: 21. doi: 10.3389/fnbeh.2016.00021.

Geurts, D., von Borries, K., Volman, I., Bukten, B., Cools, R. and Verkes, R-J. (2016). Neural Connectivity During Reward Expectation Dissociates Psychopathic Criminals from Non-Criminal Individuals with High Impulsive/Antisocial Psychopathic Traits. *Social Cognitive and Affective Neuroscience* 11: 1326–1334.

Giacino, J., Ashwal, S., Childs, N., Cranford, R., Jennett, B., Katz, D. *et al.* (2002). The Minimally Conscious State: Definition and Diagnostic Criteria. *Neurology* 58: 349–353.

Gillett, G. (2009). *The Mind and its Discontents*. Second Edition. Oxford: Oxford University Press.

Giubilini, A. and Savulescu, J. (2017). Conscientious Objection in Healthcare: Problems and Perspectives. *Cambridge Quarterly of Healthcare Ethics* 26: 3–5.

Glannon, W. (2008). Moral Responsibility and the Psychopath. *Neuroethics* 1: 158–166.

Glannon, W. (2014). Neuromodulation, Agency and Autonomy. *Brain Topography* **27**: 46–54.

Glannon, W. (2015a). Research Domain Criteria: A Final Paradigm for Psychiatry? *Frontiers in Human Neuroscience* **9**: 488. doi: 10.3389/fnhum.2015.00488.

Glannon, W. (ed.) (2015b). *Free Will and the Brain: Neuroscientific, Philosophical and Legal Perspectives*. Cambridge: Cambridge University Press.

Glannon, W. (2017). Brain Implants to Erase Memories. *Frontiers in Neuroscience* **11**: 584. doi: 10.3389/fnins.2017.00584.

Glannon, W. (2018). Brain Implants: Implications for Free Will. In Rommelfanger and Johnson, 319–334.

Glannon, W. and Ineichen, C. (2016). Philosophical Aspects of Closed-Loop Neuroscience. In El Hady, 259–270.

Glenn, A. and Raine, A. (2009). Psychopathy and Instrumental Aggression: Evolutionary, Neurobiological and Legal Perspectives. *International Journal of Law and Psychiatry* **32**: 253–258.

Glenn, A., Raine, A. and Schug, R. (2009). The Neural Correlates of Moral Decision-Making in Psychopathy. *Molecular Psychiatry* **14**: 5–6.

Glenn, A. and Raine, A. (2014a). Neurocriminology: Implications for the Punishment, Prediction and Prevention of Criminal Behavior. *Nature Reviews Neuroscience* **15**: 54–57.

Glenn, A. and Raine, A. (2014b). *Psychopathy: An Introduction to Biological Findings and their Implications*. New York: New York University Press.

Glover, J. (1984). *What Sort of People Should There Be?* Harmondsworth: Penguin.

Glover, J. (2006). *Choosing Children: Genes, Disability and Design*. Oxford: Oxford University Press.

Gold, A. and Lichtenberg, P. (2014). The Moral Case for the Clinical Placebo. *Journal of Medical Ethics* **40**: 219–224.

Goldapple, K., Segal, Z., Garson, C., Lau, M., Bieling, P., Kennedy, S. and Mayberg, H. (2004). Modulation of Cortico-Limbic Pathways in Major Depression: Treatment-Specific Effects of Cognitive Behavior Therapy. *Archives of General Psychiatry* **61**: 34–41.

Goldstein, R., Craig, A., Bechara, A., Garavan, H., Childress A.R., Paulus, M. *et al.* (2009). The Neurocircuitry of Impaired Insight in Drug Addiction. *Trends in Cognitive Sciences* **13**: 372–380.

Goodman, W. (2011). Electroconvulsive Therapy in the Spotlight. *New England Journal of Medicine* **364**: 1785–1787.

Goodman, W., Grice, D., Lapidus, K. and Coffey, B. (2014). Obsessive-Compulsive Disorder. *Psychiatric Clinics of North America* **37**: 257–267.

Gottesman, I. and Gould, J. (2003). The Endophenotype Concept in Psychiatry: Etymology and Strategic Intentions. *American Journal of Psychiatry* **160**: 636–645.

Grady, C. (2015). Enduring and Emerging Challenges of Informed Consent. *New England Journal of Medicine* **372**: 855–862.

Graham, G. (2013). *The Disordered Mind: An Introduction to Philosophy of Mind and Mental Illness*. Second Edition. New York: Routledge.

Grahn, P., Mallory, G., Khurram, O., Berry, B., Hachmann, J., Bieber, A. *et al.* (2014). A Neurochemical Closed-Loop Controller for Deep Brain Stimulation: Toward

Individualized Smart Neuromodulation Therapies. *Frontiers in Neuroscience* **8**: 1–11. doi: 10.3389/fnins.2-014.00169.

Grant, P., Huh, G., Perivoliotis, P., Stolar, N. and Beck, A. (2012). Randomized Trial to Evaluate the Efficacy of Cognitive Therapy for Low-Functioning Patients with Schizophrenia. *Archives of General Psychiatry* **69**: 121–127.

Greely, H. (2008). Neuroscience and Criminal Justice: Not Responsibility but Treatment. *Kansas Law Review* **56**: 1103–1138.

Greenberg, B., Gabriels, L., Malone, D., Rezai, A., Friehs, G., Okun, M. *et al.* (2010). Deep Brain Stimulation of the Ventral Internal Capsule/Ventral Striatum for Obsessive-Compulsive Disorder: Worldwide Experience. *Molecular Psychiatry* **15**: 64–79.

Greenberg, B., Rauch, S. and Haber, S. (2010). Invasive Circuitry-Based Neurotherapeutics: Stereotactic Ablation and Deep Brain Stimulation for OCD. *Neuropsychopharmacology* **35**: 317–336.

Gregory, S., ffytche, D., Simmons, A., Kumari, V., Howard, M., Hodgins, S. *et al.* (2012). The Anti-Social Brain: Psychopathy Matters. *Archives of General Psychiatry* **69**: 962–972.

Grisso, T., Appelbaum, P. and Hill-Fotouhi, C. (1997). The MacCAT-T: A Clinical Tool to Assess Patients' Capacities to Make Treatment Decisions. *Psychiatric Services* **48**: 1415–1419.

Grossman, N., Bono, D., Dedic, N., Kodandaramaiah, S., Rudenko, A., Suk, H. *et al.* (2017). Noninvasive Deep Brain Stimulation via Temporally Interfering Electric Fields. *Cell* **169**: 1029–1041.

Gustafson, H., Nordstrom, A. and Nordstrom, P. (2015). Depression and Subsequent Risk of Parkinson Disease: A Nationwide Cohort Study. *Neurology* **84**: 2422–2429.

Hafner, H. (2004). Schizophrenia: Still Kraepelin's Dementia Praecox? *Epidemiology and Psychological Sciences* **13**: 99–112.

Hall, K., Loscalzo, J. and Kaptchuk, T. (2015). Genetics and the Placebo Effect: The Placebome. *Trends in Molecular Medicine* **21**: 285–294.

Hamani, C., Holtzheimer, P., Lozano, A. and Mayberg, H. (eds.) (2016). *Neuromodulation in Psychiatry*. Oxford: Wiley Blackwell.

Hare, R. (2003). *Hare Psychopathy Checklist—Revised (PCL-R)*. Second Edition. Toronto: Multi-Health Systems.

Hariz, M. (2014). Afterword. In Leveque, 323–324.

Hariz, M. (2016). History of Invasive Brain Stimulation in Psychiatry: Lessons for the Current Practice of Neuromodulation. In Hamani, Holtzheimer, Lozano and Mayberg, H., 1–14.

Harris, J. (2007). *Enhancing Evolution: The Case for Making Better People*. Princeton, NJ: Princeton University Press.

Hartwig, F., Borges, M., Horta, B., Bowden, J. and Smith, G. (2017). Inflammatory Biomarkers and Risk of Schizophrenia: A 2-Sample Mendelian Randomization Study. *JAMA Psychiatry* **74** (12): 1226–1233.

Hebb, A., Zhang. J., Mahoor, M., Tsiokos, C., Matlack, C., Chizeck, H. *et al.* (2014). Creating the Feedback Loop: Closed-Loop Neuromodulation. *Neurosurgery Clinics of North America* **25**: 187–204.

Hippocrates (400BCE/1961). *On the Sacred Disease*. Boston, MA: Loeb Classical Library of Harvard University Press.

Hirschtritt, M., Bloch, M. and **Mathews, C.** (2017). Obsessive-Compulsive Disorder: Advances in Diagnosis and Treatment. *Journal of the American Medical Association* **317**: 1358–1367.

Hirschtritt, M. and **Kroenke, K.** (2017). Screening for Depression. *Journal of the American Medical Association* **318**: 745–746.

Hoekzema, E., Barba-Muller, E., Pozzobon, C., Picado, M., Lucco, F. Garcia-Garcia, D. *et al.* (2017). Pregnancy Leads to Long-Lasting Changes in Human Brain Structure. *Nature Neuroscience* **20**: 287–296.

Hohne, N., Poidinger, M., Merz, F., Pfister, H., Bruckl, T., Zimmerman, P. *et al.* (2014). Increased HPA Axis Response to Psychosocial Stress in Remitted Depression: The Influence of Coping Style. *Biological Psychology* **103**: 267–275.

Holtzheimer, P. and **Maybeg, H.** (2010). Deep Brain Stimulation for Treatment-Resistant Depression. *American Journal of Psychiatry* **167**: 1437–1444.

Holtzheimer, P. and **Mayberg, H.** (2011). Stuck in a Rut: Rethinking Depression and its Treatment. *Trends in Neurosciences* **34**: 1–9.

Holtzheimer, P., Kelley, M., Gross, R., Filkowski, M. Garlow, S. Barrocas, A. *et al.* (2012). Subcallosal Cingulate Deep Brain Stimulation for Treatment-Resistant Unipolar and Bipolar Depression. *Archives of General Psychiatry* **69**: 150–158.

Holtzheimer, P., Husain, M., Lisanby, S., Taylor, S., Whitworth, L., McClintock, S. *et al.* (2017). Subcallosal cingulate deep brain stimulation for treatment-resistant depression: A multisite, randomized, sham-controlled trial. *The Lancet Psychiatry* **11**: 839–849.

**Home Office and Department of Health and Social Security** (1975). *Report of the Committee on Mentally Abnormal Offenders.* London. Her Majesty's Stationery Office.

Horng, S. and **Miller, F.** (2003). Ethical Framework for the Use of Sham Procedures in Clinical Trials. *Critical Care Medicine* **31**: S126–130.

Horodyckid, C., Canney, M., Vignot, A., Boisgard, R., Drier, A., Huberfeld, G. *et al.* (2017). Safe Long-Term Repeated Disruption of the Blood-Brain Barrier Using an Implantable Ultrasound Device: a Multiparametric Study in a Primate Model. *Journal of Neurosurgery* **126**: 1351–1361.

Horvath, J., Perez, J., Forrow, L., **Fregni, F.** and **Pascual-Leone, A.** (2013). Transcranial Magnetic Stimulation: Future Prospects and Ethical Concerns in Treatment and Research. In Chatterjee and Farah, 209–234.

Horvath, J., Forte, J. and **Carter, O.** (2015). Evidence that Transcranial Direct Current Stimulation (tDCS) Generates Little-to-No Reliable Neurophysiologic Effect Beyond MEP Amplitude Modulation in Heathy Human Subjects: A Systematic Review. *Neuropsychologia* **66**: 213–236.

Hosking, J., Kastman, E., Dorfman, H., Samanez-Larkin, G., Baskin-Somers, A., Kiehl, K. *et al.* (2017). Disrupted Prefrontal Regulation of Striatal Subjective Value Signals in Psychopathy. *Neuron* **95**: 221–231.

Howes, O. and **McCutcheon, R.** (2015). Inflammation and the Neural Diathesis-Stress Hypothesis for Schizophrenia: A Reconceptualization. *Translational Psychiatry* **7**: e2014. doi: 10.1038/tp.2016.278.

Howes, O., McCutcheon, R., Owen, M. and **Murray, R.** (2017). The Role of Genes, Stress and Dopamine in the Development of Schizophrenia. *Biological Psychiatry* **81**: 9–20.

Hume, D. (1888/1978). *A Treatise of Human Nature*. Second Edition, ed. P.H. Nidditch. Oxford: Oxford University Press.

Hurlemann, R. and Scheele, D. (2016). Dissecting the Role of Oxytocin in the Formation and Loss of Social Relationships. *Biological Psychiatry* 79: 185–193.

Husain, M., Rush, A., Fink, M., Knapp, R., Petrides, G., Rummans T. *et al*. (2004). Speed of Response and Remission in Major Depressive Disorder with Acute Electroconvulsive Therapy (ECT): A Consortium for Research in ECT (CORE) Report. *Journal of Clinical Psychiatry* 65: 485–491.

Hyde, C., Nagle, M., Chao, T., Chen, X., Paciga, S., Wendland J. *et al*. (2016). Identification of 15 Genetic Loci Associated with Risk of Depression in Individuals of European Descent. *Nature Genetics* 48: 1031–1036.

Hyman, S. (2005). Addiction: A Disorder of Learning and Memory. *American Journal of Psychiatry* 162: 1414–1422.

Hyman, S. (2013). Psychiatric Drug Development: Diagnosing A Crisis. *Cerebrum* 5 (March–April). http://www.ncbi.nlm.nih/gov/pmc/articles/PMC3662213/?report=reader

Illes, J. and Racine, E. (2005). Imaging or Imagining? A Neuroethics Challenge Informed by Genetics. *American Journal of Bioethics* 5: 5–18.

Ineichen, C., Glannon, W., Temel, Y., Baumann, C. and Suruku, O. (2014). A Critical Reflection of the Technological Development of Deep Brain Stimulation (DBS). *Frontiers in Human Neuroscience* 8: 730. doi: 10.3389/fnhuman.2-014.00730.

Insel, T. (2010). Rethinking Schizophrenia. *Nature* 468: 187–193.

Insel, T. (2013). *Transforming Diagnosis*. Available at: http://www.numh.nih.gov/about/director/2013/transforming-diagnosis.html.

Insel, T., Cuthbert, B., Garvey, M., Heinssen, R., Pine, D., Quinn, K. *et al*. (2010). Research Domain Criteria (RDoC): Toward a New Classification Framework for Research on Mental Disorders. *American Journal of Psychiatry* 167: 748–751.

Insel, T. and Wang, P. (2010). Rethinking Mental Illness. *Journal of the American Medical Association* 303: 1970–1971.

Iuculano, T. and Cohen Kadosh, R. (2013). The Mental Cost of Cognitive Enhancement. *Journal of Neuroscience* 33: 4482–4486.

Jacob, J. (2015). Anxiety Disorders Affect 4.3 Million Working US Adults. *Journal of the American Medical Association* 314: 330.

James, W. (1956). *The Will to Believe*. New York: Dover.

Jameson, J. and Longo, D. (2015). Precision Medicine—Personalized, Problematic and Promising. *New England Journal of Medicine* 313: 1–6.

Jamison, K.R. (2014). To Know Suicide: Depression Can Be Treated, But It Takes Competence. *New York Times*, April 16. http://www.nytimes.com/2014/08/16/opinion/depression-can-be-treated-but-it-takes-competence.html.

Jamison, K.R. (2017). *Robert Lowell, Setting the River on Fire: A Study of Genius, Mania and Character*. New York: A.A. Knopf.

Jarvis, S. and Schultz, S. (2015). Prospects for Optogenetic Augmentation of Brain Function. *Frontiers in Systems Neuroscience* 9. doi: 10.3389fnsys.2017.00157.

Javitt, D. and Freedman, R. (2015). Sensory Processing Dysfunction in the Personal Experience and Neuronal Machinery of Schizophrenia. *American Journal of Psychiatry* 172: 17–31.

Joffe, R. (2011). Hormone Treatment of Depression. *Dialogues in Clinical Neuroscience* **13**: 127–132.

Johnson, L.S. and **Rommelfanger, K.** (eds.) (2018). *The Routledge Handbook of Neuroethics.* New York: Routledge.

Johnston, M. (1992). Constitution Is Not Identity. *Mind* **101**: 89–106.

Jones, O., **Wagner, A., Faigman, D.** and **Raichle, M.** (2013). Neuroscientists in Court. *Nature Reviews Neuroscience* **14**: 730–736.

Jonsen, A., **Winslade, W.** and **Siegler, M.** (2010). *Clinical Ethics A Practical Approach to Ethical Decisions in Clinical Medicine.* Seventh Edition. New York: McGraw Hill.

Kagan, S. (2012). *Death.* New Haven, CT: Yale University Press.

Kamm, F.M. (2002). Genes, Justice and Obligations to Future People. *Social Philosophy & Policy* **19**: 350–388.

Kamm, F.M. (2007). *Intricate Ethics: Rights, Responsibilities and Permissible Harm.* Oxford: Oxford University Press.

Kandel, E. (1998). A New Intellectual Framework for Psychiatry. *American Journal of Psychiatry* **155**: 457–469.

Kandel, E., **Markram, H., Matthews, P., Yuste, R.** and **Koch, C.** (2013). Neuroscience Thinks Big (and Collaboratively). *Nature Reviews Neuroscience* **14**: 659–664.

Kane, J., **Robinson, D., Schooler, N., Mueser, K., Penn, D., Rosenheck, R.** *et al.* (2016). Comprehensive Versus Usual Community Care for First-Episode Psychosis: 2-Year Outcomes from the NIMH RAISE Early Treatment Program. *American Journal of Psychiatry* **173**: 362–372.

Kane, R. (1996), *The Significance of Free Will.* New York: Oxford University Press.

Kant, I. (1785/1964). *Groundwork of the Metaphysics of Morals,* trans. H.J. Paton. New York: Harper & Row.

Kant, I. (1786/1965). *Metaphysical Elements of Justice,* trans. J. Ladd. Indianapolis: Bobbs-Merrill.

Kaptchuk, T., **Friedlander, E., Kelley, J., Sanchez, N., Kokkotou, E., Singer, J.** *et al.* (2010). Placebos without Deception: A Randomized Controlled Trial in Irritable Bowel Syndrome. *PLoS One* **5**: e15591. doi: 10.1371/journal.pone.0015591.

Kaptchuk, T. and **Miller, F.** (2015). Placebo Effects in Medicine. *New England Journal of Medicine* **373**: 8–9.

Kelly, B. and **McLoughlin, D.** (2002). Euthanasia, Assisted Suicide and Psychiatry: A Pandora's Box. *British Journal of Psychiatry* **181**: 278–279.

Kendler, K. (2006). Reflections on the Relationship between Psychiatric Genetics and Psychiatric Nosology. *American Journal of Psychiatry* **163**: 1138–1146.

Kendler, K. (2016). Phenomenology of Schizophrenia and the Representativeness of Modern Diagnostic Criteria. *JAMA Psychiatry* **73**: 1082–1092.

Kendler, K. and **Parnas, J.** (eds.) (2012). *Philosophical Issues in Psychiatry II: Nosology.* Oxford: Oxford University Press.

Kendler, K. and **Parnas, J.** (eds.) (2014). *Philosophical Issues in Psychiatry III: The Nature and Sources of Historical Change.* Oxford: Oxford University Press.

Kendler, K. and **Parnas, J.** (eds.) (2017). *Philosophical Issues in Psychiatry IV: Psychiatric Nosology DSM-5.* Oxford: Oxford University Press.

Kesey, K. (1962). *One Flew Over the Cuckoo's Nest.* New York: Penguin.

Keshavan, M., Kennedy, J and Murray, R. (2004). *Neurodevelopment and Schizophrenia.* Cambridge: Cambridge University Press.

Keshavan, M., Giedd, J., Lau, J., Lewis, D. and Paus, T. (2014). Changes in the Adolescent Brain and the Pathophysiology of Psychotic Disorders. *The Lancet Psychiatry* 1: 549–558.

Kestle, J. (2015). Industry-Sponsored Research. *Journal of Neurosurgery* 122: 136–138.

Kim, J. (1998). *Mind in a Physical World: An Essay on the Mind-Body Problem and Mental Causation.* Cambridge, MA: MIT Press.

Kim, J. (2010). *Philosophy of Mind.* Third Edition. New York: Westview Press.

Kim, S., De Vries, R., Parnami, S., Wilson, R., Kim, H.M., Frank, S. *et al.* (2015). Are Therapeutic Motivation and Having One's Doctor as Researcher Sources of Therapeutic Misconception? *Journal of Medical Ethics* 41: 391–397.

Kim, S., De Vries, R. and Peteet, J. (2016). Euthanasia and Assisted Suicide of Patients with Psychiatric Disorders in the Netherlands 2011 to 2014. *JAMA Psychiatry* 73:362–368.

Kim, W. and Cho, J. (2017). Encoding of Discriminative Fear Memory by Input-Specific LTP in the Amygdala. *Neuron* 95: 988–990.

Kim, W., Sharim, J., Tenn, S. Kapreelian, T., Bordelon, Y., Agasaryan, A. *et al.* (2018). Diffusion Tractography Imaging-Guided Frameless Linear Accelerator Stereotactic Radiosurgical Thalamotomy for Tremor: Case Report. *Journal of Neurosurgery* 128: 215–221.

Kimsma, G. (2006). Euthanasia for Existential Reasons. *Lahey Clinic Medical Ethics* 13: 1–2, 12.

Kimsma, G. (2012). Assessment of Unbearable and Hopeless Suffering in Evaluating :A Request to End Life. In Youngner and Kimsma, 333–350.

Kindt, M., Soeter, M. and Vervliet, B. (2009). Beyond Extinction: Erasing Human Feat Responses and Preventing the Return of Fear. *Nature Neuroscience* 12: 256–258.

Kinon, B., Potts, A. and Watson, S. (2011). Placebo Responses in Clinical Trials with Schizophrenia Patients. *Current Opinion in Psychiatry* 24: 107–113.

Kircher, T. and David, A. (eds.) (2003). *The Self in Neuroscience and Psychiatry.* Cambridge: Cambridge University Press.

Kirmayer, L., Lemelson, R. and Cummings, C. (eds.) (2015). *Re-Visioning Psychiatry: Cultural Phenomenology, Critical Neuroscience and Global Mental Health.* New York: Cambridge University Press.

Kirsch, I., Deacon, B., Huedo-Medina, T., Scobona, A., Moore, T. and Johnson, B. (2008). Initial Severity and Antidepressant Benefits: A Meta-Analysis of Data Submitted to the Food and Drug Administration. *PLoS Medicine* 5: e45. doi: 10.1371/journal.pmed.0050045.

Kiverstein, J. and Clark, A. (2009). Introduction: Mind Embodied, Embedded, Enacted: One Church or Many? *Topoi* 28: 1–7.

Klaming, L. and Haselager, P. (2013). Did My Brain Implant Make Me Do It? Questions Raised by DBS Regarding Psychological Continuity, Responsibility for Actions and Mental Competence. *Neuroethics* 6: 527–539.

Kleinman, A. (1988). *Rethinking Psychiatry: From Cultural Category to Personal Experience.* New York: Free Press.

Ko, J., Feigin, A., Mattis, P., Tang, C., Ma, Y., Dhawan, V. *et al.* (2014). Network Modulation Following Sham Surgery in Parkinson's Disease. *Journal of Clinical Investigation* 124: 3656–3666.

Kok, R. and **Reynolds, C.** (2017). Management of Depression in Older Adults: A Review. *Journal of the American Medical Association* **317**: 2114–2122.

Kokkinou, M. Ashok, A. and Howes, O. (2018). The Effects of Ketamine on Dopaminergic Function: Meta-Analysis and Review of the Implications for Neuropsychiatric Disorders. *Molecular Psychiatry* **23**: 59–69.

Kong, C., **Dunn, M.** and **Parker, M.** (2017). Psychiatric Genomics and Mental Health Treatment: Setting the Ethical Agenda. *American Journal of Bioethics* **17**: 3–12.

Kopell, B. and **Rasouli, J.** (2016). Comments (on the paper by De Ridder, Vanneste, Gillett *et al*,). *Neuromodulation* **19**: 248.

Kopelman, M. (2002). Disorders of Memory. *Brain* **25**: 2152–2190.

Kraepelin, E. (1896/1913). *Psychiatrie: Ein Lehrbuch fur Studirende und Aerzte.* Leipzig. Verlag von Johann Ambrosius Barth. (*A Textbook of Psychiatry for Students and Doctors*).

Kramer, P. (1993). *Listening to Prozac.* New York: Penguin.

Kramer, P. (2005). *Against Depression.* New York: Viking.

Kramer, P. (2016). *Ordinarily Well: The Case for Antidepressants.* New York: Farrar, Straus and Giroux.

Kroes, M., **Tendolkar, I.,** van Wingen, G., van Waarde, J., **Strange, B.** and **Fernandez, G.** (2014). An Electroconvulsive Therapy Procedure Impairs Reconsolidation of Episodic Memories in Humans. *Nature Neuroscience* **17**: 204–206.

Labonte, B., **Suderman, M.,** Maussion, G., **Lopez, J-P.,** Navarro-Sanchez, L. Yerko, V. *et al.* (2013). Genome-Wide Methylation Changes in the Brains of Suicide Completers. *American Journal of Psychiatry* **170**: 511–520.

Lapidus, K., **Kopell, B.,** Ben-Haim, S., **Rezai, A.** and **Goodman, W.** (2013). History of Psychosurgery: A Psychiatrist's Perspective. *World Neurosurgery* **80**: s27, e1–16.

Laureys, S., **Celesia, G.,** Cohadon, F., **Lavrijson, J.,** Leon-Carrion, J., **Sannita, W.** *et al.* (2010). Unresponsive Wakefulness Syndrome: a New Name for the Vegetative State of Apallic Syndrome. *BMC Medicine* **8**: 68.

Laxton, A., **Tang-Wai, D.,** McAndrews, M., **Zumsteg, D.,** Wennberg, R., **Keren, R.** *et al.* (2010). A Phase I Trial of Deep Brain Stimilation of Memory Circuits in Alzheimer's Disease. *Annals of Neurology* **68**: 521–534.

LeDoux, J. (2015). *Anxious: Using the Brain to Understand and Treat Fear and Anxiety.* New York: Viking.

Lee, S., **Ripke, S.,** Neale, B., **Faraone, S.,** Purcell, S., **Perlis, R.** *et al.,* **Cross-Disorder Group of the Psychiatric Genomics Consortium** (2013). Genetic Relationship between Five Psychiatric Disoders Estimated from Genome-Wide SNPs. *Nature Genetics* **45**: 984–994.

Leichsenring, F. and **Leweke, F.** (2017). Social Anxiety Disorder. *New England Journal of Medicine* **376**: 2255–2264.

Leveque, M. (ed). (2014). *Psychosurgery: New Techniques for Brain Disorders.* Heidelberg: Springer.

Levy, N. and **Clausen, J.** (eds.) (2014), *Handbook of Neuroethics.* Berlin: Springer.

Liao, M. (ed.) (2016). *Moral Brains: The Neuroscience of Morality.* Oxford: Oxford University Press.

Lidstone, S., **Schulzer, M.,** Dinelle, K., **Mak, E.,** Sossi, V., **Ruth, T.** *et al.* (2010). Effects of Expectation on Placebo-Induced Dopamine Release in Parkinson Disease. *Archives of General Psychiatry* **67**: 857–865.

Lidz, C., Appelbaum, P., Grisso, T. and Renaud, M. (2004). Therapeutic Misconception and the Appreciation of Risks in Clinical Trials. *Social Science and Medicine* **58**: 1689–1697.

Linden, D. (2014). *Brain Control: Developments in Therapy and Implications for Society*. London: Palgrave Macmillan

Linden, D., Habes, I., Johnston, S., Linden, S., Tatineni, R., Subramaniab, L. *et al.* (2012). Real-time Self-Regulation of Emotion Networks in Patients with Depression. *PLoS One* **7**: e38115. doi:. 10.1371/journal.pone.0038115.

Lipsman, N., Giacobbe, P., Bernstein, M and Lozano, A. (2012). Informed Consent for Clinical Trials of Deep Brain Stimulation in Psychiatric Disease: Challenges and Implications for Trial Design. *Journal of Medical Ethics* **38**: 107–111.

Lipsman, N. and Glannon, W. (2013). Brain, Mind, and Machine: What Are the Implications of Deep Brain Stimulation for Perceptions of Personal Identity, Agency and Free Will? *Bioethics* **27**: 465–470.

Lipsman, N., Woodside, D., Giacobbe, P., Hamani, C. Carter, J., Norwood, S. *et al.* (2013). Subcallosal Cingulate Deep Brain Stimulation for Treatment-Refractory Anorexia Nervosa: A Phase 1 Pilot Trial. *The Lancet* **381**: 1361–1370.

Lipsman, N., Schwartz, M., Huang, Y., Lee, L., Sankar, T., Chapman, M. *et al.* (2013). MR-Guided Focused Ultrasound Thalamotomy for Essential Tremor: A Proof-of-Concept Study. *Lancet Neurology* **12**: 462–468.

Lipsman, N. and Lozano, A. (2015). Implications of Functional Neurosurgery and Deep Brain Stimulation for Free Will and Decision-Making. In Glannon, 191–204.

Lipsman, N., Lam, E., Volpini, M., Sutandar, K., Twose, R., Giacobbe, P. *et al.* (2017). Deep Brain Stimulation of the Subcallosal Cingulate for Treatment-Refractory Anorexia Nervosa: 1-Year Follow-Up of an Open-Label Trial. *The Lancet Psychiatry* **4**: 285–294.

Lipsman, N., Meng, Y., Bethune, A., Hung, Y., Lam, B. Masellis, M. *et al.* (2018). Blood-Brain Barrier Opening in Alzheimer's Disease Using MR-Guided Focused Ultrasound. *Nature Communications* **9**: 2336. doi: 10.1038_s41467-018-04529-6.ris.

Lisanby, S. (2007). Electroconvulsive Therapy for Depression. *New England Journal of Medicine* **357**: 1939–1945.

Lisanby, S. (2017). Noninvasive Brain Stimulation for Depression—The Devil Is in the Dosing. *New England Journal of Medicine* **376**: 2593–2594.

Lisanby, S., Maddox, J., Prudic, J., Devanand, D. and Sackheim, H. (2000). The Effects of Electroconvulsive Therapy on Memory of Autobiographical and Public Events. *Archives of General Psychiatry* **57**: 581–590.

Lonergan, M., Oliveira-Figueroa, L., Pitman, R. and Brunet, A. (2013). Propranolol's Effects on the Consolidation and Reconsolidation of Long-Term Emotional Memory in Healthy Participants: A Meta-Analysis. *Journal of Psychiatry and Neuroscience* **38**: 222–231.

Lott-Schwartz, H. (2012). Jump Start Your Brain. *Boston Magazine*. June 1. http://www.boston-magazine.com/news/article/2012/06/01/jump-start-your-brain/.

Louis, E. (2016). Treatment of Medically Refractory Essential Tremor. *New England Journal of Medicine* **375**: 792–793.

Lozano, A. (2017). Waving Hello to Noninvasive Deep-Brain Stimulation. *New England Journal of Medicine* **377**: 1096–1098.

Lozano, A., Mayberg, H., Giacobbe, P., Hamani, C., Craddock, R. and Kennedy, S. (2008). Subcallosal Cingulate Gyrus Deep Brain Stimulation for Treatment-Resistant Depression. *Biological Psychiatry* **64**: 461–467.

Lozano, A. and Lipsman, N. (2013). Probing and Regulating Dysfunctional Circuits Using Deep Brain Stimulation. *Neuron* **77**: 406–424.

Luaute, J., Maucort-Boulch, L., Tell, F., Quelard, T., Sarraf, J., Iwaz, D. *et al.* (2010). Long-Term Outcomes of Chronic Minimally Conscious and Vegetative States. *Neurology* **75**: 246–252.

Lyon, J. (2017). Chess Study Revives Debate Over Cognition-Enhancing Drugs. *Journal of the American Medical Association* **318**: 784–786.

Mackay, E., Dalman, C., Karlsson, H. and Gardner, R. (2017). Association of Gestational Weight Gain and Maternal Body Mass Index in Early Pregnancy with Risk for Nonaffective Psychosis in Offspring. *JAMA Psychiatry* **74**: 339–349.

Macklin, R. (1999). The Ethical Problems with Sham Surgery in Clinical Research. *New England Journal of Medicine* **341**: 992–996.

Magrassi, L. Maggione, G., Pistarini, C., Perri, C., Bastianello, S., Antonio, G. *et al.* (2016). Results of a Prospective Study (CATS) on the Effects of Thalamic Stimulation in Minimally Conscious and Vegetative State. *Journal of Neurosurgery* **125**: 972–981.

Maibom, H. (2008). The Mad, the Bad and the Psychopath. *Neuroethics* **1**: 167–184.

Maiese, M. (2016). *Embodied Selves and Divided Minds*. Oxford: Oxford University Press.

Mallet, L., Polosan, M., Jaafari, N., Baup, N., Welter, M., Fontaine, D. *et al.* (2008). Subthalamic Nucleus Stimulation in Severe Obsessive-Compulsive Disorder. *New England Journal of Medicine* **359**: 2121–2134.

Malloy-Diniz, L., Marques de Miranda, D. and Grassi-Oliveira, R. (2017). Executive Functions in Psychiatric Disorders. *Frontiers in Psychology/Frontiers in Psychiatry* **8**: 1461. doi: 10:3389/978-2-88945-306-1.

Mantione, M., Nieman., D., Figee, M. and Denys, D. (2014). Cognitive-Behavioral Therapy Augments the Effects of Deep Brain Stimulation in Obsessive-Compulsive Disorder. *Psychological Medicine* **44**: 3515–3522.

Markram, H., Meier, K., Lippert, T., Grillner, S., Frackowak, R., Dehaene, S. *et al.* (2011). Introducing the Human Brain Project. *Procedia Computer Science* **7**: 39–42.

Maslen, H., Douglas, T., Cohen Kadosh, R. Levy, N. and Savulescu, J. (2012). *Mind Machines: The Regulation of Cognitive Enhancement Devices*. Oxford Martin Policy Paper, Institute of Science and Ethics. https://www.oxfordmartin.ox.ac.uk.downloads/briefs/2012.

Maslen, H., Pugh, J. and Savulescu, J. (2015). The Ethics of Deep Brain Stimulation for the Treatment of Anorexia Nervosa. *Neuroethics* **8**: 215–230.

Maxmen, A. (2017). Psychedelic Compound in Ecstasy Moves Closer to Approval to Treat PTSD. *Nature* April 28. doi: 10.1038/nature.2017.21907.

Mayberg, H. (2009). Targeted Electrode-Based Modulation of Neural Circuits for Depression. *Journal of Clinical Investigation* **119**: 717–725.

Mayberg, H. (2014). Neuroimaging and Psychiatry: The Long Road from Bench to Bedside. *Hastings Center Report* **44** (2): 31–36.

Mayberg, H., Lozano, A., Voon, V. McNeely, H. Seminowicz, D., Hamani, C. *et al.* (2005). Deep Brain Stimulation for Treatment-Resistant Depression. *Neuron* **45**: 651–660.

Mayberg, H., Silva, J. Brannen, S., Tekell, J., Mahurin, R., McGinnis, R. and Jerabek, P. (2002). The Functional Neuroanatomy of the Placebo Effect. *American Journal of Psychiatry* **159**: 728–737.

McCormack, R. and Flechais, R. (2012). The Role of Psychiatrists and Mental Disorder in Assisted Dying Practices Around the World: A Review of the Legislation and Official Reports. *Psychosomatics* **53**: 319–326.

McCormack, R. and Price, A. (2014). Psychiatric Review Should Be Mandatory for Patients Requesting Assisted Suicide. *General Hospital Psychiatry* **36**: 7–9.

McGrath, C., Kelley, M., Holtzheimer, P., Dunlop, B., Craighead, W., Franco, A. *et al.* (2013). Toward a Neuroimaging Treatment Selection Biomarker for Major Depressive Disorder. *JAMA Psychiatry* **70**: 821–829.

McHugh, P. and Slavney, P. (1998). *The Perspectives of Psychiatry*. Second edition. Baltimore, MD: The Johns Hopkins University Press.

McLaughlin, B. and Beckerman, A. (eds.) (2009). *The Oxford Handbook of Philosophy of Mind*. Oxford: Oxford University Press.

McMahan, J. (2002). *The Ethics of Killing: Problems at the Margins of Life*. Oxford: Oxford University Press.

Mele, A. (1995). *Autonomous Agents: From Self-Control to Autonomy*. New York: Oxford University Press.

Melloni, M., Urbistondo, C., Sedeno, L., Gelormini, C., Kichic, R and Ibanez, A. (2012). The Extended Frontal-Striatal Model of Obsessive-Compulsive Disorder: Convergence from Event-Related Potentials, Neurophysiology and Neuroimaging. *Frontiers in Human Neuroscience* **6**: 259. doi: 10.3389/fnhum.2012.00259.

Meng, Y., Suppioah, S., Mithani, K., Solomon, B., Schwartz. M. and Lispman, N. (2017). Current and Emerging Brain Applications of MR-Guided Focused Ultrasound. *Journal of Therapeutic Ultrasound* **5**: 16. doi: 10.1188/s40349-017-005-z.

Merkel, R., Boer, G., Fegert, J., Galert, T., Hartmann, D. Nuttin, B. *et al.* (2007). *Intervening in the Brain: Changing Psyche and Society*. Berlin and Heidelberg: Springer

Merkow, M., Burke, J., Ramayya, A., Sharan, A., Sperling, M. and Kahana, M. (2017). Stimulation of the Human Medial Temporal Lobe Between Learning and Recall Selectively Enhances Forgetting. *Brain Stimulation* **10**: 645–650.

Metzinger, T. (2003). *Being No One: The Self-Model Theory of Subjectivity*. Cambridge, MA: MIT Press.

Meynen, G. (2010). Free Will and Mental Disorder: Exploring the Relationship. *Theoretical Medicine and Bioethics* **31**: 429–443.

Meynen, G. (2012). Obsessive-Compulsive Disorder, Free Will and Control. *Philosophy, Psychiatry & Psychology* **19**: 323–332.

Meynen, G. (2015). How Mental Disorders Can Compromise the Will. In Glannon, 125–145.

Meynen, G. (2016). Neurolaw: Recognizing Opportunities and Challenges for Psychiatry. *Journal of Psychiatry and Neuroscience* **41**: 3–5.

Micieli, R., Lopex-Rios, A., Aguilar, R., Posada, L. and Hutchison, W. (2017). Single-Unit Analysis of the Human Posterior Hypothalamus and Red Nucleus during Deep Brain Stimulation for Aggressivity. *Journal of Neurosurgery* **120**: 1158–1164.

Mikell, C., Sinha, S. and Sheth, S. (2016). Neurosurgery for Schizophrenia: An Update on Pathophysiology and a Novel Therapeutic Target. *Journal of Neurosurgery* 124: 917–928.

Mill, J.S. (1859/1978). *On Liberty*, ed. E. Rapaport. Indianapolis, IN: Hackett.

Mill, J.S. (1863/1998). *Utilitarianism*, ed. R. Crisp. Oxford: Oxford University Press.

Miller, A., Meletic, V. and Raison, C. (2009). Inflammation and its Discontents: The Role of Cytokines in the Pathophysiology of Major Depression. *Biological Psychiatry* 65: 732–741.

Miller, A. and Raison, C. (2016). The Role of Inflammation in Depression: From Evolutionary Imperative to Modern Treatment Target. *Nature Reviews Immunology* 16: 22–34.

Miller, F. (2015). Treatment-Resistant Depression and Physician-Assisted Death. *Journal of Medical Ethics* 41: 885–886.

Miller, F. and Appelbaum, P. (2018). Physician-Assisted Death for Psychiatric Patients— Misguided Public Policy. *New England Journal of Medicine* 378: 883–885.

Misiak, B., Frydecka, D. and Rybakowski, J. (2016). Endophenotypes for Schizophrenia and Mood Disorders: Implications from Genetic, Biochemical, Cognitive, Behavioral and Neuroimaging Studies. *Frontiers in Psychiatry* 7: 83. doi: 10.3389/fnpsyt.2016.00083.

M'Naghten Case (1843/1975). 8 Eng. Rep. 718, 722. Cited in the Report of the Committee on Mentally Abnormal Offenders. London: Her Majesty's Stationery Office.

Model Penal Code (1985). *Official Draft and Commentaries*. Philadelphia, PA: American Law Institute.

Mollenhauer, B. and Weintraub, D. (2017). The Depressed Brain in Parkinson's Disease: Implications for an Inflammatory Biomarker. *Proceedings of the National Academy of Sciences* 114: 3004-3005.

Morgan, H. (1990). Dostoevsky's Epilepsy: A Case Report and Comparison. *Surgical Neurosurgery* 33: 413–416.

Morse, S. (2006). Brain Overclaim Syndrome and Criminal Responsibility: A Diagnostic Note. *Ohio State Journal of Criminal Law* 3: 397–412.

Morse, S. (2008). Psychopathy and Criminal Responsibility. *Neuroethics* 1: 205–212.

Morse, S. (2011a). Lost in Translation: An Essay on Law and Neuroscience. In Freeman, 529–562.

Morse, S. (2011b). Genetics and Criminal Responsibility. *Trends in Cognitive Sciences* 15: 378–380.

Morse, S. (2015). Neuroscience, Free Will and Criminal Responsibility. In Glannon, 251–286.

Morsella, E., Godwin, C. Jantz, T., Krieger, S. and Gazzaley, A. (2015). Homing in on Consciousness in the Nervous System: An Action-Based Synthesis. *Behavioral and Brain Scicences* 38: 1–106.

Moum, S., Orice, C., Limotai, N., Oyama, G., Ward, H., Jacobson, C. *et al.* (2012). Effects of STN and GPi Deep Brain Stimulation on Impulse Control Disorders and Dopamine Dysregulation Syndrome. *PLoS One* 7: e20768. doi: 10.1371/journal.pone.0029768.

Muller, S. and Walter, H. (2010). Reviewing Autonomy: Implications of the Neurosciences and the Free Will Debate for the Principle of Respect for the Patient's Autonomy. *Cambridge Quarterly of Healthcare Ethics* 19: 205–217.

Muller, S. and Christen, M. (2011). Deep Brain Stimulation in Parkinsonian Patients—
Ethical Evaluation of Cognitive, Affective and Behavioral Sequelae. *American Journal of
Bioethics-Neuroscience* 2: 3–13.

Muller, S., Riedmuller and van Oosterhout, A. (2015). Rivaling Paradigms in Psychiatric
Neurosurgery: Adjustability Versus Quick Fix Versus Minimal Invasiveness. *Frontiers in
Integrative Neuroscience* 9: 27. doi: 10.3389/fnint.2015.00027.

Muller, V., Cieslik, E., Serbanescu, I., Laird, A., Fox, P. and Eickhoff, B. (2017). Altering
Brain Activity in Unipolar Depression Revisited: Meta-Analyses of Neuroimaging
Studies. *JAMA Psychiatry* 74: 47–55.

Myers, J. (2017). Holding the Self and the World Together: Robert Lowell, Mania and
Having to Write. *Journal of the American Medical Association* 318: 988–989.

Nader, K. and Einarsson, E. (2010). Memory Reconsolidation: An Update. *Annals of the
New York Academy of Sciences* 1191: 27–41.

Nader, K., Schafe, G. and LeDoux, J. (2000). Fear Memories Require Protein Synthesis in
the Amygdala for Reconsolidation after Retrieval. *Nature* 408: 722–726.

Nagel, T. (1991). *Equality and Partiality*. Oxford: Oxford University Press.

Naqvi, N., Rudrauf, D., Damasio, H. and Bechara, A. (2007). Damage to the Insula
Disrupts Addiction to Cigarette Smoking. *Science* 315: 531–534.

Nash, J. (2002). "60 Minutes" Interview with Mike Wallace, March 17. https://www.cbsnews.
com/news/john-nash-60-minutes-beautiful-mind/2002/03/17

National Institute of Mental Health (2011). Research Domain Criteria (RDoC). http://
www.nimh.nih.gov/research-priorities/rdoc/index.shtml

Naudts., K., Ducatelle, C., Kovacs, J., Laurens, K., Van Den Eynde, F. and Van Heeringen,
C. (2006). Euthanasia: The Role of the Psychiatrist. *British Journal of Psychiatry*
188: 405–409.

Naughton, M., Clark, G., O'Leary, O., Cryan, J. and Dinan, T. (2014). A Review of
Ketamine in Affective Disorders: Current Evidence of Clinical Efficacy, Limitations of
Use, and Pre-Clinical Evidence on Proposed Mechanisms of Action. *Journal of Affective
Disorders* 156: 24–35.

Nesse, R. (2000). Is Depression an Adaptation? *Archives of General Psychiatry* 57: 14–20.

Nestler, E. (2014). Epigenetic Mechanisms of Depression. *JAMA Psychiatry* 71: 454–456.

Nitsche, M., Boggio, P., Fregni, F. and Pacual-Leone, A. (2009). Treatment of Depression
with Transcranial Direct Current Stimulation (tDCS): A Review. *Experimental
Neurology* 219: 14–19.

Northoff, G. (2011). *Neuropsychoanalysis in Practice: Brain, Self and Objects*. Oxford: Oxford
University Press.

Northoff, G. (2014a). *Unlocking the Brain: Volume II: Consciousness*. Oxford: Oxford
University Press.

Northoff, G. (2014b). *Minding the Brain: A Guide to Philosophy & Neuroscience*.
London: Palgrave Macmillan.

Northoff, G. (2015). How the Self Is Altered in Psychiatric Disorders. In Kirmayer,
Lemelson and Cummings, 81–116.

Northoff, G. (2016). *Neuro-Philosophy and the Heathy Mind: Learning from the Unwell
Brain*. New York: W.W. Norton and Company.

Nugent, A., Miller, F., Henter, I. and Zarate, C. (2017). The Ethics of Clinical Trials Research in Severe Mood Disorders. *Bioethics* 31: 443–453. .

Nutt, A. (2015). Did John Nash's Schizophrenia Boost His 'Beautiful Mind'? *Washington Post* May 26. https://www.washingtonpost.com/news/to-your-health/wp/2015/05/26/did-john-nashs-schizophrenia-boost-his-beautiful-mind/?utm_term.aO13aa2278f

Nuttin, B. Cosyns, P., Demeulemeester, H., Gybels, J. and Meyerson, B. (1999). Electrical Stimulation in Anterior Limbs of Internal Capsules in Patients with Obsessive-Compulsive Disorder. *The Lancet* 354: 1526.

Nyholm, S. and O'Neill, E. (2016). Deep Brain Stimulation, Continuity Over Time and the True Self. *Cambridge Quarterly of Healthcare Ethics* 25: 847–858.

Oakley, D. and Halligan, P. (2017). Chasing the Rainbow: The Non-Conscious Nature of Being. *Frontiers in Psychology* 8: 1924. doi. 10.3389/fpsyg.2017.01924

Olbert, C. and Gala, G. (2015). Supervenience and Psychiatry: Are Mental Disorders Brain Disorders? *Journal of Theoretical and Philosophical Psychology* 35: 203–219.

Olie, E. and Courtet, P. (2016). The Controversial Issue of Euthanasia in Patients with Psychiatric Illness. *JAMA Psychiatry* 316: 656–657.

Osler, M., Rozing, M., Christensen, G., Andersen, P. and Jorgensen M. (2018). Electroconvulsive Therapy and Risk of Dementia in Patients with Affective Disorders: A Cohort Study. *The Lancet Psychiatry* 5: 348–356.

Owen, A. (2008). Disorders of Consciousness. *Annals of the New York Academy of Sciences* 1124: 225–238.

Owen, A., Coleman, M., Boly, M., Davis, M., Laureys, S. and Pickard, J. (2006). Detecting Awareness in the Vegetative State. *Science* 313: 1402.

Owen, M., Sawa, A. and Mortensen, P. (2016). Schizophrenia. *The Lancet* 388: 86–97.

*Oxford English Dictionary (OED)* (2003). Third Edition. Oxford: Oxford University Press.

Palm, U., Schiller, C., Fintescu, Z., Obermeier, M., Keeser, D., Reisinger, E. *et al.* (2012). Transcranial Direct Current Stimulation in Treatment-Resistant Depression: A Randomized, Double-Blind Placebo-Controlled Study. *Brain Stimulation* 5: 242–251.

Parfit, D. (1984). *Reasons and Persons*. Oxford: Clarendon Press.

Parnas, J. (2003). Self and Schizophrenia: A Phenomenological Perspective. In Kircher and David, 217–241.

Parsons, R. and Ressler, K. (2013). Implications of Memory Modulation for Post-Traumatic Stress and Fear Disorders. *Nature Neuroscience* 16: 146–153.

Paus, T., Keshavan, M. and Giedd, J. (2008). Why Do Many Psychiatric Disorders Emerge During Adolescence? *Nature Reviews Neuroscience* 9: 947–957.

Patterson, P. (2011). *Infectious Behavior: Brain-Immune Connections in Autism, Schizophrenia and Depression*. Cambridge, MA: MIT Press.

Penfield, W. and Rasmussen, T. (1950). *The Cerebral Cortex of Man: A Clinical Study of Localization of Function*. New York: Macmillan.

Pepper, J., Hariz, M. and Zrinzo, L. (2015). Deep Brain Stimulation Versus Anterior Capsulotomy for Obsessive-Compulsive Disorder: A Review of the Literature. *Journal of Neurosurgery* 122: 1028–1037.

Perry, J. (ed.) (2008). *Personal Identity*. Second Edition. Berkeley and Los Angeles, CA: University of California Press.

Petersen, T. and **Kragh, K.** (2016). Should Violent Offenders Be Forced to Undergo Neurotechnological Treatment? *Journal of Medical Ethics* 43: 30–34.

**Phillips, M.** (2016). The Lobotomy Files. Part Two: One Doctor's Legacy. *Wall Street Journal.* September 11. http://projects.wsj.com/lobotomyfiles/?ch=two

**Pitman, R.** (2011). Will Reconsolidation Blockade Offer a Novel Treatment for Posttraumatic Stress Disorder? *Frontiers in Behavioral Neuroscience* 5: 11. doi: 10.3389/fnbeh.2013.00044.

**Pitman, R.** (2015). Harnessing Reconsolidation to Treat Mental Disorders. *Biological Psychiatry* 78: 819–820.

**Pitman, R.,** Sanders, K., Zusman, R., **Healy, A.,** Cheema, F.Lasko, N. *et al.* (2002). Pilot Study of Secondary Prevention of Posttraumatic Stress Disorder with Propranolol. *Biological Psychiatry* 51: 189–192.

**Pocket, S.,** Banks, W. and **Gallagher, S.** (eds.) (2006). *Does Consciousness Cause Behavior? An Investigation of the Nature of Volition.* Cambridge, MA: MIT Press.

**Post, R.** (2018). Preventing the malignant transformation of bipolar disorder. *Journal of the American Medical Association* 319: 1197–1198.

**Potter, S.,** El Hady, A. and **Fetz, E.** (2014). Closed-Loop Neuroscience and Neuroengineering. *Frontiers in Neural Circuits* 8: 1–3. doi: 10.3389/fncir.2014.00115.

**Prescott, S.,** Ma, Q and **De Koninck, Y.** (2014). Normal and Abnormal Coding of Somatosensory Stimuli Causing Pain. *Nature Neuroscience* 17: 183–191.

**Pressman, J.** (1998). *Last Resort: Psychosurgery and the Limits of Medicine.* Cambridge: Cambridge University Press.

**Proulx, C.,** Aronson, S., Milivojevic, D., **Molina. C.,** Loi, A., **Monk, B.** *et al.* (2018). A Neural Pathway Controlling Motivation to Exert Effort. *Proceedings of the National Academy of Sciences* 115: 5792–5797.

**Pycroft, L.,** Boccard, S. Owen, S., **Stein, J.,** Fitzgerald, J. Green A. *et al.* (2016). Brainjacking: Implant Security Issues in Invasive Neuromodulation. *World Neurosurgery* 92: 454–462.

**Quill, T.** (2018). Dutch Practice of Euthanasia and Assisted Suicide: A Glimpse at the Edges of the Practice. *Journal of Medical Ethics* 44: 297–298.

**Quill, T.** and **Battin, M.** (2004a). Excellent Palliative Care as the Standard, Physician-Assisted Dying as a Last Resort. In Quill and Battin, 323–333.

**Quill, T.** and **Battin, M.** (eds.) (2004b). *Physician-Assisted Dying: The Case for Palliative Care and Patient Choice.* Baltimore, MD: The Johns Hopkins University Press.

**Quill, T.,** Back, A. and **Block, S.** (2016). Responding to Patients Requesting Physician-Assisted Death: Physician Involvement at the Very End of Life. *Journal of the American Medical Association* 315: 245–246.

**Rabin, R.C.** (2017). Lawsuit Over a Suicide Points to Risk of Antidepressants. *New York Times,* September 11. https://www.nytimes.com/2017/09/11/well/mind/paxil-antidepressants-suicide.html.

**Rachels, J.** (1975). Active and Passive Euthanasia. *New England Journal of Medicine* 292: 78–80.

**Raison, C.** and **Miller, A.** (2011). Is Depression an Inflammatory Disorder? *Current Psychology Reports* 13: 467–475.

Ratcliffe, M. (2015). *Experiences of Depression: A Study in Phenomenology.* Oxford: Oxford University Press.

Ratcliffe, M. and Achim, S. (eds.) (2014). *Depression, Emotion and the Self: Philosophical and Interdisciplinary Perspectives.* Exeter: Imprint Academic.

Ratcliffe, M., Broome, M., Smith, B. and Bowden, H. (2014). A Bad Case of the Flu? The Comparative Phenomenology of Depression and Somatic Illness. In Ratcliffe and Achim, 163–181.

Rawls, J. (1971). *A Theory of Justice.* Cambridge, MA: Harvard Belknap Press.

Reardon, S. (2017). Brain Implants for Mood Disorders Tested in People. *Nature* **551**: 549–550.

Redberg, R. (2014). Sham Controls in Medical Device Trials. *New England Journal of Medicine* **371**: 892–893.

Reichenberg, A. and Mollon, J. (2016). Challenges and Opportunities in Studies of Cognition in the Prodrome to Psychosis: No Detail is too Small. *JAMA Psychiatry* **73**: 1249–1250.

Redlick, R., Almeida, J., Grotegerd, D., Opel, N., Kugel, H., Heindel, W. *et al.* (2014). Brain Morphometric Biomarkers Distinguishing Unipolar and Bipolar Depression: A Voxel-Based Morphometry-Pattern Classification Approach. *JAMA Psychiatry* **71**: 1222–1230.

Richmond, S., Rees, G. and Edwards, S. (eds.) (2012). *I Know What You're Thinking: Brain Imaging and Mental Privacy.* Oxford: Oxford University Press.

Ripke, S., Neale, B., Corvin, A., Walters, J., Farh, K., Hilmans, P. *et al.* (2014). Biological Insights from 108 Schizophrenia-Associated Genetic Loci. *Nature* **511**: 421–427.

*Rogers v. Okin.* (1979), 478 F. Supp. 1342 (D. Mass, US).

Rommelfanger, K. (2013). A Role for Placebo Therapy in Psychogenic Movement Disorders. *Nature Reviews Neurology* **9**: 351–356.

Rommelfanger, K. and Johnson, L.S. (eds.) (2018). *The Routledge Handbook of Neuroethics.* New York: Taylor & Francis.

Roskies, A. (2002). Neuroethics for the New Millennium. *Neuron* **35**: 21–23.

Roskies, A. (2006). Neuroscientific Challenges to Free Will and Responsibility. *Trends in Cognitive Sciences* **10**:419–423.

Roskies, A. (2008). Neuroimaging and Inferential Distance. *Neuroethics* **1**: 19–30.

Roskies, A. (2010). How Does Neuroscience Affect Our Conception of Volition? *Annual Review of Neuroscience* **33**: 109–130.

Roskies, A. (2013a). Brain Imaging Techniques. In S. Morse and A. Roskies, eds., *A Primer in Criminal Law and Neuroscience.* New York: Oxford University Press, 37–74.

Roskies, A. (2013b). Other Neuroscientific Techniques. In Morse and Roskies, 75–88.

Ross, H. and Young, L. (2009). Oxytocin and the Neural Mechanisms Regulating Social Cognition and Affiliative Behavior, *Frontiers in Neuroendocrinology* **30**: 534–547.

Ross, S., Bossis, A., Guss, J., Aqin-Liebes, G., Malone, T. Cohen, B., Mennenga, S. *et al.* (2016). Rapid and Sustained Symptom Reduction Following Psilocybin Treatment for Anxiety and Depression with Life-Threatening Cancer: A Randomized Controlled Trial. *Journal of Psychopharmacology* **30**: 1165–1180.

Roth, B. (2016). DREADDs for Neuroscientists. *Neuron* **89**: 683–694.

Rothenberger, A., Rhode, L. and Rothenberger, L. (2015). Biomarkers in Child Mental Health: A Bio-Psycho-Social Perspective Is Needed. *Behavior and Brain Function* **11**: 31. doi: 10.1186/s.12993-015-0076-6.

Rowlands, M. (2010). *The New Science of the Mind: From Extended Mind to Embodied Phenomenology.* Cambridge, MA: MIT Press.

Ruck, C., Karisson, A., Steele, D., Edman, G., Nyman, H., Meyerson, B., Ericson, K. *et al.* (2008). Capsulotomy for Obsessive-Compulsive Disorder; Long-Term Follow-Up of 25 Patients. *Archives of General Psychiatry* **65**: 914–922.

Rurup, M. (2012). Being "Weary of Life" as a Cause for Seeking Euthanasia or Physician-Assisted Suicide. In Youngner and Kimsma, 247–262.

Rutter, M. (2013). Biomarkers: Potential and Challenges. In Singh, Sinnott-Armstrong and Savulescu, 188–205.

Ryberg, J. (2015). Is Coercive Treatment of Offenders Morally Acceptable? On the Deficiency of the Debate. *Criminal Law and Philosophy* **9**: 619–631.

Ryberg, J. and Petersen, T. (2013). Neurotechnological Behavioral Treatment of Criminal Offenders—A Comment on Bomann-Larsen. *Neuroethics* **6**: 79–83.

Sadler, J. (2004). *Values and Psychiatric Diagnosis.* Oxford: Oxford University Press.

Sadler, J. (2009). Stigma, Conscience and Science in Psychiatry: Past, Present and Future. *Academic Medicine* **84**: 413–417.

Sadler, J., Van Staden, C.W. and Fulford, K.W.M. (eds.) (2015). *The Oxford Handbook of Psychiatric Ethics,* Volumes 1 and 2. Oxford: Oxford University Press.

Sadoff, R.L (ed.) (2015). *The Future of Forensic Psychiatry: History, Current Developments, Future Directions.* Oxford: Oxford University Press.

Sanacora, G., Mason, G., Rothman, D., Hyder, F., Ciarcia, J., Ostroff, R. *et al.* (2003). Increased Cortical GABA Concentrations in Depressed Patients Receiving ECT. *American Journal of Psychiatry* **160**: 577–579.

Sanacora, G., Frye, M., McDonald, W., Mathew, S., Turner, M., Schatzberg, A. *et al.* (2017). American Psychiatric Association (APA) Council of Research Task Force on Novel Biomarkers and Treatments. A Consensus Statement on the Use of Ketamine in the Treatment of Mood Disorders. *JAMA Psychiatry* **74**: 399–405.

Sankar, T., Chakravarty, M., Bescos, A., Lara, M., Obuchi, T., Laxton, A. *et al.* (2015). Deep Brain Stimulation Influences Brain Structure in Alzheimer's Disease. *Brain Stimulation* **8**: 645–654.

Santos, F., Costa, R., and Tecuapetla, F. (2011). Stimulation on Demand: Closing the Loop on Deep Brain Stimulation. *Neuron* **72**: 197–198.

Sapolsky, R. (2000). Glucocorticoids and Hippocampal Atrophy in Neuropsychiatric Disorders. *Archives of General Psychiatry* **57**: 925–935.

Sarpal, D., Robinson, D., Lencz, T., Argyelan, M., Toshikazu, I., Karlsgodt, K. *et al.* (2015). Antipsychotic Treatment and Functional Connectivity of the Striatum in First-Episode Schizophrenia. *JAMA Psychiatry* **72**: 5–13.

Sarrazin, S., Poupon, C., Linke, J., Wessa, M., Phillips, M., Delavest, M. *et al.* (2014). A Multicenter Tractography Study of Deep White Matter Tracts in Bipolar I Disorder: Psychotic Features and Interhemispheric Disconnectivity. *JAMA Psychiatry* **71**: 388–396.

Sass, L. (2014). Delusion and Double Book-Keeping. In Fuchs, Breyer and Mundt, 125–147.

Schacter, D. (2001). *The Seven Sins of Memory: How the Mind Forgets and Remembers.* New York: Houghton Mifflin.

Schacter, D. and **Addis, D.R.** (2007). Constructive Memory: The Ghosts of Past and Future. *Nature* **445**: 27.

Schacter, D., **Addis, D.R.,** Hassabis, D. Martin, V., **Spreng, R.** and Szpunar, K. (2012). The Future of Memory: Remembering, Imagining and the Brain. *Neuron* **76**: 677–694.

Schartner, M., Carhart-Harris, R., Barrett, A., **Seth, A.** and **Muthukumaraswamy, S.** (2017). Increased Spontaneous MEG Signal Diversity for Psychoactive Doses of Ketamine, LSD and Psilocybin. *Scientific Reports* 7: 46421. doi: 10.1038/srep46421.

Schechtman, M. (1997). *The Constitution of Selves.* Ithaca, NY: Cornell University Press.

Schechtman, M. (2014). *Staying Alive: Personal Identity, Practical Concerns and the Unity of a Life.* Oxford: Oxford University Press.

Scheinost, D., Stoica, T., Saksa, J., Papademetris, X., Constable, R., Pittenger, C. *et al.* (2013). Orbitofrontal Cortex Neurofeedback Produces Lasting Changes in Contamination Anxiety and Resting-State Connectivity. *Translational Psychiatry* 3: e250. doi: 10.1038/tp/2013.24.

Schermer, M. (2015). Reducing, Restoring or Enhancing Autonomy with Neuromodulation Techniques. In Glannon, 205–227.

Schiller, D., Monfils, M.-H., Raio, C., Johnson, D., LeDoux, J. and Phelps, E. (2010). Preventing the Return of Fear in Humans Using Reconsolidation Update Mechanisms. *Nature* **403**: 49–53.

Schlaepfer, T., Cohen, M., Frick, C., Kosel, M., Brodessor, D., Axmacher, N. *et al.* (2008). Deep Brain Stimulation to Reward Circuitry Alleviates Anhedonia in Refractory Major Depression. *Neuropsychopharmacology* 33: 368–377.

Schlaepfer, T., Bewernick, B., Kayser, S., Madler, B. and Coenen, V. (2013). Rapid Effects of Deep Brain Stimulation for Treatment-Resistant Major Depression. *Biological Psychiatry* 73: 1204–1212.

Schlaepfer, T., Bewernick, B., Kayser, S., Hurlemann, R. and Coenen, V. (2014). Deep Brain Stimulation of the Human Reward System for Major Depression—Rationale, Outcomes and Outlook. *Neuropsychopharmacology* 39: 1303–1314.

Schmaal, L., Hibar, D., Samann, P., Hall, G., Baune, B., Jahanshad, N. *et al.* (2017). Cortical Abnormalities in Adults and Adolescents with Major Depression Based on Brain Scans from 20 Cohorts Worldwide in the ENIGMA MAJOR Depressive Disorder Working Group. *Molecular Psychiatry* **22**:900–909.

Schuepbach, W., Rau, J., Knudsen, K., Volkmann, J., Krack, P. Timmerman, L. *et al.* (2013). Neurostimulation for Parkinson's Disease with Early Motor Complications. . *New England Journal of Medicine* 368: 610–622.

Schuklenk, U. and **van de Vathorst, S.** (2015a). Treatment-Resistant Major Depressive Disorder and Assisted Dying. *Journal of Medical Ethics* 41: 577–583.

Schuklenk, U. and **van de Vathorst, S.** (2015b). Physician-Assisted Death Does Not Violate Professional Integrity. *Journal of Medical Ethics* 41: 887–8.

Segall, S. (2010). *Health, Luck and Justice.* Princeton, NJ: Princeton University Press.

Seidman, L., Shapiro, D., Stone, W., Woodberry, K., Ronzio, A., Cornblatt, B. *et al.* (2016). Association of Neurocognition with Transition to Psychosis: Baseline Functioning in the Second Phase of the North American Prodrome Longitudinal Study. *JAMA Psychiatry* 73: 1239–1248.

Seung, S. (2013). *Connectome: How the Brain's Wiring Makes Us Who We Are.* New York: Houghton Mifflin Harcourt.

Shalev, A., Liberzon, I. and **Marmar, C.** (2017). Post-Traumatic Stress Disorder. *New England Journal of Medicine* **376**: 2459–2469.

Shamy, M. (2010). The Treatment of Psychogenic Movement Disorders with Suggestion Is Ethically Justified. *Movement Disorders* **25**: 260–264.

Sheehan, J., Patterson, G., **Schlesinger, D** and **Xu, Z.** (2013). Gamma Knife Surgery and Anterior Capsulotomy for Severe and Refractory Obsessive-Compulsive Disorder. *Journal of Neurosurgery* **119**: 1112–1118.

Sheth, S., Neal, J., Tangherlini, F., **Mian, M.**, Gentil, A. Cosgrove, G. *et al.* (2013). Limbic System Surgery for Treatment-Refractory Obsessive-Compulsive Disorder: A Prospective Long-Term Follow-Up of 64 Patients. *Journal of Neurosurgery* **18**: 491–497.

Shields, D., **Assad, W.** Eskandar, E., Jain, F., Cosgrove, G., Flaherty, A. *et al.* (2008). Prospective Assessment of Stereotactic Ablative Surgery for Intractable Major Depression. *Biological Psychiatry* **64**: 449–454.

Sillivan, S., Vaissiere, T. and **Miller, C.** (2015). Neuroepigenetic Regulation of Pathogenic Memories. *Neuroepigenetics* **1**: 28–33.

Singh, I. and **Rose, N.** (2009). Biomarkers in Psychiatry. *Nature* **460**: 202–207.

Singh, I., **Sinnott-Armstrong**, W. and **Savulescu, J.** (eds.) (2013). *Bioprediction, Biomarkers, and Bad Behavior: Scientific, Legal, and Ethical Challenges.* Oxford: Oxford University Press

Sitaram, R., Caria, A. and **Birbaumer, N.** (2009). Hemodynamic Brain-Computer Interfaces for Communication and Rehabilitation. *Neural Networks* **22**: 1320–1328.

Slobogin, C. (2013). Bioprediction in Criminal Cases. In Singh, Sinnott-Armstrong and Savulescu, 77–90.

Slotema, C., Blom, J., **Hoek, H.** and **Sommer, I.** (2010). Should We Expand the Toolbox of Psychiatric Treatment Methods to Include Repetitive Transcranial Magnetic Stimulation (rTMS)? A Meta-Analysis of the Efficacy of rTMS in Psychiatric Disorders. *Journal of Clinical Psychiatry* **71**: 873–884.

Snijdewind, M., van Tol, D., **Onwuteaka-Philipsen, B.** and **Willems, S.** (2018). Developments in the Practice of Physician-Assisted Dying: Perceptions of Physicians Who Had Experience with Complex Cases. *Journal of Medical Ethics* **44**: 292–296.

Soares, M., Paiva, W., Guertzenstein, E., Amorim, R., Bernado, L., **Pereira, J.** *et al.* (2013). Psychosurgery for Schizophrenia: History and Perspectives. *Neuropsychiatric Disease and Treatment* **9**: 509–515.

Soeter, M. and **Kindt, M.** (2015). An Abrupt Transformation of Phobic Behavior after a Post-Retrieval Amnesic Agent. *Biological Psychiatry* **78**: 880–886.

Solomon, A. (2001). *The Noonday Demon: An Atlas of Depression.* New York: Scribner's.

Sorrells, S., Caso, J., **Munhoz, C.** and **Sapolsky, R.** (2009). The Stressed CNS: When Glucocorticoids Aggravate Inflammation. *Neuron* **64**: 33–39.

Southwick, S., Vythilingam, M. and **Charney, D.** (2005). The Psychobiology of Depression and Resilience to Stress: Implications for Prevention and Treatment. *Annual Review of Clinical Psychology* **1**: 285–291.

Spatola, G., Martinez-Alvarez, R. and **Martinez-Moreno, N.** (2018). Results of Gamma Knife Anterior Capsulotomy for Refractory Obsessive-Compulsive Disorder: Results in a Series of 10 Consecutive Patients. *Journal of Neurosurgery.* doi: 10.3171/2018.4 JNS171525.

Spence, S. (2009). *The Actor's Brain: Exploring the Cognitive Neuroscience of Free Will.* Oxford: Oxford University Press.

Sperens, M., Hamberg, K. and **Hariz, G-M.** (2017). Are Patients Ready for "EARLYSTIM"? Attitudes towards Deep Brain Stimulation Among Female and Male Patients with

Moderately Advanced Parkinson's Disease. *Parkinson's Disease* **2017**: 1939831. doi: 10.1155/2017/193983.

Sporns, O. (2012). *Discovering the Human Connectome.* Cambridge, MA: MIT Press.

Squire, L. (ed.) (2009). *Encyclopedia of Neuroscience.* Amsterdam: Elsevier.

Starson v. Swayze. (2003). Supreme Court of Canada, 32.

Steffans, D. (2017). Late-Life Depression and the Prodromes of Dementia. *JAMA Psychiatry* **74**: 637–674.

Stein, D., Goodman, W. and Rauch, S. (2000) The Cognitive-Affective Neuroscience of Obsessive-Compulsive Disorder. *Current Psychiatry Reports* **2**: 341–346.

Stein, D., Phillips, K., Bolton, D., Fulford, K., Sadler, J. and Kendler, K. (2010). What Is a Mental/Psychiatric Disorder? From DSM-IV to DSM-V. *Psychological Medicine* **40**: 1759–1765.

Stein, M. and Sareen, J. (2015). Generalized Anxiety Disorder. *New England Journal of Medicine* **373**: 2059–2068.

Steinbock, B. (2017). Physician-Assisted Death and Severe, Treatment-Resistant Depression. *Hastings Center Report* **47** (5): 30–42.

Strakowski, S. (2014). *Bipolar Disorder.* New York: Oxford University Press.

Strawbridge, R., Young, A. and Cleare, A. (2017). Biomarkers for Depression: Recent Insights, Current Challenges and Future Prospects. *Neuropsychiatric Disease and Treatment* **13**: 1245–1262.

Strawson, G. (2010). *Freedom and Belief.* Revised Edition. Oxford: Clarendon Press.

Styron, W. (1992). *Darkness Visible:* A Memoir of Madness. New York: Vintage.

Sullivan, M. and Youngner, S. (1994). Depression, Competence and the Right to Refuse Lifesaving Medical Treatment. *American Journal of Psychiatry* **151**: 971–978.

Sulmasy, D. (2017). Tolerance, Professional Judgment and the Discretionary Space of the Physician. *Cambridge Quarterly of Healthcare Ethics* **26**: 18–31.

Sulmasy, D., Ely, E. and Sprung, C. (2016). Euthanasia and Physician-Assisted Suicide. *Journal of the American Medical Association* **316**: 1600.

Swanson, J. (2016). Mental Illness, Release from Prison, and Social Context. *JAMA Psychiatry* **316**: 1–2.

Swinburne, R. (ed.) (2012). *Free Will and Modern Science.* Oxford: Oxford University Press.

Synofzik, M. (2013). Functional Neurosurgery and Deep Brain Stimulation. In Chatterjee and Farah, 189–208.

Synofzik, M. and Clausen, J. (2011). The Ethical Differences Between Psychiatric and Neurologic DBS: Smaller than We Think? *American Journal of Bioethics-Neuroscience* **2**: 37–39

Synofzik, M., Schlaepfer, T. and Fins, J. (2012). How Happy Is Too Happy? Euphoria, Neuroethics and Deep Brain Stimulation of the Nucleus Accumbens. *American Journal of Bioethics-Neuroscience* **3**: 30–36.

Szasz, T. (1961). *The Myth of Mental Illness: Foundations of a Theory of Personal Conduct.* New York: Harper and Row.

Talbot, S., Foster, S. and Woolf, C. (2016). Neuroimmunology: Physiology and Pathology. *Annual Review of Immunology* **34**: 421–447.

Taylor, C. (1992). *The Ethics of Authenticity.* Cambridge, MA: Harvard University Press.

Teufel, C. and Fletcher, P. (2016). The Promises and Pitfalls of Applying Computational Models to Neurological and Psychiatric Disorders. *Brain* **139**: 2600–2608.

Thienpont, L., Verhofstadt, M., Van Loon, T., Distelmans, W., Audeneart, K. and De Deyn, P. (2015). Euthanasia Requests, Procedures and Outcomes for 100 Belgian

Patients Suffering from Psychiatric Disorders: A Retrospective, Descriptive Study. *BMJ Open* 5: e007454. doi: 10.1136/bmjopen-2014-007454.

Tholen, A., Berghmans, R., Huisman, J., Legemaate, J., Nolen, W., Ploak, F. *et al.* (2009). *Guidelines Dealing with the Request for Assisted Suicide by Patients with a Psychiatric Disorder*. Utrecht: Dutch Psychiatric Association, De Tijdsstroom. http://steungroeppsychiaters.nl/wp-content/uploads/

Thomson, J. (1990). *The Realm of Rights*. Cambridge, MA: Harvard University Press.

Thornicroft, G., Mehta, N., Clement, S., Evans-Lacko, S., Doherty, M., Rose, D. *et al.* (2016). Evidence for Effective Interventions to Reduce Mental-Health-Related Stigma and Discrimination. *The Lancet* 387: 1123–1132.

Titova, O., Hjorth, O., Schioth, H. and Brooks, S. (2013). Anorexia Nervosa Is Linked to Reduced Brain Structure in Reward and Somatosensory Regions: A Meta-Analysis of VBM Studies. *BMC Psychiatry* 13: 110. doi: 10.1186/1471-244x-13-110.

Tononi, G. and Koch, C. (2008). The Neural Correlates of Consciousness: An Update. *Annals of the New York Academy of Sciences* 1124: 239–261.

Trimble, M. and George, M. (eds.) (2010). *Biological Psychiatry*. Third Edition. Oxford: Wiley-Blackwell.

Tulving, E. (1985). Memory and Consciousness. *Canadian Psychology* 26: 1–12.

Tulving, E. (2002). Episodic Memory: From Mind to Brain. *Annual Review of Psychology* 53: 1–25.

Turecki, G. (2014). The Molecular Basis of the Suicidal Brain. *Nature Reviews Neuroscience* 15: 802–816.

Underwood, E. (2015). Brain Implant Trials Raise Ethical Concerns. *Science* 348: 1186–1187.

Underwood, E. (2017). Brain Implant Trials Spur Ethical Discussions. *Science* 358: 710.

Valero-Cabre, A., Amengual, J., Stengel, C., Pascual-Leone, A. and Coubard, O. (2017). Transcranial Magnetic Stimulation in Basic and Clinical Neuroscience: A Comprehensive Review of Fundamental Principles and Novel Insights. *Neuroscience and Biobehavioral Reviews* 83: 381–404.

Vandenberghe, J. (2018). Physician-Assisted Suicide and Psychiatric Illness. *New England Journal of Medicine* 378: 885–887.

Van den Hout, M. and Kindt, M. (2003). Repeated Checking Causes Memory Distrust. *Behavior Research and Therapy* 41: 301–316.

Van der Lee, M. (2012). Depression, Euthanasia and Assisted Suicide. In Youngner and Kimsma, 277–287.

Van Inwagen, P. (1983). *An Essay on Free Will*. Oxford: Clarendon Press.

Van Marle, H. (2015). PTSD as a Memory Disorder. *European Journal of Psychotraumatology* 6. doi: 10.3402/ejpt.v6_27633.

Varelius, J. (2013). Medical Expertise, Existential Suffering and Ending Life. *Journal of Medical Ethics* 40: 108–109.

Varelius, J. (2016). On the Moral Acceptability of Physician-Assisted Dying for Non-Autonomous Psychiatric Patients. *Bioethics* 30: 227–233.

Viding, E., Blair, J., Moffitt, T. and Plomin, R. (2005). Evidence for Substantial Genetic Risk for Psychopathy in 7-Year-Olds. *Journal of Child Psychology and Psychiatry* 46: 592–597.

Viding, E. and McCrory, E. (2013). Genetic Biomarker Research of Callous-Unemotional Traits in Children: Implications for the Law and Policy-Making. In Singh, Sinnott-Armstrong and Savulescu, 153–172.

Viding, E., Price, T., Jaffee, S., Trzaskowski, M., Davis, O., Meabum, E. *et al.* (2013). Genetics of Callous-Unemotional Traits in Children. *PLoS One* **8**: e65789. doi: 10.1371/journal.pone.0065789.

Vilares, I., Wesley, M., Ahn, W-Y, Bonnie, R., Hoffman, M., Jones, O. *et al.* (2017). Predicting the Knowledge Recklessness Distinction in the Human Brain. *Proceedings of the National Academy of Sciences* **114**: 3222–3227.

Vincent, N. (ed.) (2013). *Neuroscience and Legal Responsibility*. Oxford: Oxford University Press.

Vincent, N. (2014). Restoring Responsibility: Promoting Justice, Therapy and Reform Through Direct Brain Interventions. *Criminal Law and Philosophy* **8**: 21–42.

Vogeley, K. (2003). Schizophrenia as Disturbance of the Self-Construct. In Kircher and David, 361–379.

*W v. M.* (2011). EWHC, 2433 UK (Fam).

Wager, T., Atlas, L., Lindquist, M., Roy, M., Woo, C-W. and Kross, E. (2013). An fMRI-Based Neurological Signature of Physical Pain. *New England Journal of Medicine* **368**: 1388–1397.

Walter, H. (2013). The Third Wave of Biological Psychiatry. *Frontiers in Psychology* **4**: 582. doi: 10.3389/fpsyg.2013.00582.

Walter, H. and Spitzer, M. (2003). The cognitive neuroscience of agency in schizophrenia. In Kircher and David, 436–444.

Wang, S., Wacker, D., Levit, A., Che, T., Betz, R., McCorvy, J. *et al.* (2017). D4 Dopamine Receptor High-Resolution Structures Enable the Discovery of Selective Agonists. *Science* **358**: 381–386.

Wasserman, D. (2005). The Non-Identity Problem, Disability and the Role Morality of Prospective Parents. *Ethics* **116**: 132–152.

Weger, M. and Sandi, C. (2018). High-Anxiety Trait: A Vulnerable Phenotype for Stress-Induced Depression. *Neuroscience and Biobehavioral Reviews* **87**: 27–37.

Wegner, D. (2002). *The Illusion of Conscious Will*. Cambridge, MA: MIT Press.

Wehler, C. and Preskorn, S. (2016). High False-Positive Rate of a Putative Biomarker Test to Aid in the Diagnosis of Schizophrenia. *Journal of Clinical Psychiatry* **77**: e451–456.

Wertheimer, A. (1987). *Coercion*. Princeton, NJ: Princeton University Press.

Wertheimer, A. and Miller, F. (2014). There Are (STILL) No Coercive Offers. *Journal of Medical Ethics* **40**: 592–593.

Wetherell, J., Petkus, A., White, K., Nguyen, H., Kornblith, S. Andreescu, C. *et al.* (2013). Antidepressant Medication Augmented with Cognitive-Behavioral Therapy for Generalized Anxiety Disorder in Older Adults. *American Journal of Psychiatry* **170**: 782–789.

Wicclair, M. (2017). Conscientious Objection in Healthcare and Moral Integrity. *Cambridge Quarterly of Healthcare Ethics* **26**: 7–17.

Widge, A. and Moritz, C. (2016). Closed-Loop Stimulation in Emotional Circuits for Neuro-Psychiatric Disorders. In El Hady, 229–239.

Widdows, K. and Davis, N. (2014). Ethical Considerations in Using Brain Stimulation to Treat Eating Disorders. *Frontiers in Behavioral Neuroscience* **8**: 351. doi: 10.3389/fnbeh.2014.00351.

Willis, T. (1681). *An Essay on the Pathology of the Brain and Nervous Stock in which Convulsive Diseases Are Treated*. London: T. Dring.

Wind, J. and Anderson, D. (2008). From prefrontal leukotomy to deep brain stimulation: the historical transformation of psychosurgery and the emergence of neuroethics. *Neurosurgery Focus* 25.doi: 10.3171/foc/2008/25/7/e10.

Witt, K. (2017). Identity Change and Informed Consent. *Journal of Medical Ethics* **43**: 384–390.

Witt, K., Kuhn, J., Timmerman, L., Zurowski, M. and Woopen, C. (2013). Deep Brain Stimulation and the Search for Identity. *Neuroethics* **6**: 499–511.

Wittgenstein, L. (1961). *Tractatus Logico-Philosophicus*, trans. D. Pears and B. McGuinness. London: Routledge & Kegan Paul.

Wolf, S. (1990). *Freedom within Reason*. New York: Oxford University Press.

Woopen, C., Pauls, K., Kory, A., Moro, E. and Timmermann, L. (2013). Early Application of Deep Brain Stimulation—Clinical and Ethical Aspects. *Progress in Neurobiology* **110**: 74–88.

World Health Organization. (2012). *Global Burden of Mental Disorders and the Need for a Comprehensive, Coordinated Response from Research and Social Sectors at the Country Level*. Geneva: World Health Organization. http://www.who.int/mental_health/WHA65.4_resolution.pdf

World Health Organization (2016). *International Statistical Classification of Diseases and Related Health Problems*. Eleventh Revision (ICD-11). Geneva: World Health Organization. http://www.who.int/classifications/icd/revision/en/

Wrosch, C. and Miller, G. (2009). Depressive Symptoms Can Be Useful: Self-Regulatory and Emotional Benefits of Dysphoric Mood in Adolescence. *Journal of Personality and Social Psychology* **96**: 1181–1190.

Yager, J. (2015). Addressing Patients' Psychic Pain. *American Journal of Psychiatry* **172**: 939–943.

Young, L., Camprodon, J., Hauser, M., Pascual-Leone, A. and Saxe, R. (2010). Disruption of the Right Temporoparietal Junction with Transcranial Magnetic Stimulation Reduces the Role of Beliefs in Moral Judgments. *Proceedings of the National Academy of Sciences* **107**: 6753–6758

Youngner, S. and Kimsma, G. (eds.) (2012). *Physician-Assisted Death in Perspective: Assessing the Dutch Experience*. Cambridge: Cambridge University Press.

Zahavi, D. (2003). Phenomenology of Self. In Kircher and David, 56–75.

Zannas, A., Provencal, N. and Binder, E. (2015). Epigenetics of Posttraumatic Stress Disorder: Current Evidence, Challenges and Future Directions. *Biological Psychiatry* **78**: 327–335.

Zanos, P., Moadell, R., Morris, P., Georgiou, P., Fischell, J., Elmer, G. *et al.* (2016). NMDAR Inhibition-Independent Antidepressant Actions of Ketamine Metabolites. *Nature* **533**: 481–486.

Zarate, C., Singh, J., Carlson, P., Bratsche, N., Ameli, R., Luckenbaugh, D. *et al.* (2006). A Randomized Trial of N-Methyl-D-Aspartate Antagonist in Treatment-Resistant Major Depression. *Archives of General Psychiatry* **63**: 856–864.

Zeman, A. (2014). Neurology Is Psychiatry—and Vice Versa. *Practical Neurology* **14**: 136–144.

Zhang, J., Zhu, Y., Zhan, G., Fenik, P. Panossian, L., Wang, M. *et al.* (2014). Extended Wakefulness: Compromised Metabolics in and Degeneration of Locus Ceruleus Neurons. *Journal of Neuroscience* **34**: 44184431.

Zimmerman, D. (1981). Coercive Wage Offers. *Philosophy & Public Affairs* **10**: 121–145.

Zorumski, C. and Conway, C. (2017). Use of Ketamine in Clinical Practice: A Time for Optimism and Caution. *JAMA Psychiatry* **74**: 405–406.

# Index

Notes: Since abbreviations are used extensively in the text, users will find entries under the same abbreviations in the index.

Abi-Dargham, Anissa, 99
ablative neurosurgery, 138–139
abortion *see* pregnancy termination (abortion)
absolute right to noninterference, 242
access consciousness, 53
action plans
    DBS, 194–195
    free will and, 70–71
    will disorders, 68
actions
    autonomy in, 76
    behavior control *vs.*, 198
AD (Alzheimer's disease)
    *APOE4,* 304
    psychiatric disorders *vs.*, 30
Addis, Donna Rose, 65
adolescence, psychiatric disorders, 308
adolescents
    EAS, 280
    electrical stimulation techniques, 114
    prenatal interventions, 320–321
affective processes, cognition interaction, 224
agency, consciousness connection, 59
alien control (experience delusions), 79–80
ALS (amyotrophic lateral sclerosis), 255
American Psychiatric Association (APA), 16
    placebo response guidelines, 124
    *see also* DSM-5 (*Diagnostic and Statistical Manual of Mental Disorders, Fifth Edition* )
amnesia, retrograde, ECT adverse effect, 110, 111
amygdala
    DBS, 147
    gray matter volume, 101
    memory content disorders, 64–65
    oxytocin in psychopathy, 227–228
    psychopathy, 223
    structural neuroimaging in depression, 39
    underactive, 228
    ventromedial PFC connectivity, 229
amygdalotomy, 141
amyotrophic lateral sclerosis (ALS), 255
AN (anorexia nervosa)
    body perception, 58–59
    brain structural changes, 46
    cognitive/mood disturbances, 113
    consent problems for clinical trial, 163–166

diagnosis, 19
disordered self, 45–46
effective treatment, 163–164
ego-syntonic disorder as, 79, 163
proxy consent in clinical trials, 152, 164
reward processing, 58–59
reward system, 165
rTMS consent problems, 164–165
somatosensory cortex, 165
TMS, 112
anhedonia, NFB, 129
anisomycin, 97
anterior capsulotomy, 141
anterior cingulate cortex
    AN structural changes, 46
    blood flow, 302
    structural neuroimaging in depression, 39
anterior cingulotomy, 141
antidepressant drugs, 108
    CBT and, 91–92
    depression, effectiveness in, 119–120
    failure in EAS, 275
    serotonin receptors, 89
antigenic memory, 44
anti-inflammatory drugs, depression, 313
antipsychotic drugs
    adverse effects, 295
    DBS in schizophrenia research, 161
    extrapyramidal adverse effects, 89–90
    first-line treatment as, 159
antisocial behavior, psychopathy, 224
anxiety disorders
    DBS fear memory erasure, 145–146
    depression and, 18–19, 301
    depression *vs.*, 123
    fear memory system disorder as, 64
    longitudinal studies, 296
    memory dysfunction, 65–66
    noninvasive prevention, 316–317
    optogenetics, 179
    placebo effect non-responsiveness, 125
    prevalence, 291
    psilocybin, 88, 94
    psychopharmacological treatment, 96
    stress hormones, 33
    treatment-resistance, 278–279
    *see also* GAD (generalized anxiety disorder)

*APOE4,* AD, 304
Appelbaum–Grisso definition of personality
change, 172
Appelbaum, Paul, 151, 258, 266
Arbabshirani, Muhammad, 301
arterial spin labelling, 302
artists, 82
assisted suicide *see* EAS (euthanasia and
assisted suicide)
Atmanspacher, Harald, 71
autonomic nervous system, hyperactivity, 302
autonomy, 7, 75–77
DBS, 187–188
definition, 75–76
implied autonomy, 191–192
insight and, 79
moral attitudes/values, 76
necessity of, 76
personal autonomy, 75–76
psychopathy neuromodulation, 221
reflective capacity, 76–77
awareness, control *vs.* in OCD, 63

bad, mad *vs.* in psychopathy, 222–223
basal ganglia, degeneration of, 32
basolateral amygdala, anisomycin injection, 97
battery life, closed-loop devices (CLDs), 168
battery replacement surgery, DBS, 168
BBB (blood–brain barrier), 311–312
permeability and focused ultrasound,
314–315
BD (bipolar disorder)
behavior, 69–70
creativity and, 82
frontal–limbic–striatal–frontal
circuit, 69–70
genetics, 297
heritability, 293
hypomania/manic states, 48
insight in, 77
neuroimaging in pathology, 22
psychopharmacology, 89, 90
suicidal ideation, 268
symptoms in DSM-5, 19–20
type II diagnosis, 18
BD I (bipolar disorder I)
diagnosis, 18
mania from pharmaceuticals, 89
BDNF protein, schizophrenia, 314–315
behavior
alienation from in OCD, 80–81
BD, 69–70
modification in psychopathy, 230–237
psychiatric disease classification, 26
unconscious processes, regulation of, 61
behavior control, 62
action *vs.,* 198
conscious motivational states, 73

DBS, 194
degree of, 198
function restoration, 196
mechanical brain implants, 190–191
neural/mental functions, 74–75
Belgian Euthanasia Law (BEL, 2009), 255–256,
256–257
Belgium
EAS legality, 254
EAS studies, 255–257
beliefs, depression, 29
*Belmont Report* (1978), 171
Benabid, Alim-Louis, 139
beneficence, 7
Berlin School of Mind and Brain, 30, 33–34
bidirectional control, constraint as, 74
biological factors, psychiatric self, 76
biological psychiatry, 24–29
cultural effects, 28
genetics, 24–25
history of, 24–25
structure & function, 25
biomarkers, 22, 298–307
available testing, 304–305
definition, 298
effectiveness of, 299
employment, 306
ethical/social concerns, 304
functional imaging, 303
interpretation, 305
medical insurance denial, 306
neuroimaging, 301–302, 303
predictive value of, 298, 303–304, 306–307
psychological harm, 101
reliability, 305
skepticism, 302–303
social implications, 305–306
symptom clustering approach in
treatment, 100
therapy initiation, 298–299
biopsychosocial model, 7–8, 91
bipolar affective disorder treatment, 89
bipolar depression
anterior cingulate cortex blood flow, 302
early age diagnosis, 270–271
epigenetics, 268
gray matter volume reduction, 101
new treatments, 279
suicidal desires, 267, 268
bipolar disorder *see* BD (bipolar disorder)
Birbaumer, Niels, 226–227
Blair, James, 224
Blair, Karina, 224
Block, Ned, 53
blood–brain barrier *see* BBB (blood–brain
barrier)
blood oxygenation level-dependent (BOLD)
signal, 26–27

blood pressure, 302
body perception, AN, 58–59
Bomann–Larsen, Lene, 231
Bragh, John, 60
brain
    computational/mechanistic models, 38, 329–330
    inflammation from infection, 40, 44–45
    injury and EAS, 280
    mind and, 16, 36–42, 49, 328
    psychopathy, 223–225
    structure, 4
brain-jacking, 203–204
Brain Research through Advanced Innovative Neurotechnologies (BRAIN), 214–215
BROADEN trial (BROdmann Area 25 DEep brain Neuromodulation), 166, 167, 176, 213–214, 279
Broca, Paul, 34
Broome, Matthew, 269
Bublitz, Christoph, 238
bullying, 224
bundle theory, 42
buprenorphine, 276
Burckhardt, Gottlieb, 137–138
Burgess, Anthony, 239

Calhoun, Vince, 301
callous-unemotional (CU) scale, 246
Canada
    Centre for Addiction and Mental Health (Toronto), 159
    EAS legality, 254, 255
Canadian Supreme Court, psychopathy treatment, 240–241
cancer, EAS, 255
capacity
    decisional see decisional capacity
    volitional see volitional capacity
capacity for consent
    AN, 163
    assessment of, 157
    cognitive/emotional impairment, 152–153
    competence vs., 151
    DBS clinical trials, 152–153
    determination, 311
    synaptic pruning, 311
    third-party assessment, 154–155
    TM, 173
capsulotomy, 271–272
cardiac arrhythmia, 302
cardiovascular effects, antipsychotic drugs, 295
Caria, Andrea, 226–227
catatonia, 33
causal determinism, 70–71
CBT (cognitive-behavioral therapy), 158–159
    antidepressants and, 91–92
    anxiety and depression, 316–317

chronic behavioral stress, 42
    DBS and, 158–159
    failure in EAS, 275
    placebo effect vs., 119
    psychopathy, 225–226
Centre for Addiction and Mental Health (Toronto, Canada), 159
Chabot, Boudewijn, 262–263
Cherkasova, Mariya, 176
children, electrical stimulation techniques, 114
chlorpromazine, 87
chronic intractable pain, neurofeedback, 129
chronic psychological stress, 72–73
    OCD, 41–42
Churchland, Patricia, 245
cingulotomy, 271–272
circuit-level explanations, limitation of, 23
citalopram, 227
Clausen, Jens, 191
CLDs (closed-loop devices), 168
    disadvantages, 169–171
    emotion detection, 170
    identification with, 207
    imprecise programming, 170–171
    neuromodulation, 195
Cleckley, Hervey, 220
clinical trials
    benefit vs. risk, 171–172
    competency, differences in, 173
    conflict of interest, 211
    consent for see clinical trials consent
    controlled clinical trials, 93–94
    design and conduct, 171
    double-blind clinical trials, 175–176
    funding lack, 214
    microglial activity, 309–310
    primary movement disorders, 157–158
    psilocybin, 94–96
    psychological harm, risk of, 153–154
    randomized controlled trials, 174–175
    recruitment problems, 159
    risk vs. benefit, 175
    safety investigations, 310
    schizophrenia, 159–160
    sponsorship by manufacturers, 211, 212–213
    subjects, information to, 171, 173
    tDCS vs. escitalopram, 113
clinical trials consent
    capacity in see capacity for consent
    psychiatric neurosurgery, 149–156
    schizophrenia, problems with, 160
    surrogate pressure, 155–156
A Clockwork Orange (Burgess), 239
closed-loop devices see CLDs (closed-loop devices)
clozapine, 87, 90

clustered regularly interspersed short
palindromic repeats (CRISPR), 321
coercion, psychopathy treatment, 231–233
cognition
  affective processes interaction, 224
  criminal responsibility, 201
  emotional interactions *see* cognitive-
    emotional interactions
  enhancement *see* cognitive enhancement
  impairment *see* cognitive impairment
  processing in symptom clustering approach
    in treatment, 100
  suffering, 261
  symptoms *see* cognitive symptoms
cognitive behavioral therapy *see* CBT
  (cognitive-behavioral therapy)
cognitive capacity
  DBS in schizophrenia research, 161
  EAS, 284–285
  ego-syntonic disorders, 274
  phenomenology of suffering, 285
cognitive–emotional interactions, 51
  deficits, 278–279
  processing circuits, 188
cognitive enhancement
  decision-making process, 104
  psychotropic drugs, 103
  studies of, 104
  tCS, 116–117
  therapy *vs.*, 104
  TMS, 112
cognitive impairment
  capacity for consent, 152–153
  dementia association, 33
  disorders in, 113
  EAS competence, 265–266
  ECT adverse effect, 110
  frontal–limbic dysfunction, 224
  MCS, 54
  placebo effect, 120
cognitive neuroscience, 329–330
cognitive symptoms
  interpretation of, 296
  psychiatric disorders, 32
Columbia, EAS legality, 254
Coman, Alina, 45–46
compatibilism, 70–71
  causal determinism, 71
competence
  capacity for consent *vs.*, 151
  EAS, 253, 265, 269, 273–274
  legal status of, 151
  matter of degree as, 274
  trial exclusion, 158
computational models, brain, 38, 329–330
computed tomography *see* CT (computed
  tomography)
computed tomography (CT), 3

conflict of interest, clinical trials, 211
connectedness, 207–208
conscience clauses, 282
conscientious objection, treatment to, 282–283
conscious dimension, self, 43
conscious motivational states, inhibition of, 73
consciousness
  agency connection, 59
  agency in, 60–61
  definition, 59–60
  fears, aspects of, 67
  neural correlates, 53
  phenomenal consciousness, 53
  psychological process, 59–60
  too much, problems of, 61–62
consciousness disorders, 52–64
  form of consciousness, 54–55
  level/degree/state of consciousness, 54–55
  organization of consciousness, 54–55
  post-coma chronic disorders, 53–54
conscious processing, unconscious processing
  *vs.* in OCD, 63
conscious self, disturbances in, 47–48
consent
  capacity for *see* capacity for consent
  expanding applications of deep brain
    stimulation, 158–167
  proxy *see* proxy consent
  psychopathy, 230–231
constraint, 41, 73–75, 193
  bidirectional control as, 74
  neural *vs.* mental levels, 75
control
  awareness *vs.* in OCD, 63
  bidirectional, constraint as, 74
  burden of, 197–201
  criminal responsibility, 201
controlled clinical trials, 93–94
cortical association networks, positive
  schizophrenia, 57
cortical–limbic pathways, psychopathy,
  246–247
cortical–striatal dysconnectivity,
  schizophrenia, 100–101
cortical–thalamic–striatal–cortical circuit, 69
cortisol
  high circulating levels, 278
  hyperactive stress, 307
  inflammatory cytokines, 312
cost-effectiveness, psychopathy treatment *vs.*
  incarceration, 234–235
costs, neuromodulation, 211–215
Courtet, Philippe, 266
C-reactive protein, 313
creativity, psychiatric disorders in, 82
criminal actions, psychopathy excuses for,
  233–234
criminal behavior, psychopathy, 224

criminal responsibility, 201–203
CRISPR (clustered regularly interspersed short palindromic repeats), 321
Crockett, Molly, 227
Cross-Disorder Group of the Psychiatric Genome Consortium, 299
CT (computed tomography), 3
cultural effects, biological psychiatry, 28
CU (callous-unemotional) scale, 246
Cuthbert, Bruce, 20
cytokines, 44
  disease pathology, 293
  inflammatory *see* inflammatory cytokines
  proinflammatory cytokines, 307

Damasio, Antonio, 61
Davis, Nick, 106
DBS (deep brain stimulation), 136, 140–149, 142–149, 330
  ablation *vs.,* 144
  action plans, 194–195
  adverse effects, 146–147
  approved conditions, 145
  associated risks, 143–144, 144–145
  behavior control, 194
  biomarkers, 22
  burden of control, 197–201
  capacity for consent, 153–154
  case study, 193–194
  CBT and, 158–159
  disorders, 173–174
  doubly innovative trials, 156–157
  doubly interactive clinical trials, 150
  dynamic feedback systems, 168–169
  early risk of, 279
  efficacy questions, 166
  electrical stimulation techniques *vs.,* 114
  expanding applications, 158–167
  failure in EAS, 275
  fear memory erasure, 145–146
  free will, 194
  GAD, 189
  high-frequency DBS, 146
  history of, 140
  hyperdopaminergic activity, 160
  identification with, 205–206
  impulse control disorder, 200–201
  induced euphoria, 199–200
  intermediary or mediating device as, 206
  low-frequency DBS, 146
  MDD, 144, 189
  mechanism of action, 142–143
  neural ablation *vs.,* 148–149
  neurogenesis in hippocampal-entorhinal circuit, 111
  neuromodulating effects, 188–189
  NFB *vs.,* 195

OCD, 143–144, 186–188
open- *vs.* closed-loop devices, 167–171
  *see also* CLDs (closed-loop devices); OLDs (open-loop devices)
outcome definition, 148
patient autonomy, 187–188
patient awareness, 191
PD, 316
personality changes, 208–209
proxy consent, 152
psychopharmacology resistant conditions, 143
reversible effects, 147–148
risks in, 155, 229–230
schizophrenia, 159, 160, 161–162
self-identity issues, 207–208
surgical ablation *vs.,* 169
temporal interference *vs.,* 118
therapeutic potential, 176
TMS *vs.,* 143
  *see also* neuromodulation
de Cates, Angharad, 269
decisional capacity
  EAS, 252, 284–285
  psychopathy, 242
decision-making process, cognitive enhancement, 104
deep brain stimulation *see* DBS (deep brain stimulation)
degeneration, basal ganglia, 32
degrees, insight of, 77–78
de Haan, Sanneke, 62–63
Dehaene, Stanislas, 56
delirium, 54
delusions
  experience (alien control), 79–80
  false beliefs of, 79–80
  insight in, 78–79
  OCD *vs.,* 78–79
  psychotic states, 285–286
  schizophrenia, 57, 120
dementia, 54
  late-life depression & cognitive decline, 33
  schizophrenia and, 33
dementia praecox, 33
Demertzi, Athena, 259
Denys, Damiaan, 62–63
depression, 312–314
  antidepressants, 91–92, 119–120
  anti-inflammatory drugs, 313
  anxiety and, 18–19, 123, 301
  associated beliefs/emotions, 29
  BD, 18
  capacity about psychiatric treatment, 266–267
  comorbidities, 262
  DBS fear memory erasure, 145–146

depression (*Cont.*)
definitions, 99
epilepsy *vs.*, 59
fear memory system disorder as, 64
fMRI-based NFB, 129
immune dysregulation, 313–314
inflammatory cytokines, 312–313
insight in, 77
ketamine, 88
lithium, 90
major depression *see* major depression;
    MDD (major depressive disorder)
memory dysfunction, 65–66
neural dysfunction, 46–47
neurological disorders *vs.*, 30
NFB inactivity, 130
NMDAR dysfunction in, 99
noninvasive prevention, 316–317
onset of, 301
placebo effect, 119, 125
prenatal risk factors, 317–318
prevalence, 291
psilocybin, 88, 94–95
psychopharmacology, 7
resting-state hyperactivity, 57–58
schizophrenia *vs.*, 59
sleep disturbances, 103
social stress *vs.*, 265–266
stress association, 301
stress hormones, 33
suicide risk, 286
tCS, 115
TMS, 112, 115
treatability of, 276
treatment resistant *see* TRD (treatment-
    resistant depression)
unipolar depression *see* unipolar depression
De Ridder, Dirk, 68
detachment, experience of, 72–73
DeVries, Raymond, 257–258
diagnosis of psychiatric disorders, accuracy
    of, 294
*Diagnostic and Statistical Manual of Mental
    Disorders-5 (DSM-5)*, 4–5
diazepam, 87
diffusion tensor imaging (DTI),
    schizophrenia, 56
diffusion-weighted magnetic resonance
    imaging (dwMRI), 21
dignity loss, EAS motivation, 260
disabled constraint, 41
disease severity, EAS, 273–274
distributive justice, 55
DLPFC *see* dorsolateral prefrontal cortex
    (DLPFC)
DNA methylation, 66–67
dopamine
D2 receptors, 56

dysregulation, 295
PD therapy, 32–33
release in PD, 122
dopamine receptor antagonists, 87
poor selectivity, 92
dopaminergic pathways, genetics, 121
dorsolateral prefrontal cortex (DLPFC)
AN structural changes, 46
ventral striatum connectivity, 229
Dostoevsky, Fyodor, 82
double-blind clinical trials, 175–176
double bookkeeping, delusional disorders
    in, 78–79
double bookkeeping, 79–80
DREADDS (designer receptors exclusively
    activated by designer drugs), 104–105
driving, epilepsy, 54
DSM-5 (*Diagnostic and Statistical Manual of
    Mental Disorders, Fifth Edition* ), 16–24
bipolar disorder symptoms, 19–20
catatonia as psychomotor disorder, 33
development of, 16–17
free will definition, 68
inadequacies of, 49–50
insight, 80
mental disorder definition, 17
merits/limitations, 15
psychopathy, 219
RDoC and, 24, 50
RDoC *vs.*, 16, 327
schizophrenia symptoms, 17
symptom-based diagnosis, 20
use in treatment responses, 22
DSM-IV (*Diagnostic and Statistical Manual of
    Mental Disorders, Fourth Edition*)
catatonia as schizophrenia, 33
pain, 259
unbearable suffering definition, 257
DSM-IV-TR
free will definition, 68
loss of freedom, 186–189
DTI (diffusion tensor imaging),
    schizophrenia, 56
Dunn, Michael, 6
dwMRI (diffusion-weighted magnetic
    resonance imaging), 21
dynamic feedback systems, DBS, 168–169
dysfunctional inhibitory mechanisms, 73
dystonia, DBS, 145

EAS (euthanasia and assisted suicide),
    251–289
adolescents/young adults, 280
arguments for/against, 264–281
case review, 257–258
cognition, 265–266, 284–285
competence, 253, 265, 273–274
criteria, 254–258

data, 254–258
decisional capacity, 252, 284–285
definitions, 254–258
disease severity, 273–274
disease types, 255
euthanasia *vs.* suicide, 283–284
existential suffering and, 263
imminent death, 280
impulsivity, 268–269
independent psychiatrists, 256
informed patients, 253
legality, 254–255
legislation, 251
medical conditions, 254–255
motivation for, 260
motivation removal, 277–278
noncompetence, 281–287
obligations, 281–287
passive euthanasia, 286
physician-assisted suicide, 284
physicians refusal, 283
psychological suffering, 256–257
questioning of, 252
regulation of, 266
request assessment, 277
request persistence, 253, 261–262, 265, 269–
    270, 280, 282–283
requests *vs.* treatment requests, 282
rights, 281–287
stability of request, 258
suffering prolongation, 252–253
TRD, 271
treatment alternatives, 271–272
treatment failure, 253, 275, 277–278
treatment-resistant depression, 251
unbearable pain, 263–264
voluntary euthanasia, 285
waiting for new treatment, 252–253,
    253–254, 280
*see also* pain; suffering
ECT (electroconvulsive therapy), 88, 107–112
applications, 108–109
development of, 107–108
discrediting of, 25
electrical stimulation techniques *vs.*, 114
failure in EAS, 275
HPA axis regulation, 108
invasive *vs.* non-invasive treatment as,
    106–107
mechanism of action, 108–109, 110–111
nonspecific effects, 109–110
risk effects, 109
EEG (electroencephalography)
NFB, 42
*see also* NFB (neurofeedback)
ego-dystonic disorders
implied autonomy, 191–192
insight in, 78–79

*see also* MDD (major depressive disorder);
    OCD (obsessive–compulsive disorder)
ego-syntonic disorders
capacity, lack of, 162–163
cognitive capacity, 274
insight in, 78
proxy consent, 155
electrical stimulation techniques
DBS *vs.*, 114
ECT *vs.*, 114
risk effects, 114
*see also* TMS (transcranial magnetic
    stimulation)
electric stimulation, psychopathy, 229
electroconvulsive therapy *see* ECT
    (electroconvulsive therapy)
electroencephalography *see* EEG
    (electroencephalography)
electrolytic ablation, 140
acceptability, 177
electrolytic, or radiofrequency, ablation,
    271–272
electrophysiology
neural circuit dysfunction, 21
symptom clustering approach in
    treatment, 100
treatment responses, 21
Ely, E Wesley, 284
Emanuel, Ezekiel, 254
emotions
cognition interactions *see* cognitive–
    emotional interactions
depression, 29
detection in closed-loop devices, 170
frontal–limbic dysfunction, 224
impairment in capacity for consent,
    152–153
psychiatric disorders, 32
suffering, 261
symptom clustering approach in
    treatment, 100
employment, biomarkers, 306
encephalopathy, 54
endocrine factors
prenatal risk factors, 320
*see also* neuroendocrine factors
endogenous dopamine therapy, PD, 32–33
endophenotypes, 297
diagnosis in, 300
end-stage cancer, EAS, 280
environment
gene–environment interactions, 293,
    300, 301
genetic interactions, 293
prenatal risk factors, 320
psychiatric self, 76
epigenetic analysis, 316–317, 327
genetic analysis and, 300

epigenetics, 66–67
  prenatal risk factors, 320
  timing of, 301
  unipolar/bipolar depression, 268
epilepsy, 54
  DBS, 145
  depression *vs.*, 59
  driving, 54
  schizophrenia *vs.*, 59
  seizures, 59
episodic memory, 65
  long-term episodic memory, change
    to, 66–67
escitalopram, 113
essential tremor, DBS, 145
estrogen, 293
euthanasia
  suicide *vs.*, 283–284
  terminal sedation, 284
  *see also* EAS (euthanasia and assisted
    suicide)
executive function deficits,
    schizophrenia, 68–69
existential suffering, 261
  psychosocial interventions, 262
  types of, 263
exogenous neural growth factor, 315–316
experience (alien control) delusions, 79–80
extinction training, 96
extrapyramidal adverse effects,
    antipsychotics, 89–90

false beliefs, delusions as, 79–80
family members, proxy consent, 152
FDA (Food and Drug Administration), TMS/
    tCA unregulation, 115–116
fear
  conscious *vs.* nonconscious aspects, 67
  disproportionate role of memories, 65
  optogenetics, 179
fear memory erasure
  hippocampus, 96
  protein synthesis blockade, 97
  PTSD treatment, 96–97
Feinberg, Todd, 41
Figee, Martijn, 187
fight-or-flight response, 40
Fitzgerald, Michael, 34
fMRI (functional magnetic resonance
    imaging), 3
  AN structural changes, 46
  biomarkers, 301–302
  CBT response to MDD, 100
  neurobiology, 21
  NFB, 42
  positive schizophrenia subtype, 328
  predictive/diagnostic value, 303
  psychiatric disease diagnosis, 26–27

psychopathy, 224–225
  real-time neural activity, 27
  study meta-analyses, 27–28
  *see also* NFB (neurofeedback)
focused ultrasound *see* FUS (focused
    ultrasound)
Food and Drug Administration (FDA), TMS/
    tCA unregulation, 115–116
forced treatment, psychopathy, 233–234, 235–
    236, 237–240
Foster, Simmie, 44
Frankfurt, Harry, 76, 231–232
freedom of thought objection, 237–245
Freehand device, 214–215
Freeman, Walter, 138
free response, 40
free will
  access of, 72
  action plans and, 70–71
  DBS, 194
  definitions, 68
  internal concept, 72
  OCD, 70
  psychoses and, 81
  structural aspects, 4
Freud, Sigmund, 24
frontal–limbic dysfunction
  cognitive defects, 224
  emotional deficits, 224
  psychopathy, 224
frontal–limbic pathway, 308
frontal–limbic–striatal–frontal circuit, 69–70
frontal lobotomy, 138–139
frontal-striatal-limbic pathways, 108–109
frontal–temporal–parietal pathway, 308
frontal–thalamic–striatal–frontal circuit, 70
Fuchs, Thomas, 63–64
functional imaging, biomarkers, 303
functional magnetic resonance imaging *see*
    fMRI (functional magnetic resonance
    imaging)
functional neuroimaging, structural
    neuroimaging combination, 301–302
function restoration, behavior control, 196
FUS (focused ultrasound), 140–141
  BBB permeability, 314–315
  failure in EAS, 275
  low-intensity FUS, 146

GABA (gamma-aminobutyric acid), 99
GABAergic neurons, optogenetics, 178
GABAergic pathways, 278, 303
GAD (generalized anxiety disorder)
  action dysfunctions, 191
  cognitive/emotional impairment, 152–153
  DBS, 189
  DBS and CBT, 159
  diagnosis, 18–19

fear processing, 75
hyperactive fear system, 99–100
mental state in, 23
neural ablation surgery, 141
NFB, 129–130
placebo effect, 119
worry symptoms, 66
*see also* anxiety disorders
Gage, Phineas, 3–4
Gala, Gary, 39
Gallagher, Shaun, 190–191
gamma aminobutyric acid (GABA), 99
Gamma Knife radiosurgery *see* GKR (Gamma Knife radiosurgery)
gene–environment interactions, 293, 300, 301
generalized anxiety disorder *see* GAD (generalized anxiety disorder)
genetic(s), 5–6, 298–307
  BD, 297
  behavior link, 300
  biological psychiatry, 24–25
  biomarkers, 299
  diagnosis, 6
  environment interactions, 293
  gene–environment interactions, 293, 300, 301
  phenotypic abnormalities, 297
  placebo effect, 121–122, 127–128
  polymorphisms and disease, 292–293
  prenatal risk factors, 320
  schizophrenia, 297
  symptom clustering approach in treatment, 100
genetic analysis, 327
  epigenetic analysis and, 300
  neuroimaging and, 310
genetic testing, prenatal interventions, 321
GKR (Gamma Knife radiosurgery), 140, 271–272
  acceptability, 177
  invasive *vs.* non-invasive treatment as, 106
Glenn, Andrea, 223–224
global neural network theory, 52
globus pallidus, stimulating techniques, 189
glutamate
  depression, 99
  signaling pathway, 278, 312–313
Gold, Azgad, 125
Goodman, Wayne, 110
Graham, George, 29–30
Grahn, Peter, 168
grand mal seizures, 59
gray matter volume, 303, 308
  schizophrenia, 68–69
Griesinger, Wilhelm, 24
Grisso, Thomas, 151
Grossman, Nir, 117
growth factor, 315–316

Halligan, Peter, 60
hallucinations
  psychotic states, 285–286
  schizophrenia, 51, 57, 120
haloperidol, 87
Hariz, Marwan, 149
heart rate, 302
hemispatial neglect following stroke, 54
HIFUS (high-intensity focused ultrasound), 140–141, 271–272
  acceptability, 177
high-frequency DBS, 146
high-intensity focused ultrasound *see* HIFUS (high-intensity focused ultrasound)
hippocampal-entorhinal circuit, neurogenesis by DBS, 111
hippocampus
  atrophy in, 23, 33, 307
  fear memory erasure, 96
  gray matter volume, 101
  memory formation, 66–67
  structural neuroimaging in depression, 39
Hippocrates, 34
Holtzheimer, Paul, 99
homeostasis, psychiatric disease, 40
Hospital Santa Creu i Sant Pau (Spain), 159
HPA (hypothalamic–pituitary–adrenal) axis, 23
  dysregulation, 278
The Human Brain Project (2013), 330
Human Connectome Project, 330
Hume, David, 42
Hyman, Steven, 101–102
hyperactive stress
  cortisol, 307
  norepinephrine, 307
hyperactivity
  subgenual cingulate, 188
  unregulated hyperactivity, 75
hyperdopaminergic activity, DBS in, 160
hyper-reflectivity, OCD, 62
hypertension, 302
hypomania, BD, 18, 48
hypothalamic–pituitary–adrenal axis *see* HPA (hypothalamic–pituitary–adrenal) axis

ICD-11 (*International Statistical Classification of Diseases and Related Health Problems*), 17
  RDoC *vs.,* 20–21
identification
  mechanical brain implants with, 205–206
  neuromodulation, 204–210
identity
  personal *see* personal identity
  relational identity, 209
  self-identity *see* self-identity
imipramine, 87

imminent death, EAS, 280
immune self, 43–44
immune system
    dysregulation in depression, 313–314
    modulating drugs, 309
    prenatal risk factors, 320
    *see also* neuroimmunology
implied autonomy, ego-dystonic disorders,
    191–192
imprecise programming, closed-loop devices,
    170–171
impulse control disorders, 73
    DBS, 200–201
    reward system inhibition failure, 193
incarceration
    psychopathy treatment as, 237–240
    treatment cost-effectiveness *vs.* in
      psychopathy, 236–237
independent psychiatrists, EAS, 256
inflammation, modulation of, 308
inflammatory cytokines, 312, 314
    depression, 312–313
information
    EAS, 253, 265
    filtering in schizophrenia, 57
    integration theory, 52–53
    placebo effect, 126–128
innate immune response, 314
innovation, neuromodulation, 211–215
Insel, Thomas, 6, 20
insight, 77–83
    autonomy and, 79
    definitions, 77
    degrees of, 77–78
    interoception, 77
    OCD and, 80–81
instrumental aggression, 224
insula, 46
integration problems, schizophrenia, 56–57
internal concept, free will, 72
*International Statistical Classification of*
    *Diseases and Related Health Problems*
    *see* ICD-11 (*International Statistical*
    *Classification of Diseases and Related*
    *Health Problems*)
interoception, insight, 77
interpretation, biomarkers, 305
invasive treatments, 105–106
    non-invasive treatments *vs.*, 105–107
irritability, longitudinal studies, 296

Jamison, Kay Redfield, 260
Jarvis, Sarah, 178–179
Johns Hopkins University Hospital, 159
Justice, 7

Kagan, Shelly, 269–270
Kandel, Eric, 25

Kant's Categorical Imperative, 173
Kaptchuk, Ted, 118
Kesey, Ken, 108
ketamine, 7, 87–88, 92–94
    abuse in, 93
    antisuicidal treatment, 276
    clinical trial lack of funding, 214
    limitations of, 93
    MDD, 278
    patient selection, 93
    psilocybin *vs.*, 95–96
Kim, Scott, 157, 257–258
Kimsma, Gerrit, 261
Kleinman, Arthur, 28
Kong, Camilla, 6
Kopell, Brian Harris, 135
Kragh, Kristian, 239–240
Kraepelin, Emil, 20

lamotrigine, 89
late-life depression, dementia association, 33
Laureys, Steven, 259
LeDoux, Joseph, 67
legal questions, psychopathy, 221–223
Lichtenberg, Pesach, 125
life fatigue, 263
light scattering, optogenetics, 180
Lima, Almeida, 138
limbic leucotomy, 141
limbic system
    PFC link, 67
    psychopathy, 223
Linden, David, 205
Lipsman, Nir, 187
Lisanby, Sarah, 108–109
lithium, 87, 90
loneliness, 263
    EAS requests, 261–262
longitudinal studies, 296
loss of control, EAS motivation, 260
Lowell, Robert, 48–49, 83
low-frequency DBS, 146
low-intensity FUS, 146
Lozano, Andres, 187
Luxembourg, EAS legality, 254

MacCat-CR assessment tool, 155
MacCat-T assessment tool, 155
mad, bad *vs.* in psychopathy, 222–223
magnetic resonance imaging *see* MRI
    (magnetic resonance imaging)
magnetic stimulation, psychopathy, 229
major depression, 264
    functional neuroimaging, 39
    genetics, 299
    neuroimaging, 69
    structural neuroimaging, 39
    *see also* MDD (major depressive disorder)

major depressive disorder *see* MDD (major depressive disorder)
major psychiatric disorders, prenatal interventions, 323
mania
  BD, 18, 48
  lithium, 90
*The Mask of Sanity* (Cleckley), 220
materialist theory of mind, RDoC, 37
maternal malnutrition, 317, 319
maternal smoking, OCD, 318–319
matter of degree, competence as, 274
Mayberg, Helen, 28, 99, 166–167
MCS (minimally conscious state), 53–54
  cognitive/motor function limitation, 54
  consciousness level/degree/state, 54–55
  disorder self-awareness, 55–56
MDD (major depressive disorder)
  action dysfunctions, 191
  antidepressants, response variation, 125–126, 135
  brain-level explanations, 92
  capacity for consent, 153–154
  CBT, 100, 159
  cognitive/emotional impairment, 113, 152–153
  comorbidities, 264
  DBS, 140, 144, 159, 173–174, 189
  diagnosis, 17–18
  electrical stimulation therapy, 188
  emergence of, 321
  hyperactive fear system, 99–100
  ketamine, 278
  mental state in, 23
  mesolimbic hypodopaminergic state, 69
  neural ablation, 272
  neural ablation surgery, 141
  NFB, 129–130
  PD connection, 32
  psychopharmacology non-response, 104–105
  seizure disorder and, 272
  self-focus, 58
  *see also* major depression
MDMA (3,4-methylenedioxymethamphetamine), 7
MDMA therapy
  adverse effects, 98
  clinical trial lack of funding, 214
  PTSD, 98–99
mechanical brain implants
  behavioral standards, 203
  behavior control, 190–191
  brain-jacking, 203–204
  enabling tool as, 206
  identification with, 205–206
  manufacturers' obligations, 200
  neurosurgeons' obligations, 200

obligation to operate, 198–199
patient uneasiness, 204–205
*see also* DBS (deep brain stimulation)
mechanistic models, brain, 38, 329–330
mechanistic theory of mind, 38
*Medical Devices: Guidelines Document – Classification of Medical Devices* (EC), 115–116
medical insurance denial, biomarkers, 306
memory
  content disorders, 64–67
  episodic *see* episodic memory
  erasure therapy, 96–98
mental constraint, neural constraint *vs.*, neuromodulating techniques, 192–193
mental disorders
  definitions, 29
  diagnostic criteria analysis, 39
  DSM-5 definition, 17
  neurobiology, 4
  types of, 17
  *see also* psychiatric diseases/disorders
mental enhancement, psychotropic drugs, 103
mental functions, behavior control, 74–75
mental suffering, 270–271
mental symptoms, psychiatric disorders, 32
Merkel, Reinhard, 238
mesolimbic hypodopaminergic state, MDD, 69
mesolimbic pathways, hyperdopaminergic activity in schizophrenia, 159–160
mesolimbic tracts, positive subtype of schizophrenia, 69
metabolic effects, antipsychotic drugs, 295
metabolic hyperactivity, low-intensity DBS/FUS, 146
3,4-methylenedioxymethamphetamine (MDMA), 7
  therapy in *see* MDMA therapy
methylphenidate, 104
Meynen, Gerben, 80–81
microglia
  disease pathology, 293
  infections of, 40, 44–45
microglial activity
  clinical trials, 309–310
  elevated activation, 307
  PET, 309
  psychosocial stress, 312
Miller, Andrew, 312
Miller, Franklin, 118, 276–277
mind
  brain *vs.*, 328
  disorders, psychiatric disorders as, 327–328
minimally conscious state *see* MCS (minimally conscious state)
Mitchell, David, 224
M'Naghten Test, 201
modafinil, 104

Mollon, Josephine, 295–296
Moniz, Egas, 138
monoamine hypothesis of depression, 99
mood disorders, 113
  DBS clinical trials, 152–153
  improvement, 195
  longitudinal studies, 296
mood improvement, TMS, 112
moral attitudes/values, autonomy, 76
"moral bad" attribution, psychiatric
    disorders, 5–6
Model Penal Code, 201
moral reasoning
  cognitive/affective processes
      interaction, 224
  psychopathy, 224
Morsella, Ezequiel, 60
Morse, Stephen, 202, 234
Mortensen, Preben, 6
Moritz, Chet, 170
motivation
  EAS for, 260
  improvement, 195
motor capacity, 51–52
motor functions
  autonomy in, 76
  limitation in MCS, 54
motor symptoms, psychiatric disorders, 32
MRI (magnetic resonance imaging), 3
  biomarkers, 301–302
  diffusion-weighted magnetic resonance
      imaging, 21
  frontal–thalamic–striatal–frontal circuit, 70
  neurobiology, 21
  positive schizophrenia subtype, 328
  see also fMRI (functional magnetic
      resonance imaging)
Muller, Sabine, 149
multifactorial nature, psychiatric
    disorders, 292
multiple sclerosis, EAS, 255

Nash, John, 81–83
National Institute of Mental Health (NIMH),
    Research Domain Criteria see RDoC
    (Research Domain Criteria)
negative rights, 282
neocortex, memory formation, 66–67
Nestler, Eric, 300–301
Netherlands
  EAS case review, 257–258
  EAS legality, 254
neural ablation, 136, 140–149
  clinical trials, 177
  DBS vs., 144, 148–149
  failure in EAS, 275
  MRI stereotactic techniques, 142
  types, 141

see also FUS (focused ultrasound); GKR
    (Gamma Knife radiosurgery); HIFUS
    (high-intensity focused ultrasound)
neural functions, behavior control, 74–75
neural mapping, temporal lobe, 145
neural prosthetics, 330
neural synchronization theory, 52
neurobiology, 20
  mental illness, 4
  placebo response, 122
  psychiatric disease, 21
neurocognition, 47
neurodegenerative disorders
  EAS, 255
  neurodevelopmental disorders from, 33
neurodevelopmental disorders, 293–294
  neurodegenerative disorders
      development, 33
  pharmacotherapy resistance, 135–136
neuroendocrine factors, 307–317
  neuroimmune factor interactions, 43
neurofeedback see NFB (neurofeedback)
neurogenesis, hippocampal-entorhinal circuit
    by DBS, 111
neuroimaging, 3, 298–307
  accuracy concerns, 27–28
  AN structural changes, 46
  biomarkers, 301–302, 303
  depression, 39
  disease diagnosis/prediction, 26
  functional imaging, 303
  functional studies in depression, 39
  genetic analysis and, 310
  genetic biomarkers, 299
  limitations of, 39
  major depression, 69
  neural circuit dysfunction, 21
  neurological vs. psychiatric disorders, 31–32
  neuromodulating techniques, 25
  psychopathy, 219, 247–248
  structural and functional neuroimaging,
      301–302
  symptom clustering approach in
      treatment, 100
  see also CT (computed tomography); fMRI
      (functional magnetic resonance
      imaging); MRI (magnetic resonance
      imaging); PET (positron emission
      tomography)
neuroimmunology, 293, 307–317
  modulating drugs, 314
  neuroendocrine factors interactions, 43
  psychiatric disorders, 309
  see also immune system
neurological disorders
  permanent degenerative effects, 253–254
  prenatal events, 23
  psychiatric disorders vs., 29–30

psychological factors, 329
social factors, 329
neurology
  consciousness, 53
  neural constraint *vs.* mental constraint, 192–193
  psychiatry overlap, 30–35, 35–36, 329
  psychotropic drugs, effects of, 297
neuromodulation, 185–217
  adverse effects, 186, 208, 214
  agents of, 189–197
  autonomy, fear of loss, 191–192
  behavior changes and conflict, 209–210
  benefit identification, 210
  clinical trial sponsorship, 211
  control, fear of, 190–192
  control restoration, 186–189
  costs, 211–215
  identification and personal identity, 204–210
  innovation, 211–215
  manufacturer insolvency, 213
  manufacturers' obligations, 200
  mechanisms of action, 211–212
  moral/legal implications, 198, 199–200
  neural *vs.* mental constraint, 192–193
  neuroimaging, 25
  psychopathy, 221, 234–235
  social justice, 211–215
  *see also* BROADEN trial (BROdmann
      Area25 DEep brain Neuromodulation);
      DBS (deep brain stimulation); neural
      ablation
neuropeptide signaling pathway, 312–313
neurophenomenology, 37, 47
neuropsychological disorders, 31
neurosurgeon, obligations of, 200
neurosurgery
  sham surgery RCTs, 174–175
  structural *vs.* psychiatric neurosurgery, 136
  *see also* psychiatric neurosurgery
neurotransmitters
  imbalance of, 87
  receptors as psychopharmacology
      targets, 92
Newborn Epigenetics Study (Duke University),
    318–319
NFB (neurofeedback), 128–132
  brain–mind/mind–brain interactions, 195–196
  DBS *vs.*, 195
  definition, 128–129
  electroencephalography, 42
  fMRI, 42, 226–227
  potential harm, 130
  psychopathy, 226–227
  social justice issues, 131
  treatable conditions, 129–130

*see also* EEG (electroencephalography);
    fMRI (functional magnetic resonance
    imaging)
*N*-methyl-D-aspartate receptors (NMDARs)
  antagonist *see* ketamine
  dysfunction in, 99
  dysregulation, 278
  schizophrenia, 56
nonconsciousness, fears, aspects of, 67
nonconsequentialist reasons, psychopathy
    treatment, 243–245
non-invasive treatments
  definitions, 106
  invasive treatments *vs.*, 105–107
  prevention of anxiety and depression, 316–317
nonmaleficence, 7
nonreductive materialism, 37, 41
non-treatment risks, 105
norepinephrine
  hyperactive stress, 307
  inflammatory cytokines, 312
Northoff, Georg, 4, 46–47
nucleus accumbens lesioning, 142

Oakley, David, 60
OCD (obsessive–compulsive disorder), 62–64
  action dysfunctions, 191
  antidepressants and CBT, 92
  awareness *vs.* control, 63
  behavior, alienation from, 80–81
  capacity for consent, 153–154
  capsulotomy, 141–142
  CBT and antidepressants, 92
  CBT and DBS, 159
  chronic psychological stress, 41–42
  cognitive/emotional impairment, 152–153
  conscious *vs.* unconscious processing, 63
  DBS, 140, 143–144, 173–174, 186–188
  DBS and CBT, 159
  delusional disorders *vs.*, 78–79
  diagnosis, 19
  emergence of, 321
  free will, 70
  hyper-reflectivity, 62
  insight and, 80–81
  interference by consciousness, 61
  mechanisms, 62
  neural ablation, 141, 272
  new treatments, 279
  nucleus accumbens lesioning, 142
  pharmacotherapy resistance, 135
  placebo effect, 119
  prenatal risk factors, 317–318, 318–319
  psychiatric assessment, 273
  seizure disorder and, 272
  suicidal desires, 267
  suicidal risk, 272–273

Olbert, Charles, 39
OLDs (open-loop devices)
 identification with, 207
 neuromodulation, 195
 technical disadvantages, 167–168
Olie, Emilie, 266
*One Flew Over the Cuckoo's Nest,* 108
open-loop devices *see* OLDs (open-loop devices)
optogenetics, 178–181
 animal models, 179
 applications, 179
 definition, 178
 limited applications, 180
 risks, 179
 safety, 180
 theoretical advantage, 178
orbitofrontal cortex, psychopathy, 223
organic brain dysfunctions, 20
Owen, Michael, 6
oxytocin, 227–228

pain, 258–264
 mechanism, 258–259
 neural networks, 259
 perception of, 259
 unbearable and EAS, 263–264
palliative care, EAS motivation, 260–261
panic
 DBS fear memory erasure, 145–146
 fear memory system disorder as, 64
 memory dysfunction, 65–66
 psychopharmacological treatment, 96
panic disorders, 66
 NFB, 129–130
 optogenetics, 179
 placebo effect, 119
Papez circuit model, 139
paranoid schizophrenia, 81–82
parental responsibility, prenatal
 interventions, 322
parietal cortex, AN structural changes, 46
parietal lobe, TMS in psychopathy, 229
Parker, Michael, 6
Parkinson's disease *see* PD (Parkinson's
 disease)
Parnas, Josef, 60, 295
paroxetine, 87
Parsons, Ryan, 96
PAS (physician-assisted suicide), euthanasia
 *vs.,* 284
passive euthanasia, 286
PD (Parkinson's disease)
 consent issues, 35–36
 DBS, 173–174, 316
 dopamine release, 122
 endogenous dopamine therapy, 32–33
 MDD connection, 32
 movement control, 191

movement disorders, DBS, 145
 neuromodulating techniques, 189
 PET, 122
 psychiatric disorders *vs.,* 30
 symptoms, 32
Penfield, Wilder, 145
Pepper, Joshua, 149
perception of risk, ethical issues, 148–149
persistent self, 43
personal autonomy, 75–76
personal identity
 definitions, 207–208
 relational identity *vs.,* 209
 structural aspects, 4
personality changes
 clinical trials, 172
 DBS, 208–209
personality, depression and, 262
PET (positron emission tomography), 3
 biomarkers, 301–302
 microglial activity, 309
 neurobiology, 21
 PD and dopamine release, 122
 positive schizophrenia subtype, 328
 predictive/diagnostic value, 303
 real-time neural activity, 27
 study meta-analyses, 27–28
Peteet, John, 257–258
Petersen, Thomas Sobirk, 239–240
petit mal seizures, epilepsy, 59
PFC (prefrontal cortex)
 atrophy in, 23, 33, 307
 dorsolateral *see* dorsolateral prefrontal
 cortex (DLPFC)
 impulse control disorders, 73
 limbic system link, 67
 psychopathy, 223
 reward system inhibition failure, 193
 sensorimotor impairment, 153
 structural neuroimaging in
 depression, 39
 tCS stimulation, 116
 ventrolateral prefrontal cortex, 223
 ventromedial *see* ventromedial PFC
phenomenal consciousness, 53
phenotypic abnormalities, genetics, 297
phobias
 DBS fear memory erasure, 145–146
 fear memory system disorder as, 64
 memory dysfunction, 65–66
physical suffering, 261
physician-assisted suicide (PAS), euthanasia
 *vs.,* 284
Pitman, Roger, 96
placebo
 cognitive/mental enhancement by
 psychotropic drugs, 103–104
 deceptive *vs.* nondeceptive use, 124–125

placebo effect/response, 118–128
  biochemical mechanism, 128
  CBT *vs.,* 119
  definition, 118–119
  disorders used in, 119–120
  ethical justification, 123–125
  genetics, 121–122, 127–128
  information disclosure, 126–127
  information withholding ethics, 127–128
  neurobiological & psychological
      processes, 122
  pharmacology response variation, 126
  psychiatric neurosurgery trials,
      174–175, 176
  weak or no response, 123
PMDs (psychogenic movement disorders)
  placebo response, 122–123
  psychosocial stress, 32–33
positive rights, 281–282
positron emission tomography *see* PET
      (positron emission tomography)
post-traumatic stress disorder *see* PTSD (post-
      traumatic stress disorder)
potential people *vs.* real people in pregnancy
      termination (abortion), 321–324
prediction
  psychiatric disorders, accuracy of, 294
  value of biomarkers, 298
prefrontal cortex *see* PFC (prefrontal cortex)
pregnancy termination (abortion), 320, 321
  real *vs.* potential people, 321–324
prenatal events, neuropathology, 23
prenatal interventions, 317–324
  adolescents, 320–321
  genetic testing, 321
  major psychiatric disorders, 323
  parental responsibility, 322
  *see also* pregnancy termination (abortion)
prenatal stress, 318–319
primary movement disorders, trial
      participation, 157–158
prodromal phase interventions, 294–298
  adverse drug effects, 295
prodromal symptoms, disease conversion,
      296–297
progesterone, 293
proinflammatory cytokines, 307
*Project for a Scientific Psychology* (Freud), 24
prosocial behavior, oxytocin effects, 228
protein synthesis blockade, fear memory
      erasure, 97
proxy consent, 311
  AN clinical trials, 164
  DBS in schizophrenia research, 162
  family members, 152
psilocybin, 7, 88, 94–96
  clinical trial lack of funding, 214
  ketamine *vs.,* 95–96

psychiatric assessment, OCD, 273
psychiatric diseases/disorders
  adolescence, 308
  autoimmune/endocrine interactions, 40
  behavior classification, 26
  competence, 267
  creativity in, 82
  debilitating effects of, 330
  definitions, 15
  development, 295
  disordered/divided self, 45
  evolutionary reasons, 28–29
  homeostasis, 40
  information processing disruption, 36–37
  mental state, effect on, 35
  mind disorders as, 327–328
  "moral bad" attribution, 5–6
  multifactorial nature, 292
  neurobiology, 21
  neuroimaging, diagnosis by, 26
  neuroimmune interactions, 293
  neurological disorders *vs.,* 29–30
  onset of, 301, 328
  psychosocial stress, 35
  self-identity issues, 208
  suicidal ideation, 252, 268
  therapy, expectations of, 277
  treatment, 267, 278
  *see also* mental disorders
psychiatric neurosurgery, 135–186
  benefits definition, 165–166
  clinical trial consent, 149–156
  history, 137–140
  rationale for, 136
  researchers' obligations, 171–177
  risks in, 136–137, 150–151
  stereotactic techniques, 139
  structural neurosurgery *vs.,* 136
  therapeutic misconception, 156–158
psychiatric nosology, 5
psychiatric self, 42, 49
  continuous nature, 45
  definitions, 76
psychiatry
  biological *see* biological psychiatry
  neurology overlap, 30–35, 35–36, 329
psychic pain, 259
psychogenic movement disorders *see*
      PMDs (psychogenic movement
      disorders)
psychology
  neurological disorders, 329
  placebo response, 122
  psychiatric self, 76
  psychotropic drug effects, 297
  schizophrenia, 91
  suffering and EAS, 256–257
psychomotor disorder, catatonia as, 33

psychopathy, 5, 219–250
  antisocial behavior, 224
  brain abnormalities, 223–225
  capacity in, 222
  children in, 247–248
  cortical–limbic pathways, 246–247
  definitions, 219–220
  DSM-5, 17
  ethical and legal questions, 221–223
  excuses for criminal actions, 233–234
  fear response diminishment, 228
  fMRI, 224–225
  frontal–limbic dysfunction, 224
  heritability of, 246
  lack of insight into condition, 244–245
  mad vs. bad, 222–223
  moral reasoning, 224
  neuroimaging, 219
  prevention of, 245–248
  reasoning/decisional capacity, 242
  traits in childhood, 245–246
  treatment see psychopathy treatment
Psychopathy Checklist-Revised, 219
psychopathy treatment, 221–222, 225–230
  adherence to, 242–243
  behavior modification, 230–237
  coercion in, 231–233
  consent to trials, 230–231
  cost-effectiveness vs. incarceration, 236–237
  electric stimulation, 229
  forced treatment, 233–234, 235–236,
      237–240
  freedom of thought objection, 237–245
  incarcaration cost-effectiveness vs., 236–237
  indirect vs. direct, 238
  legal cases, 240–241
  magnetic stimulation, 229
  neuromodulation, 221, 234–235
  psychopharmacology, 220, 238–240
  psychotherapy, 247
  refusal, 235
  right to refusal, 241
  serotonin, 227
  violation of freedom as, 240
  see also antipsychotic drugs
psychopharmacology, 7, 89–105
  anti-inflammatory drugs in depression, 313
  benefit vs. risk, 88, 90
  clinical trial lack of funding, 214
  diagnosis in, 89
  discrediting of, 25
  history of, 87–88
  identification of, 98–99
  non-response to, 87, 104–105
  psychopathy treatment, 220, 238–240
  reconsolidation blockade, 96
  research goals, 90
  resistant disorders, 150

social justice, 102–103
  symptom clustering approach, 99–100
  see also antidepressant drugs; antipsychotic
      drugs; psychotropic drugs
psychoses
  delusions vs. hallucinations, 285–286
  disorders of consciousness as, 60
  free will and, 81
  ultra high risk of, 310–311
psychosocial interventions
  existential suffering, 262
  loneliness, 262
psychosocial stress
  inflammatory cytokines, 312
  microglia activation, 312
  psychiatric disease, 35
  psychogenic movement disorders, 32–33
Psychosurgery Report and Recommendations
      (1977), 171
psychotropic drugs, 239–240
  adverse effects, 297
  cognitive/mental enhancement, 103, 107
  early use negative effects, 306
  new research, 103
  response rate, 55
  risks of, 299
  sleep disturbances, 103
  social justice, 102–103
PTSD (post-traumatic stress disorder)
  DBS fear memory erasure, 145–146
  diagnosis, 19
  fear memory dysfunction, 64, 65–66
  MDMA therapy, 98–99
  mental paralysis, 65
  neural ablation surgery, 141
  optogenetics, 179
  psychopharmacology, 7, 96–97
publicly funded healthcare, NFB cost,
      131–132

quality of life
  EAS choice, 265
schizophrenia, 291

radiofrequency ablation, 140
  acceptability, 177
Raine, Adrian, 223–224
Raison, Charles, 312
randomized controlled trials (RCTs), 174–175
Rasouli, Jonathan, 135
Ratcliffe, Matthew, 72
rationality, suicide, 270
RDoC (Research Domain Criteria), 4, 16–24
  aims of, 20–21
  biological/non-biological factor
      explanations, 23–24
  biological psychiatry structure &
      function, 25

drawbacks of, 22–23
DSM-5 and, 24, 50
DSM-5 vs., 16, 327
ICD-11 vs., 20–21
materialist theory of mind, 37
merits/limitations, 15
real people vs. potential people in pregnancy
    termination (abortion), 321–324
reasoning capacity, psychopathy, 242
reconsolidation blockade,
    psychopharmacology, 96
Redberg, Rita, 175–176
Redfield Jamison, Kay, 48–49
reductive materialism, 37, 38
reflective capacity, autonomy, 76–77
refusal, right of in treatment, 241
Reichenberg, Abraham, 295–296
relational identity, personal identity vs., 209
repetitive transcranial magnetic stimulation
    see rTMS (repetitive transcranial
    magnetic stimulation)
repetitive transcranial magnetic stimulation
    (rTMS), 112
requests for EAS, 253, 258, 261–262, 265,
    269–270, 280
Research Domain Criteria see RDoC (Research
    Domain Criteria)
respiratory paralysis, tCS adverse effects, 115
Ressler, Kerry, 96
resting-state activity, schizophrenia, 56–57
resting-state hyperactivity, depression, 57–58
retrograde amnesia, ECT adverse effect,
    110, 111
reward system
    AN, 58–59, 165
    impulse control disorders, 193
    psychopathy, 224–225
    unregulated hyperactivity, 75
Riedmuller, Rita, 149
Rietveld, Erik, 62–63
right temporal lobe, TMS in psychopathy, 229
right to refusal, psychopathy treatment, 241
risk perception, ethical issues, 148–149
Ritter, Michael, 299
Robert Lowell: Setting the River on Fire
    (Redfield Jamison), 48–49
Rogers v. Okin, 240
Rommelfanger, Karen, 122–123
Rose, Nikolas, 305–306
Roskies, Adina, 2–3
Rotter, Stefan, 71
rTMS (repetitive transcranial magnetic
    stimulation), 112
    AN consent problems, 164–165
    failure in EAS, 275
    psychotropic drugs vs., 134–135
    seizures, caused by, 114
Rutter, Michael, 305

Sawa, Akira, 6
Schacter, Daniel, 64, 65
schizophrenia
    BDNF protein, 314–315
    biomarkers, 300
    brain inflammation, 40
    catatonia as, 33
    clozapine, 90
    cognitive/mood disturbances, 113
    conscious disorder as, 60
    cortical-striatal dysconnectivity, 100–101
    DBS research, 161–162
    DBS trials, 159
    delusions, 57, 120
    dementia and, 33
    depression vs., 59
    development of, 308
    epilepsy vs., 59
    executive function deficits, 68–69
    genetics, 297, 299
    gray matter volume, 68–69
    hallucinations, 51, 57, 120
    information filtering, 57
    insight in, 77
    integration problems, 56–57
    neural dysfunction, 46–47
    neuroimaging in pathology, 21–22, 56,
        100–101
    neuroimmune interactions, 293
    neurological disorders vs., 30
    new clinical trials, 159–160
    NMDAR dysfunction in, 99
    paranoid schizophrenia, 81–82
    pharmacotherapy resistance, 135
    placebo response, 120–121
    positive subtype, 56–57, 69, 328
    prenatal risk factors, 317–318
    prevalence, 291
    psychological dimension, 91
    psychopharmacology, 90–91
    resting-state activity, 56–57
    self–world relationship, 58
    social dimension, 91
    suicidal desires, 267, 286
    symptoms, 17
    TMS, 112
Schug, Robert, 223–224
Schuklenk, Udo, 251–252
Schultz, Simon, 178–179
seizures
    comorbidities, 272
    epilepsy, 59
selective serotonin reuptake inhibitors see
    SSRIs (selective serotonin reuptake
    inhibitors)
selectivity, memory erasure therapy, 97–98
self
    awareness of see insight

self (*Cont.*)
 conscious dimension, 43
 disordered/divided in psychiatric
  disorders, 45
 identification of, 42–43
 persistent self, 43
 psychiatric self *see* psychiatric self
 unconscious dimension, 43
 world, relation to, 58
self-focus, MDD, 58
self-identity
 neuromodulation, 204–210
 psychiatric disorders, 208
sensory gating impairment, 297
serotonin, 227
 oxytocin combination, 229
 receptors and antidepressants, 89
serotonin and norepinephrine reuptake
  inhibitors *see* SNRIs (serotonin and
  norepinephrine reuptake inhibitors)
sertraline, 87
severe brain injury, EAS, 280
sham surgery, RCTs for psychiatric
  neurosurgery, 174–175
Singh, Ilina, 305–306
Sitaram, Ranganatha, 226–227
sleep disturbances
 depression, 103
 longitudinal studies, 296
SNRIs (serotonin and norepinephrine
  reuptake inhibitors), 87, 91
 adverse effects, 91
social factors, 72–73
 biomarkers, 304, 305–306
 neurological disorders, 329
 schizophrenia, 91
social harm, psychopathy, 219–220
social isolation, EAS requests, 261–262
social justice
 neuromodulation, 211–215
 NFB, 131
 psychopharmacology, 102–103
 psychotropic drugs, 102–103
social stress, depression *vs.*, 265–266
somatic diseases
 pain, 259–260
 psychotropic drugs, 297
somatosensory cortex, AN, 165
Spence, Sean, 74
Spring, Charles, 284
SSRIs (selective serotonin reuptake
  inhibitors), 91
 adverse effects, 89, 91
 cognitive/mental enhancement, 103
 overdose on, 98
 psychopathy, 227
*Starson v. Swayze*, 240–241
Steinbrock, Bonnie, 252–253

stigma, psychiatric disorders, 5–7
Stoessi, A Jon, 176
stress
 chronic *see* chronic psychological stress
 depression association, 301
 hyperactive stress *see* hyperactive stress
 psychosocial *see* psychosocial stress
 social stress *vs.* depression, 265–266
stress hormones, 33
stroke, psychiatric disorders *vs.*, 30
structural neuroimaging, function
  neuroimaging combination, 301–302
structural neurosurgery, psychiatric
  neurosurgery *vs.*, 136
subcaudate tractotomy, 141
subgenual cingulate, hyperactivity, 188
substance abuse, depression and, 262
subthalamic nucleus, stimulating
  techniques, 189
suffering, 258–264
 assessment fairness, 264–265
 cognitive components, 261
 definition, 259
 emotional components, 261
 phenomenology of, 285
 physical disease absence, 263
 prolongation and EAS, 252–253
 psychological suffering, 256–257
 severity and symptom severity, 274
 unbearable, 257
 volitional components, 261
suicide
 depression in, 260, 286
 euthanasia *vs.*, 283–284
 ideation, 267–268
 mental disorder impulse, 276
 morality and rationality, 270
Sullivan, Mark, 266–267
supervenience, 39–40
surgical ablation, DBS *vs.*, 169
Sutorius, Philip, 263
Switzerland, EAS legality, 254
symptoms
 amelioration, psychiatric neurosurgery
  benefits, 165–166
 severity *vs.* suffering severity, 274
synapse elimination (pruning), 308, 310
 excessive, 311
Szasz, Thomas, 25

Talairach, Jean, 139
Talbot, Sebastien, 44
tCS (transcranial current stimulation), 88–89
 adverse effects, 115
 escitalopram *vs.*, 113
 ethical questions, 113
 failure in EAS, 275
 invasive *vs.* non-invasive treatment as, 106

regulation of, 113–114
self-use problems, 115
temporal interference (TI), 117–118
    DBS *vs.,* 118
temporal lobe, neural mapping, 145
terminal sedation, euthanasia, 284
testosterone, disease pathology, 293
Thienpont, Lieve, 255–257
third-party assessment, capacity for consent,
    154–155
thoughts, unconscious processes,
    regulation of, 61
thyroid hormone, 302
TI *see* temporal interference (TI)
TMS (transcranial magnetic stimulation), 10,
    88–89, 112–117, 172
    application, 112–113
    DBS *vs.,* 143
    ethical questions, 113
    failure in EAS, 275
    invasive *vs.* non-invasive treatment as, 106
    procedure length, 114–115
    proxy consent, 152
    psychopathy, 229
    regulation of, 113–114
    repetitive *see* rTMS (repetitive transcranial
        magnetic stimulation)
    self-use problems, 115
Tourette syndrome, DBS, 145
tractotomy, subcaudate, 141
transcranial current stimulation *see* tCS
    (transcranial current stimulation)
transcranial magnetic stimulation *see* TMS
    (transcranial magnetic stimulation)
TRD (treatment-resistant depression), 6–7,
    278–279
    DBS new treatment targets, 279
    EAS, 251, 271, 273–274
    incidence, 275–276
    suicidal desire, 286
treatment, 87–133, 292
    associated risks, 105
    conscientious objection to, 282–283
    EAS requests *vs.,* 282
    neuroimaging/electrophysiology, 21
    non-responsiveness in depression, 6–7
    non-reversal of pathology, 292
    resistance in EAS, 253
    waiting for in EAS, 252–253
    *see also* psychopharmacology
treatment-resistant depression *see* TRD
    (treatment-resistant depression)
trephination, 137
trials *see* clinical trials
Tulving, Endel, 65

ultra high risk of psychosis, 310–311
unbearable pain, EAS, 263–264

unbearable suffering, 257
unconscious dimension, self, 43
unconscious processing
    conscious processing *vs.* in OCD, 63
    thoughts & behavior regulation, 61
Underwood, Emily, 212–213
unipolar depression
    early age diagnosis, 270–271
    ECT, 108–109
    epigenetics, 268
    gray matter volume reduction, 101
    new treatments, 279
    suicidal desires, 267, 268
unregulated hyperactivity, reward system, 75
US (ultrasound) *see* FUS (focused ultrasound);
    HIFUS (high-intensity focused
    ultrasound)
USA, EAS legality, 254
US National Commission for the Protection
    of Human Subjects of Biomedical
    and Behavioral Research, *Belmont
    Report,* 171

van de Vathorst, Suzanne, 251–252
van Gogh, Vincent, 82
van Koningsbruggen, Martin, 106
van Oosterhout, Ansel, 149
Varelius, Jukka, 286
VBM (voxel- based morphometry), 101
    neurobiology, 21
    positive schizophrenia subtype, 328
vegetative state *see* VS (vegetative state)
venlafaxine, 87
ventral striatum, dorsolateral prefrontal cortex
    connectivity, 229
ventrolateral prefrontal cortex,
    psychopathy, 223
ventromedial cortex, 39
ventromedial PFC
    amygdala connectivity, 229
    psychopathy, 223
Viding, Essi, 245–246
viral infections, 318, 319
Vogeley, Kai, 60
volitional capacity, 51
    phenomenology of suffering, 285
volitional components, suffering, 261
voluntariness, EAS competence, 265
voluntary euthanasia, 285
voxel- based morphometry *see* VBM (voxel-
    based morphometry)
VS (vegetative state), 53–54
    level/degree/state of
        consciousness, 54–55

waiting for treatment, EAS, 252–253
Wallace, Mike, 81–82
Walter, Henrik, 24–25

Watts, James, 138
WHO (World Health Organization), mental
    health burden, 1
Widge, Alik, 170
will
  definitions of, 51–52
  disorders of, 67–75
Willis, Thomas, 34
Woolf, Clifford, 44

working memory, disease pathogenesis, 297
world, self, relation to, 58
worry symptoms, GAD, 66

young adults, EAS, 280
Youngner, Stuart, 266–267

Zeman, Adam, 31, 34–35
Zrinzo, Ludvic, 149